STRESS
LESS

STRESS
LESS

The New Science That Shows
Women How to Rejuvenate
the Body and the Mind

Thea Singer

HUDSON
STREET
PRESS

HUDSON STREET PRESS
Published by Penguin Group
Penguin Group (USA) Inc., 375 Hudson Street, New York, New York 10014, U.S.A. • Penguin Group (Canada), 90 Eglinton Avenue East, Suite 700, Toronto, Ontario, Canada M4P 2Y3 (a division of Pearson Penguin Canada Inc.) • Penguin Books Ltd., 80 Strand, London WC2R 0RL, England • Penguin Ireland, 25 St. Stephen's Green, Dublin 2, Ireland (a division of Penguin Books Ltd.) • Penguin Group (Australia), 250 Camberwell Road, Camberwell, Victoria 3124, Australia (a division of Pearson Australia Group Pty. Ltd.) • Penguin Books India Pvt. Ltd., 11 Community Centre, Panchsheel Park, New Delhi – 110 017, India • Penguin Books (NZ), 67 Apollo Drive, Rosedale, North Shore 0632, New Zealand (a division of Pearson New Zealand Ltd.) • Penguin Books (South Africa) (Pty.) Ltd., 24 Sturdee Avenue, Rosebank, Johannesburg 2196, South Africa

Penguin Books Ltd., Registered Offices: 80 Strand, London WC2R 0RL, England

First published by Hudson Street Press, a member of Penguin Group (USA) Inc.

First Printing, October 2010
10   9   8   7   6   5   4   3   2   1

Ⓗ REGISTERED TRADEMARK — MARCA REGISTRADA
HUDSON
STREET
PRESS

LIBRARY OF CONGRESS CATALOGING-IN-PUBLICATION DATA

Singer, Thea.
    Stress less : the new science thast shows women how to rejuvenate the body and the mind / Thea Singer.
        p. cm.
    Includes bibliographical references and index.
    ISBN 978-1-59463-060-6
    1. Stress management for women. I. Title.
    RA785.S546 2010
    616.9'800821—dc22

                            2010022829

Printed in the United States of America
Set in Goudy Old Style   •   Designed by Eve L. Kirch

PUBLISHER'S NOTE
Every effort hasd been made to ensure that the information contained in this book is complete and accurate. However, neither the publisher nor the author is engaged in rendering professional advice or services to the individual reader. The ideas, procedures, and suggestions contained in this book are not intended as a substitute for consulting with your physician. All matters regarding your healt require medical supervision. Neither the author nor the publisher shall be liable or responsible for any loss or damage allegedly arising from any information or suggestion in this book.

While the author has made every effort to provide accurate telephone numbers and Internet addresses at the time of publication, neither the publisher nor the author assumes any responsibility for errors, or for changes that occur after publication. Further, publisher does not have any control over and does not assume any responsibility for author or third-party websites or their content.

To Henry and Sophie Rose,
for keeping me forever young.

CONTENTS

Contents

ACKNOWLEDGMENTS

My thanks first to the scientists who generously opened up their worlds—and their labs—to me, sharing their remarkable research, tirelessly answering my questions, and drawing pictures to bring this or that physiological mechanism to life. I don't have room to name all of them here, so I will limit myself to those whose work launched this book. I trust that the dozens of others will know how grateful I am for their enthusiasm for this project and for trusting me to translate their complex discoveries for the wider public.

I am indebted to Elizabeth H. Blackburn, Elissa S. Epel, and Jue Lin at the University of California, San Francisco, not just for lighting the fire that sparked this book, but also for their continued encouragement, numerous leads (to papers and colleagues), and patience in breaking down even the most difficult concepts. Calvin B. Harley, a pioneer in telomere biology, provided historical insight. Thank you to Robert M. Sapolsky at Stanford University; Bruce S. McEwen at the Rockefeller University; Mary F. Dallman, professor emeritus at UCSF; Cheryl D. Conrad at Arizona State University; Sonia Lupien at the University of Montreal; and UCLA's Teresa E. Seeman and Shelley E. Taylor, for giving me the scientific foundation necessary to understand the new science of stress, as well as continuing to push the envelope themselves with their current research. Judith Campisi and Gordon J. Lithgow, both at California's Buck Institute for Age Research, gave me new perspective on the telomere story, as did the University of Washington's Matt R. Kaeberlein and the University of Michigan's Richard A. Miller.

Writing a book can be quite a stressful experience—in both the good and bad sense of the word. I know firsthand how the support of friends and family goes a terrifically long way in counteracting the latter. My heartfelt thanks to Brad Mindich and the *Boston Phoenix* for providing me with a room of my own at an incredibly difficult time. To my oldest friends: Susan Lewin, whose wisdom inspired me and who caught me when I fell. To Beverly Ehrich, Bonnie Piegari, Sue Cahn, and Amy Faxon, who showed me how resilient I can be. To my writer/editor friends, who read drafts of chapters and helped me maintain much-needed perspective: Jane Dornbusch, Emily Terry, Lisa Fowler, Maureen Dezell, Leigh Buchanan, Susan Senator, Beth Teitell, and Sasha Helper. And deep thanks, too, to David H. Freedman, who, with several books under his belt, offered guidance from the beginning, and to George Johnson, Amanda Cook, and Bill Patrick, all of whom, at the eleventh hour, pulled me through.

I offer a special thanks to my agent, Liza Dawson, who believed in me as a book author more than I believed in myself, and continues to nurture that possibility. Much gratitude to Hudson Street Press, for plucking my article on Liz and Elissa's studies out of O, *The Oprah Magazine* and asking me to expand it into a book, and then shepherding the project through. I could not have pulled together the myriad details in these pages without the razor-sharp skills of Jackie Houton, Dara Steinberg, and Linda Kinstler. I owe a debt of gratitude to Elena Vizvary, Lindsey Vizvary Galveo, Ricky Galveo, and Sam Einhorn, who meticulously checked every fact in this book for nothing more than lattes and a home-cooked meal, and to Connie Procaccini, who turned around miles of taped interviews in record time.

Thank you, too, to all those in my life who kept the chaos at bay, enabling me to concentrate on researching and writing, including Joe Depa, Marvin Brainin, Rochelle Friedman, Carol Gross, and the Elizabeths of Gabriel's.

Finally, a huge thanks to my family: my sisters Paula and Candy, my stepdaughter, Lexi, and my two loves: Henry and Sophie. The last two spent too many hours without me as I slaved away in my basement hovel and took over the family room with my endless stacks of papers and books. I am grateful for your forbearance, for cheering me on, and for keeping me fed.

FOREWORD

Can chronic stress age us? The clues for answering that question are finally all in one place and together they tell a compelling story. Thea Singer has synthesized the disparate scientific literatures on stress and aging, and the conclusion is intriguing: Stress is the new biological clock (that is the real title of this book!). But exactly how does stress speed the clock up, or, better yet, how might we turn it back?

This is a scholarly work hidden underneath a breezy, funny conversation about life and how our bodies work. The title is, of course, the publisher's way of getting you to open this book. It worked, didn't it?

There are many books about stress, but this is the only one I know of that drills down so deeply into mechanistic studies, and at the same time widely covers the most important ways that stress targets the body and mind. Thea Singer takes us into the labs and minds of scientists across the globe to show us how it all works, especially explaining how stress is relevant to aging.

This book covers a topic I am obsessed with: telomeres—the very tips of our chromosomes, and a marker of cell aging. It describes some of our research group's studies on how stress may affect telomeres, leading to their shortening. So I may be biased in my enthusiasm for the topic. But as you will see, telomeres are both fascinating and important to human health and aging, and we are even developing a company to measure telomeres.

In this book, you will be taken through fifty years of stress research, and delve into some of the most interesting new discoveries. We re-searchers tend to be, by nature and by the politics of funding, stuck in our own disciplines, narrowly focusing on one aspect of stress. Thea Singer is meticulous about getting the science accurate, making it un-derstandable, and connecting it with the other studies, knitting together the fabric of the stress-aging field. In fact, she uncovers connections that even most researchers did not see.

Hear snippets of real lives, experiments, and some solid tips on what to do to prevent stress damage to your body and mind. Don't expect a new diet or quick fixes. Rather, expect to never view your body, and spe-cifically the mind-body connection, the same again.

Chronic, ongoing stress can be toxic to our bodies. Yet these effects can be invisible for years and years. Many of us are so used to living with high stress levels that we aren't even aware that our bodies are under stress—and that our biological aging is speeding far ahead of our chrono-logical age.

Stress science is inevitably complex. While there is a lot of media coverage on the negative effects of stress, there is little explanation of the *why*. Stress researchers spend their time understanding the complex-ity, and many are loathe to make statements to the press that simplify and potentially mislead. Thea Singer explains complex mechanistic studies that the media can't bear to summarize, given the short sound bites they are allotted.

You may ask: Do I have time to read about this complexity? Your hands are likely full managing your stressful life. But then ask yourself: Can I afford not to? This book gives you the opportunity to become a stress expert, not just by living the stress of life, but by understanding good versus bad stress, and applying the knowledge to your own daily life. If you dare, you can assess your own life stress—as well as your at-titudes and behaviors driving that stress—by taking the scientifically validated tests within this book. These self-assessments make the book deeply personal. Your new awareness of the hidden sources and effects of stress may be stressful itself, but in the end it will be empowering. If you really understand, for example, what sleep debt is doing to your brain, hormones, and gut, you just might prioritize sleep more.

Thea Singer covers intricate details of how the stress response works, from the brain and nerves to hormones and immune cells, but in an understandable way. Once you get the enjoyable crash course in physiology, you will see into the hidden pathways of how stress gets under the skin to speed the clock on life. This book explains, for example, how some types of stress can make cells healthier and boost our response to vaccinations, while other types can lead to damage and accelerated cell aging. Thea Singer also uncovers the mysteries of stress: Why is it that short-term stress can boost memory but chronic stress dulls it? Why does exercise appear to be the "fountain of youth," but when you do too much of it . . . well, you should have chosen the couch! How is meditation so beneficial? What are negative thoughts doing to the brain and cells? And what does love have to do with it?

It has been said that stress is 10 percent what happens to us in life—the uncontrollable part—and 90 percent how we react to those circumstances. Surprisingly, we usually have more control and options than we feel we do. After reading this book, you may find yourself thinking about your telomeres when you encounter a stressful situation—that is a good thing! It can help you make the decision: Should I exercise or get right to work? There is still so much we don't know about biological aging, but the emerging picture is hopeful: There seems to be a lot we can do to slow our cellular aging, even in mid- and late life.

I hope this book serves as a wake-up call about how stress affects us as individuals and a society. Large segments of our society feel high stress with too little control, with fleeting awareness of the present moment. And large forces—including societal factors like widespread financial stress—are causing true survival stress, not just our brains' tendency to over-interpret danger signals. These huge, contextual factors, including our income level or the neighborhood we live in, appear to shape our lives, our level of stress arousal, our health, and may be ultimately linked to our telomere length.

I believe that just as stress is invisible, so are the interconnections between us all, rich and poor. Might policy, public health, and science converge to inspire a program of "societal stress reduction"? This book opens the door to the possibility, introducing initiatives such as Experience Corps. May this book take us a step closer not only to our personal health and longevity, but to strive for a healthier society, where we are more socially connected and compassionate to those around us, where there are more safety nets, where even those with few resources can also have a chance to slow down the stress-aging clock.

Elissa Epel, Ph.D.

Associate Professor, Department of Psychiatry, University of California, San Francisco

Director, UCSF Center for Obesity Assessment, Study, and Treatment

Associate Director, Center for Health and Community

San Francisco, April 15, 2010

INTRODUCTION

Stress—The New Biological Clock

How You Can Turn It Back

Every stress leaves an indelible scar, and the organism pays for its survival after a stressful situation by becoming a little older.

—Hans Selye, M.D., Ph.D., D.Sc., "Emphasis," paper from
Smith, Kline, and French, Winter 1969

Margie E. Lachman's office at Brandeis University, where she is a professor and the chair of the Department of Psychology, is enormous and sunlit. Impressionist oil paintings on loan from the school's famous Rose Art Museum illuminate the walls, and gifts from students—glass flowers, a model of a Vietnamese "longevity" turtle—rest alongside a blue and yellow tin of Lucy's Predic-a-Mints, of *I Love Lucy* fame. Lachman, a cheerful, wholesome-looking woman with rectangular glasses and dark wavy hair swept up in a silver barrette, clearly mixes whimsy with her academic rigor.

Lachman specializes in the area of life span development, including the sense of control we feel we have (or don't have) in adulthood and old age. She was one of the original investigators on the massive study Midlife in the United States (MIDUS I), launched in 1995 to explore the health and well-being of more than seven thousand Americans, and she continues as an investigator on the study's ten-year follow-up, MIDUS II.

I'm talking with Lachman to try to understand why we baby-boomer women may be the most stressed-out beings on the planet. "Stress is highest in young adulthood and midlife," Lachman writes in the scientific paper that brought me here. These adults, she continues, "experienced more frequent overload stressors, especially involving children and financial risk."

Why might that be? For starters, midlife in general presents unprecedented challenges, say social scientists, leaving us more vulnerable to day-to-day stressors from the get-go. It's at midlife that we become aware of our mortality. Our bodies are no longer under our control the way they once were: no more reversing Friday night's chocolate-cake binge with one day of Boca burgers and egg whites. Our health—and that of our partners—is increasingly precarious. "We find that a lot of people, as they get older, think that aging is just this inevitable, irreversible process of decline," Lachman tells me, noting that such thinking can work against us. Lachman knows whereof she speaks: She's a baby boomer herself—one of the forty-two million women between the ages of forty and fifty-nine living in the United States, according to U.S. Census Bureau data from 2005. It's a group that comprises more than 14 percent of the total American population. "The beliefs that people hold regarding aging really do have an impact in terms of how they behave and how they react and what the actual outcomes are," she says. "People who feel that they are not in control of aging actually look different from people who feel that they are."

No control. It lies at the heart of everything stressful, to a greater or lesser degree. The economy is in terrible shape. We (and our graying mates) are losing our jobs—maybe even struggling to hold on to our homes. We are caring for growing children with one hand and aging parents with the other, while also trying to save for those kids' college and our own retirement. A survey from the Pew Research Center on the "Sandwich Generation" presents the stark stats: A quarter of women—particularly those between the ages of thirty and fifty—reported caring for a parent or other older relative. A whopping 54 percent of those in such a caregiving role said it caused them "at least some stress," and 20 percent of that group said they were under "a lot of stress."

Also adding to the burden is the fact that most of us work outside the home for economic reasons, even as we continue to do the lion's share of housekeeping and child care (we're expected to bring home the bacon *and* fry it up in a pan, to paraphrase the old Enjoli perfume ad). Compounding the pressure is that our workplaces are often unsupportive of our multiple roles. If we work on our own as consultants, as more and more of us do as companies shrink, we also have to deal with the loss of work camaraderie and hours of social isolation. (And no, Facebook, virtual office that it can be, does not replace that chat by the watercooler.)

And unlike other generations, we cut ourselves little slack. Boomer women essentially invented the Superwoman syndrome—we would do it all, for everyone, and do it well. Now, at midlife, we're taking stock, questioning whether we've achieved what we could or "should" have—and invariably beating ourselves up for falling short. Baby-boomer women "even made parenting a competitive sport," notes Cornell University's Elaine Wethington, a medical sociologist specializing in stress and midlife, in an article in the university's publication *Human Ecology*. "It wasn't enough to have and raise children. They had to have perfect children."

Such demands can have a steep price: One of Wethington's recent studies shows that a quarter of American women have had at least one episode of depression—a rate twice that of men.

It's not just the major stressors that do us in—job loss, death of loved ones, long-term debt. The daily hassles—family fights, traffic, work deadlines—take their toll, too, piling up like bumper-to-bumper cars on a weak bridge. David M. Almeida, Ph.D., a developmental psychologist at Pennsylvania State University, has subjects in his studies fill out daily stress diaries over various periods of time so he can assess how overloads occur. In a weeklong study, he and colleague Melanie C. Horn, Ph.D., found that young adults and those at midlife reported more days with stressors, more days with multiple stressors, and more frequent "overload stressors" than older folks did. More support for Lachman's contention. I wasn't surprised.

"It's at midlife when we are pulled in many directions in terms of being responsible for others, from our own children to our aging parents," says Almeida. "It's also a time when we're more likely to be in management positions at work. All of these things expose us to more 'danger' events, the most prevalent types of stressors." Danger events, he explains, are those that lead us to worry about the future—for example, hearing that the company's revenues are down just when your son goes off to college, or that your mother, two hundred miles away in New Jersey, has been taken to the emergency room by ambulance. "We're in the driver's seat, which supposedly would give us more control," he says. "But we also have more responsibility."

<center>~~~~~</center>

Such repeated stress frazzles us. It makes us snap at our partners and kids—even growl at the dog. It keeps us awake at night and clouds our professional judgment. We've known for years that it puts us at greater risk for any number of diseases. What we didn't know until now is that it actually physically ages us, all the way down to the DNA in our cells.

It was through such stressed women (they were caring for their chronically ill children) that 2009 Nobel Prize–winning cell biologist Elizabeth H. Blackburn, Ph.D., and health psychologist Elissa S. Epel, Ph.D., both at the University of California, San Francisco, made the groundbreaking discovery from which this book sprang: that chronic stress literally gnaws at our DNA—its tips, or telomeres, to be precise—speeding up the rate at which our cells age by an alarming *ten years or more.*

The implications are clear: For us midlifers, stress has become the new biological clock.

Yet, as the research in this book will also show, there's good news to go along with that shocking discovery—ways that we can slow, and even turn back, that relentless timepiece. For the Epel and Blackburn findings also reveal that what matters in cell aging is the level of *perceived* stress, which means that the antidote lies, significantly, in our own hands—or, more precisely, in our minds and our behaviors.

Of course, no scientist would ever suggest that we *eliminate* stress, whether psychological or biological. Indeed, as stress guru Bruce S. McEwen, Ph.D., puts it, if we got rid of stress, "we'd be dead." Director of the neuroendocrinology laboratory at Rockefeller University in New York City, McEwen has been a leader in the study of stress for decades, training generations of young scientists who make up a veritable who's who of stress researchers.

Temporary, or acute, stress, in fact, can be very good for us. Exercise is a prime example (see Chapter 5). Researchers such as Gordon J. Lithgow, Ph.D., at California's Buck Institute for Age Research, have shown that acute stress can even extend life span. Lithgow, a lanky, enthusiastic man with a broad forehead and inquisitive eyes, studies stress and aging in that most elemental of beings, single-celled worms (*C. elegans*). He's shown that acute stressors—say, increased temperature for several hours—enable the worms to live up to 30 percent longer than their nonheated peers. How so? The added heat perturbs the homeostasis, or internal constancy, of the worm's single cell. The cell in response kicks out what are called heat shock proteins, which, in a process called hormesis (more on this in Chapter 4), causes the cell to metaphorically thicken its skin, making it better able to withstand future insults that could contribute to its demise. (We have homeostatic systems, too, as you may recall from high school biology. An example is body temperature: We operate at full throttle only when it's near that constant 98.6 degrees Fahrenheit.)

Why do we care about stress in, of all things, worms? Scientists in search of so-called longevity genes—such as the University of Michigan's Richard A. Miller, Ph.D.; the University of Washington's Matt R. Kaeberlein, Ph.D.; and Harvard's David A. Sinclair, Ph.D.*—rely heavily

---

* Sinclair is the man who put red wine—or at least resveratrol, a natural substance therein—on the longevity-gene map.

on the fact that many cellular responses to stress are conserved through-out evolution. Worms may not be us, but the mechanistic lessons from worms may, they believe, apply to us.

Distinctions also split psychosocial stress—the heart-quickening, stomach-tensing kind we automatically associate with the word *stress*. Many scientists break psychosocial stress into two categories and limn how our bodies and brains respond differently to each. There's challenge stress (good for you), which refers to situations we find demanding but for which we have the resources to cope. Waiting in Whistler at the top of the mountain to slalom to Olympic gold—that's challenge stress, as is (yes!) sex (see Chapter 3). In contrast, threat stress (very bad) refers to situations that are overwhelming, in which we feel helpless in the face of the onslaught. Caring for a chronically ill child, as the subjects in Black-burn and Epel's research were doing, qualifies as threat stress.

Stanford University neurobiologist Robert M. Sapolsky, Ph.D., an-other giant in the stress-research world and author of the acclaimed *Why Zebras Don't Get Ulcers*, elaborates. "Our goal isn't to have a life with no stress—anyone ranging from a developmental psychologist to a geron-tologist knows that," he wrote in an e-mail before our first meeting. "The idea is to have the right amount of stress. So what's the right amount? Generally, it's for challenges/stressors that are moderate in severity and transient in duration. And what does that define? *Stimulation*. 'Moderate in severity'—it's not for nothing that three-minute roller-coaster rides aren't so severe that they rip your internal organs loose. 'Transient'—it's not for nothing that roller-coaster rides aren't three weeks long. Another way of framing what good stress is: circumstances where you voluntarily relinquish a degree of control and predictability in a setting that overall is benevolent. You're willing to let yourself be utterly out of control as to when the scary thing happens on the movie screen—because you know that the murderer is going to stay on the screen."

McEwen, for his part, refines the psychosocial stress categories even further. Challenge stress, he says, encompasses both positive stress, in which you have good self-esteem and relish the chance to rise to the challenge, and tolerable stress, in which "something bad happens, but you have good social support and self-esteem, so you have the tools—economic, personal, and so on—to weather the storm." Finally, there is toxic stress. "That's the really bad stuff, where you don't have adequate resources," he explains. "Maybe you're poor, maybe you don't have good social support, maybe you've been abused as a child." These are the folks who may not be able to rebound, and for whom pathology—major depression, for example—may develop. Blackburn and Epel's caregivers with the shortest telomeres fit there.

~~~~~

Where do *you* fall on that stress spectrum? To help you find out, I've provided a targeted test at the start of each chapter in this book; use the tests together to develop your own stress profile. Questions they'll help you answer include: What is my personal stress level? Which behaviors of mine increase my stress level and which ones reduce it? How should I change my lifestyle to bring about the latter so I can slow the aging process? These are not cobbled-together pseudoscientific scales but the actual tests used in scientific studies on stress and the behaviors that inform stress: diet, exercise, psychological outlook, social support, sleep, and more. Indeed, many of them come directly from the studies cited in these pages.

The discussions following the tests delve deep into Blackburn and Epel's groundbreaking research on stress and aging, as well as that of dozens of other scientists whose hours spent bent over pipettes and petri dishes, crunching numbers from intricate surveys, and analyzing the behavior and brain changes of subjects from rats to people provide crucial new insights into our understanding of stress and how it ages us. They also explore the latest science showing how to manage our stress so we can slow the aging process.

Driving this approach is my own understanding of the mind-set of so many midlife women like me: The how-tos of combating stress are not enough—and not only because we are, constitutionally, it seems, dedicated to understanding the why of things, avidly researching our own health concerns both online and in print. It's also because, for us, meaning begets action. We act not blindly but with definite intention based on reliable, concrete information we've dug up ourselves. We are knowledge *seekers*. Our old mantra, "Don't trust anyone over thirty," has become "Don't trust the experts alone to tell us what we need to know."

And so, be prepared to take a collaborative journey inside your body and brain to learn what makes your stressed self tick—and how you personally can slow that clock. The study of how stress contributes to our cells' aging—which Blackburn and Epel opened the door to—is incredibly new. But be assured: By the time you finish this book, you, too, will be comfortably batting around the word *telomere* at cocktail parties and the gym, and making the lifestyle choices, based on rigorous science, that speak specifically to you. My intent is not to lay out an ironclad program for you to rigorously follow, but rather to let you, the intelligent and informed reader, pick and choose your strategies for reducing stress. After all, lack of control and unpredictability *induce* stress. What all of us need, now more than ever, is to trust our own good minds to make our own wise choices.

As Margie Lachman told me: "You can't stop aging, but you can slow or compensate for it—you can prevent certain changes, or at least minimize them." That's what control is about. And control over stress and aging is what this book will teach you, on your own terms.

STRESS
LESS

CHAPTER 1

The Old Science of Stress

Turning and turning in the widening gyre
The falcon cannot hear the falconer;
Things fall apart; the centre cannot hold . . .

—William Butler Yeats, "The Second Coming," 1920

In 2006, Melody Morrow's company, a large Miami-based distributor of electronic components, crashed—literally: a botched computer conversion dried up inventory, turning the company to ash—and in June 2007 it was sold to a private investment group for a song. As the company tanked, Melody, then forty-one and the single mother of three, took repeated pay cuts and watched her position contract from global sales manager to regional salesperson and her client base evaporate. "The phones," says the nine-year sales veteran, shivering, "went totally silent."

Still, she was grateful to have a job at all, even if she did have to start from scratch, rebuilding accounts. Or trying to. The ascent felt like clambering up an ice-covered mountain in skis. She just didn't have the knack for closing deals with new suppliers or even pulling old ones back into the fold. A year and a half later, her job status was just as precarious. "Today, as a matter of fact, I thought I was going to get the ax," she says.

Some days, she would come home and just sob. "I'd think, 'I can't do this,'" she continues. "It's like the weight of the world."

Finances had always been tight for Melody, but through careful budgeting and an aversion to credit cards, she'd managed to squeak by, keeping up with the payments on her three-bedroom house in Palm Harbor, Florida—even without the weekly $650 in child support her ex-husband was supposed to pay. She was the polar opposite of the folks caught up in the subprime mortgage mess that crested in 2008, losing their homes to foreclosure because they'd borrowed more than they could afford.

Or so she thought.

As her income shrank, Florida hurricanes sent her homeowners insurance soaring, and her property taxes soon followed. Unbeknownst to employees, the new management canceled the company's health insurance—right when Melody was in the midst of treatment for precancerous cells on her cervix. She wonders if, somehow, all the stress had anything to do with the cells' development.

By March 2008, Melody had fallen so far behind in the monthly payments on her $220,000 mortgage that she put the house up for sale by owner. No one came calling.

And then an "angel," she says, entered the picture.

Real-estate agent Stephanie Akhavan was sent by the mortgage company to list the house. But, says Melody, she did much more than that; she psychically led her to safety. "I could barely move or talk about the house," she says, recalling her deepening depression. "When Stephanie talked to me, I'd just sob. She knew I couldn't sell the house—physically, because of my job, and mentally. So she talked for me."

Finally, in October, two months after she was officially served with a foreclosure notice, Melody got an offer on the house: $140,000—a shortfall of $80,000. By then, she'd been watching in horror as neighbors backed up U-Hauls to their own underwater properties and simply fled. "If the mortgage broker didn't take that offer," says Melody, "we could have been out on the street."

"I got out from under, but I knew in my heart I was leaving with nothing," she says. "The new floor, the painting, the blood, sweat, and tears that I had in mowing that grass, front and back, every weekend, and trimming and edging—blisters on my hands and my feet." She breaks down again. "Leaving my home that I worked so hard for. That was so awful."

Now Melody and her two younger daughters rent a two-bedroom

condo in a large complex about five miles from the old house. Most of the other residents are elderly.

"Sometimes my girls were very angry and would yell at me and say, 'How did you get us into this position? I hate you!'" she says. Other times, they would lend a hand: Her seventeen-year-old daughter, for instance, got a job in a nursing home to help make ends meet.

Melody and her daughters still have no health insurance; the acquiring company's premiums are too high. No one has been to the doctor for more than a year. Melody just can't afford the follow-up to have those precancerous cells checked.

Still, for her, the emotional price far outweighs the monetary one. "The guilt. If there's anything that I can say to you, it's guilt—guilt for everything. It's, you know, how did this happen? You feel like you've failed your family. But I also feel like I've failed in my job because I'm not where I need to be."

What Is Your Debt Stress?

In the current economy, nearly everyone struggles with financial challenges. Worry about money may be one of the greatest stressors going—and any amount of debt compounds the pressure. Take this test to learn how much your debt is stressing you out.

In answering the questions below, consider your *overall* debt, including any debt on credit cards, store credit, mortgages, home-equity loans, car loans, and any other outstanding loans.

1. Overall, how often do you worry about the total amount you owe in overall debt? Would you say you worry

   (a) All of the time
   (b) Most of the time
   (c) Some of the time
   (d) Hardly ever
   (e) Not at all

2. How much stress does the total debt you are carrying cause you? It is

    (a) A great deal of stress
    (b) Quite a bit
    (c) Some stress
    (d) Not very much
    (e) No stress at all

3. Now, thinking ahead over the next five years, how much of a problem, if any, will the total debt you have taken on be for you? Will it be

    (a) An extreme problem
    (b) A large one
    (c) Medium
    (d) Small
    (e) No problem at all?

4. How concerned are you that you will never be able to pay off these debts? Are you

    (a) Very concerned
    (b) Quite concerned
    (c) Somewhat concerned
    (d) Not very concerned
    (e) Not at all concerned?

Calculating your score:

Each (a) answer is worth 4 points, each (b) is worth 3 points, each (c) is worth 2 points, each (d) is worth 1 point, each (e) is worth 0 points. Add your total points together and multiply the sum by 6.25.

Interpreting your score the *Stress Less* way*:

0–10 points: No debt stress
11–23: Low debt stress
24–36: Medium debt stress
37–55: Medium-high debt stress
56–75: High debt stress
76–100: Extreme debt stress

* The *Stress Less* interpretation was developed by the author, not the scientists.

~~~

We've heard it so often, for so many years, that it's like a drumbeat of doom: Stress, when it's chronic or repeated, can make us sick—or at the very least lay the groundwork for any number of diseases to take hold.

But what is it, literally, that stress is doing to our bodies and our brains to bring us, healthwise, to our knees? Exactly how does it throw our systems—cardiovascular, immune, neurological, gastrointestinal, and so on—so disastrously out of whack?

For years we've been hearing warnings about the veritable dictionary of diseases that can be the end result of such "systemic dysregulation": from allergies and atherosclerosis to chronic fatigue syndrome, cognitive impairment, and type 2 diabetes; from high blood pressure and high cholesterol to heart attacks and infections; from obesity to ulcers. As long ago as 1993, stress guru Bruce McEwen gave the process a name: allostatic load. Many of these diseases rely on a slow accumulation of damage, and so appear more frequently as we age, earning them the label "diseases of aging," along with cancer and forms of dementia such as Alzheimer's.

How can a psychological construct, something "all in our heads," have such devastating physiological effects? To hear stress researchers tell it, the fact that it's all in our heads is exactly the point—a no-brainer, if you will. The brain, says McEwen, is the "key organ of stress." It decides not only what's stressful but also just how our bodies will respond to those threats, real or imagined. "I have made the claim that stress begins in the brain, giving the statement the same ring of scientific certainty as the idea that the earth revolves around the sun," writes McEwen bluntly in his book *The End of Stress as We Know It.* And these days, with our minds ruminating over everything from how we'll keep our jobs and pay the mortgage to how we'll tutor our kids in Think Math while dashing to the hospital to consult with doctors about an aging parent's pneumonia, the threats never cease.

What follows is a brief (mechanistic) history of stress—the platform on which the new science in the rest of this book rests. The basics are important; to understand the revolutionary, you've got to get the fundamentals under your belt.

~~~~~~

Picture, if you will, Melody Morrow hunched over in the bathroom stall at work, her head in her hands, choking back sobs. Her heart is racing and her hands are clammy, and not just because they're catching tears. This go-round in the Ladies', Melody just may throw up.

Why is her body in such an uproar?

In fact, all of her physical reactions are happening for a reason— it's just that they've gone overboard. Melody Morrow is experiencing a stress response (it's an actual scientific term) that simply won't quit. Here are the discoveries that uncovered how it works.

1911: Fight or Run!

The stress response occurs in two phases. Both depend on the release of hormones, or chemical messengers, generally secreted by the glands of the endocrine system, which is one of the three control systems of the body (the immune and the nervous system are the other two).

The endocrine system comprises our glands, the hormones they secrete, and the tissues the hormones target. Oddly, the designation *hormone* (from the Greek, meaning "to excite") derives not from the messenger's makeup or how it acts on cells but from the fact that it travels a distance through the bloodstream in order to act at all. In fact, the same chemical messenger can be dubbed a hormone in one context and something else in another. Dopamine, for example, part of the brain's pleasure circuit, is a hormone when it travels from the hypothalamus, a gland deep in the brain, to the pituitary, a gland in the brain a distance away; but it's a neurotransmitter when it springs from a nerve cell, or neuron, and alters the electrical activity of an adjacent nerve cell.

Fight-or-flight, so dubbed by American physiologist Walter B. Cannon in the early 1900s, is the first phase of the stress response. It describes our body's immediate internal events—those of any animal, actually—when a predator threatens life and limb. These events evolved to save us—to get our asses in gear when we were being charged by, say, a moose, so we could either kill the predator or flee to safety. Indeed, if Melody were a prehistoric hunter-gatherer in Siberia rather than a twenty-first-century woman huddled on a toilet in Miami, she'd be a prime example of evolutionary adaptation.

But she's not. And here's why:

Consider that hunter-gatherer stalking the alpine tundra in search of dinner, spear in hand. His brain, as always, is in charge of all thoughts and actions, and directs the goings-on beneath it via the spinal cord and the peripheral nerves, chains of neurons that branch out of the spine to all the muscles and organs in the body.

This peripheral nervous system comprises two main components: the voluntary (somatic) nervous system and the involuntary (autonomic) nervous system. The somatic nervous system reaches into skeletal muscles—in the thighs, feet, arms—and to external sensory receptors, such as the skin. It is what enables the hunter-gatherer to consciously (hence the "voluntary") clamber through the soil, skirting dwarf shrubs. The autonomic nervous system, on the other hand, snakes out to blood vessels, organs—heart, lungs, stomach, larynx, genitals, for instance—and glands. Of the two, it is the main player in the stress response.

The autonomic nervous system also branches into two parts: the sympathetic and the parasympathetic nervous systems (SNS and PNS). Both originate in the brain stem and innervate the same organs and glands, but they have opposing effects: The sympathetic system turns on in reaction to stress; the parasympathetic system permits recovery from the sympathetic system's doings, bringing things back to baseline.

So here's the hunter-gatherer, creeping through the moss and lichen. Suddenly, he spies the moose, whose conjured image alone has set him salivating. Now his mouth goes dry. All systems shift to red alert: *This* is fight-or-flight.

The processes needed *right now* to save his skin (oxygen to lungs, fuel to skeletal muscles, razor-sharp attention) rev up; those that can wait for another day (reproduction, digesting that roe-deer leg, bulking up biceps) put on the brakes. Through a private circuit of the sympathetic nervous system, his cerebral cortex—the 0.1-inch-thick mantle of neuron-rich gray matter overlaying his entire brain and the center of higher functions (vision, hearing, speech)—tells his hypothalamus, a tooth-shaped structure deep inside, to zip a message to his adrenal glands, the pair of which sit atop his kidneys. The message—*Eek! A moose!*—lands smack in the center of the adrenals (in a section called the medulla), which respond by shooting epinephrine (also called adrenaline), the first of the major stress hormones, into his bloodstream. The endings of all the other nerves of the sympathetic nervous system quickly shoot out the second fight-or-flight hormone, norepinephrine (also called noradrenaline). Both epinephrine and norepinephrine are classified as catecholamines, chemical messengers derived from the amino acid tyrosine—a useful bucket to dump them into, if you're looking for a way to classify them quickly.

This is the sympathetic-adrenal-medullary (SAM) axis kicking into gear. Within seconds, the hunter-gatherer's breathing quickens as the epinephrine dilates the bronchial tubes in his lungs to make space for more oxygen. His blood pressure rises as the hormone charges his heart so it can pump that extra oxygen as well as epinephrine-released fuel (glucose, the simplest sugar, our cells' primary energy store; plus simple fats and amino acids) from the liver, fat cells, and muscles to the parts of the body that need them most: the brain (*Must stay focused! Make a map of every tree I can climb!*) and the skeletal muscles, particularly the large muscles of the legs (*Must charge or run away!*).

Blood vessels leading to necessary body parts open up, too, to allow safe passage of the oxygen-and-nutrient-laden blood. Meanwhile, the blood vessels returning to the heart and those supplying the skin constrict. This vise on the veins to the heart means that blood crashes more forcefully into the chamber, adding oomph to its discharge—picture waves rebounding off a seawall in a hurricane. A constriction of the arteries to the skin slows down bleeding should the hunter-gatherer get attacked or trip over a rock as he scrambles to safety. The epinephrine also stimulates production of fibrinogen—the protein source of fibrin, the main ingredient of blood clots—from the liver to doubly ensure that the hunter-gatherer doesn't bleed to death if he's injured.

Meanwhile, the parasympathetic nervous system does the opposite: It shuts off until the crisis is over, so the activities it stimulates—salivation, digestion, growth, sexual arousal, which would only get in the way—can't interfere.

So that's phase one; it strikes within seconds. But bringing home the moose meat takes longer than that. It's time for Plan B, which can extend the body's hyper-readiness for minutes or even hours.

Enter the glucocorticoid boost.

1930s: Kind of a GAS

Identified in the 1930s by Hungarian-born endocrinologist Hans Selye, the glucocorticoid boost was originally saddled with the clunky moniker General Adaptation Syndrome (GAS) when Selye stumbled—almost literally—across it in his lab at McGill University, in Montreal.

Glucocorticoids are a class of steroid—fat-soluble compounds derived from cholesterol that do everything from clear brain cobwebs (estrogen does that) to spark PMS (progesterone does that). Cortisol—the same stuff that's the active ingredient, in synthetic form (hydrocortisol), of creams for skin rashes and other inflammatory processes—is the glucocorticoid that plays the leading role in the stress response. (The rat version of the hormone is called corticosterone, a word worth knowing, since much wisdom about stress comes from stressing and then minutely examining rats.)

Tooling around in his lab, Selye was out to discover a new hormone in the placenta when GAS overwhelmed him. Not the overwhelming gas pains of indigestion—something less noticeable but more pernicious: For several months, he'd been injecting one group of rats daily with an ovarian extract—and another group with saline, a spleen extract, or kidney extract, to serve as a control. The plan was that the ovarian-pumped critters would exhibit interesting symptoms attributable to a new hormone, which Selye would then isolate, tell the world about, and make his scientific name. But curiously, *all* the rats, regardless of extract, got the same symptoms: swollen adrenals, shrunken lymph nodes, and peptic ulcers.

Selye had a flash: Perhaps it wasn't the *substance* he was injecting that sparked the symptoms but the rats' common *reaction* to their treatment—that is, being grabbed, prodded, and ultimately stabbed with a needle.

To test his hypothesis, Selye injected other rat groups with toxins, such as a formaldehyde solution, or subjected them to physical challenges: exposure to cold, forced exercise, immobilization. Again and again he found the same bloated adrenals, wrung-out nodes, and stomach ulcers—regardless of the insult. He labeled the common response the General Adaptation Syndrome, and in his first paper on the phenomenon, published in 1936, he described it as "a generalized effort of the organism to adapt itself to new conditions." Later, he dubbed those new conditions stressors.

From a mechanistic perspective, Selye's discovery cut out the sympathetic nervous system, and added the pituitary gland to the hypothalamus-adrenals mix to form the second stress axis: the hypothalamus-pituitary-adrenal (HPA) axis, which during chronic or repeated stress becomes its own axis of evil. Linguistically, he codified the entire stress response (which is what we call GAS today), laying out a neat trajectory from fight-or-flight (good thing) to glucocorticoid boost (good thing) to what can happen if both reactions stay on consistently (very, very bad)—as they did for Selye's rats and Melody Morrow.

Now, let's go back to that hunter-gatherer poised in mid-fight-or-flight on the Siberian tundra. The catecholamines, with all their attendant effects, are flowing. Now his cerebral cortex, still on high alert, signals his hypothalamus, but this time tells it to secrete two substances—corticotropin-releasing hormone (CRH) and arginine vasopressin (AVP)—through a teensy circulatory system that links the hypothalamus to the pituitary gland, which dangles beneath the hypothalamus like a grape.

The pituitary—the so-called master gland of the endocrine system—has been variously described as similar in size and shape to an almond or a garbanzo bean, but the grape comparison better conjures the arbor effect. (Truth be told, pictures of the gland, which has both a posterior and an anterior segment, most remind me of a pair of testes, but educational materials don't go there.) CRH and AVP spark the pituitary to pour another hormone, adrenocorticotropin hormone (ACTH), into the bloodstream; it speeds through the vessels to the adrenal glands, atop the kidneys. Here, instead of activating the center, or medulla, of the glands, as the sympathetic nervous system did to release the catecholamines in fight-or-flight, ACTH activates the layers of tissue that *cover* the glands—the adrenal cortex. On the spot, the adrenal cortex cranks out the second major stress hormone—the glucocorticoid known as cortisol in humans (corticosterone in rats)—and releases it into the circulation.

In non-emergency situations, cortisol follows the body's circadian rhythms, set by the body's inner clock, which is also located in the hypothalamus. The clock—and hence cortisol—responds to light and dark, day and night, among other signals (such as temperature). Optimally, our cortisol is highest in the early morning, dips in the afternoon, and drops low at night. There's a logical pattern here: Cortisol kicks in to mobilize stored energy—specifically, glucose—for anything from climbing out of bed to slaying a moose for supper.

Let loose in the hunter-gatherer's bloodstream, cortisol gets to work: It meets up with the catecholamines and the hormone glucagon, which is released by the pancreas during stress, to aid them in breaking down glycogen—daisy chains of glucose molecules stored in the liver and muscles—to keep the easily absorbed glucose coming. It stimulates the liver to make *new* glucose from amino acids that have been sent through the blood from non-exercising muscles—a process called gluconeogenesis. The liver is, in a sense, an emergency chef, keeping the energy rations coming. Cortisol, guard-like, also ensures that the food goes only where it's supposed to: It blocks the glucose from entering fat and non-essential muscle tissue so that it will be available for, say, the hunter-gatherer's now fired-up brain or pounding feet.

The rising cortisol levels spur the hormone to do its final job: to tell the hypothalamus to stop the presses, so to speak—that is, to stop secreting CRH, which in turn stops the flow of ACTH from the pituitary gland, which puts the kibosh on any further cortisol being released from the adrenals. "It's a circular system," says Stafford L. Lightman, Ph.D., director of the UK's Henry Wellcome Laboratories, whose team is working to understand this negative feedback loop better. The point is to keep cortisol levels within an appropriate range. As we age, the feedback loop weakens—sadly, as do many of our body's checks and balances—leaving cortisol levels higher longer.

～～～

That's what happens when all goes well: The stress response turns on to help us meet a challenge (stun a moose, dive at the Olympics, ace that job interview) and turns off when the crisis is over. The hunter-gatherer slings hunks of the dead moose over his shoulder and heads home—his heart, brain, liver, and so on returned to baseline. That's *good* stress. Indeed, without stress of the challenge sort, as Bruce McEwen says in the introduction, "we'd be dead."

But for folks such as Melody Morrow (and too often for you and me), with our Sandwich Generation multitasking lives and our anticipation of threats that haven't struck and possibly never will (Will I get canned today? Will my dad have another heart attack? Forgot that phone number again—do I have early onset Alzheimer's?), the stress response either stays on, period, or repeatedly flares, sending us again and again into revved-up mode. With cortisol bathing our cells and glucose pouring into our bloodstream for no physiological reason, all hell can break loose. The worry may be all in our heads, but our bodies (including our brains) pay the price.

Let's tunnel down into three major systems to see what that price can be. (For the inside story on the key organ of stress, the brain, see Chapter 3.)

Your Immune System on Stress

You've likely noticed that when you're chronically stressed, you get colds more frequently, allergies kick in, or perhaps those latent cold sores (herpes simplex type 1) sprout in your mouth. That's because there's an incredibly strong link between the nervous, endocrine, and immune systems. The peripheral nerves of the autonomic nervous system reach deep into organs and glands, such as lymph nodes and bone marrow that manufacture or store immune-system cells (white blood cells, or leukocytes). Indeed, an entire field, psychoneuroimmunology, has evolved to study the interactions between these three systems.

The Background Basics

Coursing through our bloodstream all the time are immune-system watchdog cells called macrophages. They are part of the innate immune system—the body's first line of defense—and they operate in a relatively short time frame (minutes to hours). These cells scan for foreign invaders—bacteria, viruses, parasites, fungi—and race to the point of entry (the skin, say, or mucous membranes of the mouth or nose) to gobble up the trespassers. Other innate-system cells, including neutrophils and natural killer cells, travel to the site, too, and release toxic substances and pro-inflammatory messenger proteins called cytokines, including the interleukins and tumor necrosis factor-alpha

(TNF-α), which promote wound healing. Innate-system cells also secrete generalized antibodies, small protein molecules that freeze invaders in their tracks. Nothing custom made, mind you, but sufficient to trap garden-variety bugs. They're backed up by brigades of C-reactive proteins—fluid-filled molecules produced by the liver—which seep out of the blood vessels and charge to areas of infection or injury. Hence the swelling and inflammation that accompany everything from, say, a torn cuticle to a sprained ankle.

After their fine microbe meal, the macrophages hoist vestiges of their kill (a.k.a. antigens) to their surfaces like a moose head over a mantel—it's a visible call to arms—and head to the lymph nodes or spleen. The display sparks the acquired immune system, the second, more sustained line of defense. Its weapons include T cells, which are made in the bone marrow and mature in the thymus (hence the T), a small gland sitting just behind the breastbone; and B cells, which are made *and* mature in the bone marrow (ditto the B). The very sight of the bloody corpse on the macrophage mantel signals a subset of T cells called helpers to release interleukins, which in turn instruct regular T cells in the thymus to begin dividing like crazy to bulk up the ground troops.

The cell-division process is called mitosis, and the dividing cells are considered mitotic. The end result of cell division is to produce an exact genetic replica of the mother cell. Cells that don't divide—or postmitotic cells—include mature skeletal muscle cells, mature heart muscle cells, and mature neurons.

Next, the helper T cells secrete a cytokine called B-cell growth factor, which tells the B cells to divide and multiply like there's no tomorrow. B cells produce and launch custom antibodies into the bloodstream—protein molecules shaped to fit like a glove on a specific antigen and hold it hostage until other circulating proteins can kill it. Antibodies are smart bombs to the T cells' ground troops: They neutralize the threat—but not before they imprint it on their "memories," so they'll be at the ready to neutralize it again should it return. Ever wonder why you got chicken pox only once? It's because the antibodies that formed when you were scratching away at age six recognize any chicken-pox virus that makes its way inside you and immediately neutralize it.

If all that firepower isn't enough, allied forces are called in: The interleukins and TNF-α radio the hypothalamus to increase the body's temperature (voilà: fever) to burn the enemy to a crisp.

Adding Acute Stress to the Mix

Initially, the epinephrine rush and the cortisol influx boost the immune response. The innate immune system responds by rushing immune cells through the circulation to the skin and vulnerable muscles and tissues (*Must be prepared for injury!*) and releasing those generic antibodies into the saliva (*Capture any invader!*). The acquired system follows. In fascinating studies published in the mid-1990s, immunologist Firdaus Dhabhar, Ph.D., then a postdoc working with rats in Bruce McEwen's Rockefeller University lab, found that in small early doses, glucocorticoids actually help pull white blood cells out of the circulation and redirect them to places they might be in demand, such as the skin and lymph nodes. They also activate so-called cell-adhesion molecules, which, like glue, help the white blood cells stick to the blood vessels and tissues they've migrated to so wounds can heal faster. McEwen's lab dubbed the phenomenon stress-induced trafficking, which explains the process but sounds like something a drug dealer, not a blob of cytoplasm, would do.

Now at Stanford, Dhabhar has led additional studies showing that in mice, acute stress (restraining the animals) at the time of vaccination actually *increases* immunity over the long term by upping the numbers of memory helper T cells in the lymph nodes. In other studies, he's shown that stressing mice before operating on them to implant a sponge leads to a *200 to 300 percent higher* immune-cell infiltration around the sponge compared to nonstressed animals. So the next time your child— or you—gets stressed about receiving that flu shot, don't worry: that brief freak-out may well be boosting immune protection.

When the Stressor Turns Chronic

Chronic stress does the opposite of acute—or temporary—stress: It *suppresses* the immune system, particularly the acquired immune system, making us more susceptible to infections. Hence those colds, allergies, and herpes simplex 1 outbreaks.

Here's why: The thymus gland, where T cells mature, is very susceptible to elevated glucocorticoid levels, in both animals and people. In fact, a glut of glucocorticoids leads immune cells in the thymus to commit a kind of molecular suicide, known as apoptosis—a very orderly offing of themselves whereby cells are swallowed up by macrophages and essentially disappear. Apoptosis is programmed cell death for the good of the organism; it's supposed to kick in to, say, stop a cancerous cell from dividing. But glucocorticoids can set the process in motion, handing the white blood cell the rope and helping it climb atop a chair. How do scientists know this? They can see it: Hans Selye's chronically stressed rats also had shrunken thymus glands—evidence of loss of T cells.

Excess glucocorticoids can also suppress the production of cytokines—those messenger proteins that tell T cells to get fruitful and multiply, and that radio the locations of attacking invaders. This screws up the distribution of troops, sending them packing to the lymph nodes, for example, when there's a virus in the lungs. Glucocorticoids can also put a damper on new antibody production. Writes Robert Sapolsky in *Why Zebras Don't Get Ulcers*: "For most things that you can measure in the immune system, sustained major stressors drive the numbers down to 40 to 70 percent below baseline." *That's* suppressed.

Your Heart on Stress

The hunter-gatherer spies the moose and epinephrine charges his heart, making it beat faster and stronger. He can hear the thing banging in his ears. His blood pressure rockets. Then cortisol kicks in, shoveling

troughs of glucose through his thicker-than-usual blood (from epinephrine's release of fibrinogen, for clotting) to the muscles, brain cells, and
all other areas that click on in such an emergency.

This is all fine in the short run—necessary, in fact, if he's to get
(rather than be) dinner. But myriad studies show that if the stress response goes on too long or in repeated spikes, the wear and tear on his
heart and blood vessels can lead to terrible health consequences, from
high blood pressure to heart attack.

The Background Basics

Think of your heart as your body's generator: Through a vast system
of blood vessels (arteries and arterial capillaries) stretching from head to
toe, it pumps nutrients and oxygen to every cell in your body. Through
just as vast a system (veins and veinal capillaries), it returns the "empty"
blood plus waste, such as carbon dioxide (hence veins' darker color), to
the heart for a refill. The heart, too, has its own personal system of blood
vessels: coronary arteries (they encircle the heart like a crown), which
branch off the aorta, the largest artery in the body; and corresponding coronary veins. All of these blood vessels plus your heart make up
your cardiovascular system, a massive electric power grid sending juice
throughout a city (you). Thanks to this intense circulatory oversight,
every cell in your body has intimate access to necessary goods: white
blood cells (immune cells), red blood cells (oxygen carriers), hormones,
cytokines—anything it needs to stay alive and functioning.

The most vulnerable sites in the blood vessels are the junctures—the
points where one big vessel, say, branches into smaller ones, each of which
then branches into even smaller ones, and so on. It makes sense: The
crotch of a tree is certainly more susceptible to splitting than the trunk.
Now imagine a geyser shooting up through that trunk. Before the water
rockets off on its dual pathway—through the upper trunk and the angled-
off branch—it has to slam into the crotch. It's a perfect setup for injury.

Blood pressure, in fact, is nothing more than the force with which the blood exiting the heart presses against the smooth walls of the arteries as it travels to its destinations. Systolic pressure (the top number on a blood-pressure reading) registers the force when the heart is pumping, sending blood throughout the body. Check yours out: Anything over 140 is considered high. Diastolic pressure (the bottom number) registers the force between beats, when the heart is at rest. The tipping point here is 90. Hence, 120/80 or lower is normal blood pressure, and 140/90 or higher is high blood pressure.

Adding Acute Stress to the Mix

When epinephrine spikes the heart, the blood gushes into the arteries with greater force, pressing against the walls like there's no tomorrow and causing the leap in blood pressure. (Interesting side point: Beta-blockers work by blocking the receptors through which epinephrine acts, thereby keeping blood pressure down.) The epinephrine also, you'll recall, sets glucose, fatty acids, and amino acids free in the bloodstream to "feed" the muscles and other cells that need them. As noted previously, when danger strikes, these are good things: The heart can now pump extra oxygen and fuel to the parts of the body that need them to fight or flee.

The glucocorticoid boost then buttresses these sympathetic nervous system effects. Glucocorticoids increase blood pressure, partly by causing cells to retain more salt and water, and partly by causing vessels to constrict. They do the latter by inhibiting the synthesis of dilating substances inside the artery walls, and by sensitizing the vessels to the constricting effects of norepinephrine. Glucocorticoids also inhibit chemicals that keep blood platelets—loose cytoplasm fragments that aid clotting—from gathering in clumps. These clumps of platelets will help reduce bleeding should the hunter-gatherer be injured while fighting or fleeing.

The arteries, of course, are built to withstand these changes in the short term—unless, of course, they're damaged already, which can make the heart particularly susceptible to a shock. Once the stressor has passed, the parasympathetic nervous system takes over, slowing down the heart via the vagus nerve, a giant snaking thing with seemingly endless fibers that originates in the brain stem and extends all the way down to the colon.

The vagus nerve plays a crucial role regarding even the smallest stressors. A healthy heart normally has an irregular beat. Indeed, its rate even speeds up when you inhale—that is, the time interval between beats shortens—and it slows down when you exhale. This is heart-rate variability and is what enables us to climb out of bed in the morning without fight-or-flight kicking in. Heart-rate variability is controlled by the vagus nerve's loosening its grip so the heart can beat a bit faster as we swing our feet to the ground, and then tightening it again to slow the heart down once we're upright.

"If you have good parasympathetic balances, like the shock absorbers on the car, that helps the cardiovascular system weather these different experiences that we have," says McEwen. "The parasympathetic system also calms down inflammation—one of the big causal factors of cardiovascular disease."

When the Stressor Turns Chronic

Just imagine if the sympathetic nervous system were repeatedly or chronically turned on. Its antithesis, the parasympathetic system, would be chronically turned off. There's no calm now, even without a storm.

For starters, your heart-rate variability will be shot, and your heart rate perpetually high. Your blood pressure will be perpetually high, too (that's hypertension), which means a constant slamming of blood against junctures and vessel walls. With too much of this, the vessel lining begins to erode, just as the concrete of a seawall begins to wear away after repeated thumping by waves. Think Hurricane Ike in Galveston, Texas, September 2008. After the storm, sinkholes marred the sidewalk atop the city's renowned seventeen-foot-high seawall, and the erosion of the beach fronting the seawall left its pine pilings scarily exposed.

In arteries, such sinkholes are called lesions. Immune cells travel to the scene to tend to the damage, making the lesions sticky as inflammation sets in. Among the rescue team are so-called foam cells—macrophages loaded with fats (specifically, low density lipoproteins, a.k.a. "bad" cholesterol). As glucocorticoids continue to pour out of the adrenal glands, glucose and platelets join the fats gathering in the viscous blood and jamming into the lesions. All the gunk together can form an atherosclerotic plaque (from the Greek *athero*, or "paste," and *sclerosis*, or "hardness"). Plaques can clog arteries, making it difficult for organs, including the heart, to receive enough oxygen and nutrients, and giving blood slamming against artery walls nowhere to go but out—literally: The blood can rupture the vessel wall, resulting in a thick clot, or thrombus, to fill the gap. If that clot blocks a coronary artery, you have a heart attack; if it blocks an artery in the brain, you have a stroke.

Pounding blood and the fat-streaked artery walls can also lead to an aneurysm of the aorta, in which the aorta walls are so weakened that they bulge with each thump, and maybe even burst. The same can happen with an artery in the brain.

Less immediately dire but still forecasting doom is this scenario: Your elevated blood pressure, combined with constricted vessels (thanks to excessive glucocorticoids, as explained previously), causes the arteries to work harder to manage the passage of blood. Working harder builds up the muscles surrounding the artery walls. Thicker muscles may look good on arms when we don a sleeveless dress, but for arteries they're horrible news: The thicker the muscle, the more rigid the vessel, which means restricted blood flow to organs and tissues as well as a reduced ability to regulate blood flow. Think about it: You can regulate water passing through a hose by pinching the rubber, but you have no control over water passing through a PVC pipe. In our bodies, this rigidity is called hardening of the arteries.

Also contributing to the hardening of the arteries (as well as to joint stiffening) is the excess glucose released by the soaring glucocorticoids. How? The glucose attaches to proteins such as hemoglobin (in red blood cells) and collagen and elastin, which make up our joints' connective tissue, and through a chemical process called glycation forms "advanced glycation end products," or—in an uncharacteristic scientific play on words—AGEs. These are clunky globs that weigh down proteins, causing them to malfunction and draw adjacent molecules into a cross-linked mess. The accumulation of AGEs is a natural process, but chronic stress accelerates it (so does eating foods high in AGEs—yes, foods contain them, too). Hardening of the arteries, in turn, can lead to an enlarged heart, putting you at increased risk for heart failure, a heart attack, or sudden cardiac arrest.

Your Digestive System on Stress

Remember Hans Selye's stressed-out rats? Along with swollen adrenals and shrunken lymph nodes, the harried rodents had—yup—stomach ulcers. How many of us haven't experienced some kind of stress-related digestive turmoil? In my twenties, I had my own bout: spastic and irritable colon, they called it back then, when the colonoscope was a new toy bandied about (more precisely, within) sans sedation. At the time my doctor prescribed eating anything bland, that is, white—white rice, white bread, white-meat chicken with no skin. Roughage came from grainy psyllium husk, which turned to sludge in water if you didn't drink the tonic fast enough. Today, of course, the treatment is exactly the opposite: If you have a colon that's spasming, the reasoning goes, give it something to chew on.

Ulcers and irritable bowel syndrome (as it's now called) are just two digestive flare-ups associated with stress. There's also inflammatory bowel disease (the umbrella term for ulcerative colitis and Crohn's disease), dyspepsia, gastroesophageal reflux, constipation, "the runs," and more. If you already have one of these lovely conditions, stress can make it worse.

Here's a peek inside your gut when stress hits.

The Background Basics

You chomp on dinner, and the masticated meal travels past your throat and down the muscular hollow that is your esophagus, and lands in your stomach. There it's broken down into fats, proteins, and carbohydrates by hydrochloric acid and enzymes secreted by the stomach lining. Next the broken-down food moves to the small intestine—approximately twenty-two feet of tightly coiled tubing rich with glands that secrete more digestive enzymes. The enzymes degrade the food nutrients into individual molecules that can pass through the small-intestine wall into the bloodstream, which carries them to hungry cells in your organs and tissues. Next stop for what is now glop is the large intestine, whose biggest part is the colon. It sucks the water out of the mixture and returns it, too, to the bloodstream. Early the next morning, after the obligatory caffeine, you truck your electronic book into the bathroom and get rid of the solid waste that's left.

What keeps the food moving reliably down the gastrointestinal (GI) tract? Impulses from peripheral nerves of both the sympathetic and parasympathetic systems, and hormones. The humungous vagus nerve, part of the vagal system, sprouts two networks that land in the colon; it takes the lead in directing the contractions that shove the food through the tract.

There's actually a name for the linkage between the brain and nervous systems and GI tract: the brain-gut axis. Interestingly, according to McMaster University gastroenterologists Stephen M. Collins, M.B.B.S., and Premysl Bercik, M.D., communications on the axis go two ways: from brain to gut and vice versa. And the correspondents on the line include not just the brain, hormones, and nerves but also a multitude of microorganisms (more than 10^{14}) that call the gut home.

Adding Acute Stress to the Mix

Digestion shuts down during stress, as energy (mostly glucose) and oxygen are redirected to the muscles and organs (lungs, brain, heart) that need them most. That means the parasympathetic system, which stimulates intestinal contractions, shuts off and the sympathetic system, which releases the catecholamines, switches on. This, along with the release of CRH and other hormones in phase two of the stress response (the glucocorticoid boost), slows down the small intestine's dumping of its contents into the large intestine and increases the activity of the colon, leading more liquid to be sucked through its walls into the bloodstream. The process ensures that nature won't call while the hunter-gatherer is fleeing from what he'd hoped would be his evening meal. The glucocorticoids released during the boost also briefly inhibit the secretion of stomach acid and stimulate the production of a buffer substance, bicarbonate. The entire GI tract is temporarily on leave. Once the stressor passes, the plumbing and digestive functions start back up again.

When the Stress Is Chronic

There is an entire body of medical and popular literature on the relationship between chronic stress and gastrointestinal upheaval, whether "functional" (with no identifiable physiological cause), like my irritable bowel syndrome, or "organic" (with a detectable cause), like inflammatory diseases such as ulcerative colitis (inflammation of the mucosal lining of the large intestine) and Crohn's disease (inflammation of the lining *and* wall of the entire GI tract).

Many problems stem from the fact that when stress is chronic, normal digestion doesn't resume. Small-intestine activity remains damped down, and large-intestine activity remains ramped up. This can result in either constipation or diarrhea, both of which are symptoms of irritable bowel syndrome. And while glucocorticoids initially help protect the stomach by shutting down the production of hydrochloric acid, their repeatedly being switched on and off has the opposite effect. Why? Glucocorticoids inhibit the production of mucus (a protector) and chemicals called prostaglandins (healers) and, as described earlier, they constrict the blood vessels in the GI tract so that blood can get where it's needed fast. Repeatedly interrupted mucus and prostaglandin production means a thinner and dryer stomach lining. So when digestion—read: hydrochloric acid production—does resume in between stress-out sessions, the stage is set for an ulcer.

Not all ulcers are created equal, and there's been some controversy over their origins. Peptic ulcers strike in the stomach (gastric peptic ulcers) or the structures directly connected to the stomach: the esophagus (esophageal ulcers) and the duodenum (duodenal ulcers). The latter is the part of the GI tract leading from the stomach to the small intestine. Belief in the role of the bacterium *Helicobacter pylori* in generating peptic ulcers has gained considerable favor over the years, but questions still remain. For example, studies have shown that the bacterium exists in people with longer-term (six months or more) duodenal ulcers but not in those with ulcers that heal faster. This suggests that a) *H. pylori* doesn't cause the ulcers but may keep them active, or b) the surplus of stomach acid over the long term may provide what the bacterium needs: a comfy nest. Moreover, *H. pylori* is nearly ubiquitous in guts the world over, yet those infected with it have only a 10 to 20 percent risk of developing ulcers. Furthermore, duodenal ulcers, in particular, show up in people with no sign of the bacterium at all.

Much more straightforward in origin is the stress ulcer, also called an acute gastric ulcer, which has been linked directly to severe physical trauma, such as a burn, sepsis, or surgery. It is catalyzed by the same CRH release and vagal-system action noted previously, combined with the restricted blood supply that can accompany such trauma. Acute gastric ulcers, unlike those of the peptic variety, don't eat through the stomach wall but erode the surface of its lining.

Prolonged stress can also throw off the gut's balance of good and bad bacteria, just as antibiotics can. Microorganisms in the gut serve many functions: They protect against bacteria, viruses, and fungi; metabolize drugs; and help us absorb nutrients and fats. But because stress can change the gut's chemical environment, the place can become inhospitable to microorganisms that keep the bad guys in check.

Such stress can also increase the permeability of the intestinal walls, opening the door to antigens and other pro-inflammatory substances from past battles that have been lying dormant. The microorganism population, already topsy-turvy, can't mount the defense your body needs. The conditions are perfect for a flare-up if you're susceptible to disorders such as colitis or Crohn's.

1993: Enter Allostatic Load

Bruce McEwen—who in 1968 discovered that brain cells actually have glucocorticoid receptors, making them directly susceptible to the hormone's actions—wanted a term that would describe the price our brains and bodies pay for enduring chronic stress. In 1993 he introduced one: *allostatic load*.

Allostasis means "stability through change." It refers to the hormones and the autonomic-nervous-system regulators that our bodies call forth to maintain equilibrium in our systems—cardiovascular, immune, metabolic, and so on—as we respond to stressors. What constitutes a stressor may surprise you: Changes in your physical state—from sleeping to waking, resting to exercising, even sitting to standing—are all stressors, albeit short-lived ones. So are day-to-day external and internal experiences, such as hunger, noise, and danger.

Any number of conditions can throw those systems off kilter: stressors that don't let up, for instance, or a supersensitivity, born of genes and early environment, that keeps us from habituating to common frazzlers such as giving a speech. The result? Allostatic load: the wear and tear of stress, over time, on our various systems or, as McEwen puts it, the "cumulative physiological cost of adaptation to stress." And it's the size of our allostatic load, he says, together with our genetic makeup, that determines how we progress toward diseases ranging from hypertension and type 2 diabetes to atherosclerosis and obesity.

"Allostasis refers to the idea that when we experience a stressful challenge—whether it's getting out of bed in the morning or having harsh words with our boss or our spouse, or having something happen while driving to work—our body copes by putting out hormones and other chemicals that help us adapt and stay alive," says McEwen. "But at the same time, we recognize that if these chemicals are overactive—whether it's epinephrine increasing our blood pressure or cortisol increasing glucose—they contribute over time to disorders like hardening of the arteries, hypertension, type 2 diabetes, increased inflammation, and cognitive decline. Allostatic load refers to the cumulative burden of stress, which is an almost inevitable consequence of being alive as we're defending our bodies."

As we age, our allostatic load goes up simply because wear and tear accumulates. Think about it: Forty-five years of chemicals flowing as we adapt to stressors will take more of a toll than twenty-two years of the same. To measure the rise, UCLA's Teresa E. Seeman, Ph.D., and McEwen developed an allostatic load index that actually predicts health and mortality risk better than traditional individual measures, which may in fact not predict risk at all on their own. The measure, which relies on a sophisticated formula for analysis, has ten components, including blood pressure (for cardiovascular activity); waist-hip ratio (for metabolism and fat distribution); cholesterol (it influences atherosclerosis); and cortisol, epinephrine, and norepinephrine levels. Seeman also considers quality-of-life variables in her assessments, including social support, education, and socioeconomic status—all of which can exacerbate or counteract allostatic load, depending on whether they're high or low.

"This whole idea of allostasis and allostatic load is to get away from focusing just on the stressful *experience* and focus on people's lifestyle as well," says McEwen. "People compartmentalize. For example, they don't realize that with depression and anxiety disorder, there also very likely will be cardiovascular problems, hypertension, obesity, diabetes, maybe arthritis. There are cormorbidities."

Yet the concept—smart and accurate as it is—has not made it into either the popular or the clinical vernacular, despite its seventeen years on the scene. Why might that be? After all, we've all heard repeatedly about metabolic syndrome (a.k.a. syndrome X), which encompasses several factors: blood pressure, belly fat, triglyceride levels, HDL ("good") cholesterol, and glucose levels.* Still, those all indicate a *specific* risk, namely, for cardiovascular disease, stroke, and diabetes. It may be that the allostatic load index's greatest strength—its comprehensiveness—is what's kept it from being put into practice.

"Bruce and I have encountered a huge amount of skepticism from the different research disciplines because research has these much more narrowly focused traditions," says Seeman. "I think one of the things that people don't like about allostatic load is that it's not an indicator of specific outcomes. We've used allostatic load to predict overall mortality and we've used it to show risk for general cognitive and physical decline. If you're a researcher and what you want to do is predict who is going to have a myocardial infarction or a stroke, then our index is probably not what you're going to look for." She pauses. "That's the resistance that we're getting. People are saying, 'You're putting apples and oranges together. You have metabolism and the HPA-axis.' My argument is that yes, that does all play a role in the outcome you're interested in."

But what if there were a *simple* marker that could provide a reading of how stress affects our overall health and mortality risk, while also indicating where we stood regarding specific disorders and even aging itself? How great would that be?

Now there is such a marker: The new science of stress that follows differs not just in degree but in kind from the old science of stress described in this chapter. It takes a comprehensive approach yet is easily

---

* According to the American Heart Association and the National Heart, Lung, and Blood Institute, you have metabolic syndrome if you have three or more of these signs: blood pressure equal to or higher than 130/85 mmHg, fasting blood sugar (glucose) equal to or higher than 100 mg/dL, large waist measurement (men: 40 inches or more, women: 35 inches or more), low HDL cholesterol (men: under 40 mg/dL, women: under 50 mg/dL), triglycerides equal to or higher than 150 mg/dL.

grasped. It provides a novel, more direct way to look at the inescapable link between stress and aging. By so doing it makes plain the solution to the timeless question on so many of our minds: How can I slow—or even reverse—my aging process?

Read on for the telomere story.

~~~

CHAPTER 2

The New Science of Stress

Reality is an activity of the most august imagination.

—Wallace Stevens, 1954

In December 1995, at age thirty-nine, Lia Spiliotes took her son, James, almost two, to visit her parents at their home in Long Island, New York. Three months earlier, she'd left her husband—a wunderkind rocket scientist with a heart as cold as the zero-gravity space structures he studied—and this was the first time she'd traveled to see her parents alone with the baby.

The drive from Somerville, Massachusetts, to New York was a breeze. Not so the visit. Under the gaze of her warm but traditional Greek parents, Lia felt alternately like a burden and a failure. To escape the weight of their expectations, she took James to a beloved sailing club in nearby Sayville. Once there, she stepped out into the gravel parking lot to "check out the scoop."

She doesn't remember much else. For as she turned to fetch the baby, her loafer caught on a lip of ice and—zip!—she tasted metal, then crash-landed on grit. Her feet flew out from under her like whacked-out propeller blades, sending her entire body weight—all 272 pounds of it— smack onto her left leg. Later she'd learn that the bone had shattered so badly that the leg would have to be set three times. In the interim, she nearly lost her job at a pharmaceutical consultancy.

"At that point, after five years of marriage, I had gained an entire person and had high blood pressure and high cholesterol," says the five-foot-six Lia.

There was more to deal with than the fallout from a failing marriage. When James turned one, he'd stopped meeting developmental milestones. "He started walking at eleven months, but he'd bang into furniture," Lia says, miming his black, curly head bonking into a chair. "And he didn't have the verbal abilities at even the lowest level for his age." He avoided eye contact, was very sensitive to light, and suffered seizures in the early morning.

After what seemed like endless neuropsychological evaluations with repeatedly grim results ("Don't expect too much of him growing up," one doctor baldly told her), James got a diagnosis, kind of: pervasive development delay, not otherwise specified—a notch on the autism spectrum. The uncertainty—the "not otherwise specified" piece of it—sent Lia reeling.

"There's a whole category of kids in that middle section of the spectrum, which I call the 'miscellaneous bucket,' where when you ask the neurologists, 'So what is this all about?' they say they don't really know," she says. "It makes it very hard on parents to figure out how to help their kids develop." They're also left floundering socially, without the literature and support groups that parents of kids with an official diagnosis, such as Asperger's, have.

As the years passed, Lia careered between battling for her son and battling to maintain her own equilibrium. Arranging special-education plans to help her boy speak, finding the proper seizure medication, and coping with James's disruptive behaviors, such as biting teachers, alternated with her own binges: downing six martinis when James was staying with the ex-to-be, say, or dropping a fistful of Percocet the next morning in an effort to stop the pounding in her head.

"It's like somebody that has a chronic illness," Lia says about caring for a child labeled "unspecified." "It never leaves you. It can be quiet because things seem to be on an even keel; James is overall warm and loving." But then suddenly something snaps and James gets stuck, his thoughts derailed. "He'll say the same thing over and over: 'I have my hermit crabs.' 'When can we get the hermit crabs?' The hermit crabs, the hermit crabs. And maybe you know what kicked it off, or maybe you don't." The isolation and the not knowing—the inability to forestall or curtail, or even predict the denouement—can stretch her to the breaking point.

"The stress is incredible," she says. "By age forty-two, when James was five, I'd turned completely and utterly gray."

How Stressed Do You Feel?

The Perceived Stress Scale is a scientifically proven measure for assessing our overall level of angst. Where do you fall on the stress spectrum?

The questions below ask you about your feelings and thoughts during the last month. In each case, circle *how often* you felt or thought a certain way.

0 = Never   1 = Almost never   2 = Sometimes
3 = Fairly often   4 = Very often

1. In the last month, how often have you been upset because of something that happened unexpectedly?

    0   1   2   3   4

2. In the last month, how often have you felt that you were unable to control the important things in your life?

    0   1   2   3   4

3. In the last month, how often have you felt nervous and "stressed"?

    0   1   2   3   4

4. In the last month, how often have you felt confident about your ability to handle your personal problems? (R)

    0   1   2   3   4

5. In the last month, how often have you felt that things were going your way? (R)

0   1   2   3   4

6. In the last month, how often have you found that you could not cope with all the things that you had to do?

0   1   2   3   4

7. In the last month, how often have you been able to control irritations in your life? (R)

0   1   2   3   4

8. In the last month, how often have you felt that you were on top of things? (R)

0   1   2   3   4

9. In the last month, how often have you been angered because of things that were outside of your control?

0   1   2   3   4

10. In the last month, how often have you felt difficulties were piling up so high that you could not overcome them?

0   1   2   3   4

Calculating your score:

1. Take your responses to questions 4, 5, 7, and 8 and *reverse* each one (they are marked *R*). That is, if you circled 0, give the response the value of 4; if you circled 1, give the response the value of 3; and so on: 2 = 2, 3 = 1, 4 = 0. Add up the *reversed* values. (Reverse scoring is what makes many tests scientifically valid, as opposed to the guesswork of many popular tests.)

2. Add up your responses to the remaining questions: 1, 2, 3, 6, 9, 10.

3. Add the sums from 1 and 2 to get your total score.

Scores range from 0 to 40. The higher your score, the more stressed-out you feel.

Interpreting your score the *Stress Less* way*:

0–10: Low stress
11–20: Medium stress
21–30: High stress
31–40: Extreme stress

~~~~~

Stress and aging: an anecdotally irrefutable link. We've all seen friends become symbols of the phenomenon, like Lia; indeed, we're all running from the gray hair and sagging jowls, the papery skin and flabby bellies that would qualify us for the role ourselves. Newsmakers have put a public face—literally—on the sad trajectory. Consider the images of Beth Twitty Holloway flashing across TV screens and tabloid covers between 2005 and 2006. At daughter Natalee's 2005 high school graduation, when Beth was forty-four, the two—blond locks flowing—could have passed for sisters. But a year after Natalee's disappearance in Aruba, Beth looked as if she'd aged decades, her face gaunt, the skin on her neck pooling in hollows. Even her hair looked different—still yellow, but coarse, like hay.

But the direct biological line between stress and aging wasn't drawn in the scientific sand until 2004, when the scientific journal *PNAS* published the groundbreaking study led by cell and molecular biologist Elizabeth Blackburn and health psychologist Elissa Epel showing that chronic stress may actually gnaw away at our DNA, speeding up the rate at which our cells age by a shocking ten years or more. The finding gave scientific credence to a truth those of us over the age of twenty-five have known in our bones (and hearts and multiple other organs) for years.

What made the paper so revolutionary wasn't just that the association between stress and aging had been shown in humans rather than

---

* The *Stress Less* interpretation was developed by the author, not the scientists.

in the customary laboratory animals. It was that this was the first demonstration of a link that went from the macro (the psychosocial world, where children whine and husbands see in only black and white) to the micro (the world inside our cells, tunneling to our DNA). As such, it showed, elegantly and rigorously, that stress is associated not only with the diseases of aging—such as cardiovascular disease, cancer, and type 2 diabetes—as so many studies before it had shown, but with the actual biological aging of our cells.

The Blackburn and Epel paper was equally revolutionary in that, by its very design, it opened the door to the solution to our seemingly irrevocable decline. Using just two primary measures, the scientists showed, quantitatively, that perception is key: The amount of stress people in the study *felt* they were under, not external circumstances, correlated with how close to the end their cells might be. That means that each of us holds the antidote—the ability to slow that unsightly ripening (as Shakespeare referred to it in *As You Like It*)—in our own hands, or more precisely, in our brains and bodies.

The Rockefeller's Bruce McEwen perhaps said it best for an article I wrote for *O* magazine in 2006 on the Blackburn and Epel discovery: "Americans have been so focused on finding that magic bullet, the quick fix, the pharmacological treatment to slow aging, we don't realize there's a lot we can do to help ourselves."

"But wait," we protest. "We've tried so hard to be good: We eat right to stay slim and exercise to keep our hearts and muscles strong. What gives?"

Truth is, all along we may have been targeting the wrong villains, those we can *see*—carbs, fat, couch-potato-ness—rather than the one that gets under the skin (and the radar): stress.

The idea that chronic stress is associated with poorer health—conditions such as cardiovascular disease, type 2 diabetes, depression, gastrointestinal problems, high blood pressure, weakened immune responses, even more belly fat—is not new. Nor is it revelatory that compromised health can grind us down, making us appear—and feel—old before our time.

What was not known, however, before Blackburn and Epel's work, was just *how* stress, a psychosocial construct, went about wreaking havoc, particularly at the level of our cells—those microscopic units that alone and in intricate dances with one another perform all the fundamental processes of life.

"This was not about fruit flies; it was about humans," says Robert Sapolsky, his blue eyes flashing above his bush of a beard as he explains the significance of the Blackburn and Epel study. The noted Stanford neurobiologist wrote a commentary on the study that appeared in *PNAS* a week after the paper's publication. "These were not humans getting irradiated in Nagasaki; these were humans with stressors that were heavily—not entirely, but heavily—psychosocial. And you could put all the pieces together. All the steps are in there."

~~~~~~

Elizabeth Blackburn is sitting to my right at the round maple table in the corner of her office in Genentech Hall, a mammoth structure of beige brick and glass at the University of California, San Francisco. We are discussing her latest experiments: investigations into how psychological states such as stress and depression might affect the rate at which our cells age, and the relationship between diseases of aging and cancer. The odd thing is, she's not sitting on a chair. This 2009 winner of the Nobel Prize in Physiology or Medicine and Morris Herzstein professor of biology and physiology at UCSF is comfortably perched—even bouncing a bit—atop a large gray exercise ball.

Blackburn's uncommon mix of accessibility and rigor, down-to-earthness and brilliance, comes as no surprise to me. The first time we met, four years ago, she offered me tea and cookies—and pillows for my back—as we chatted in her room at the Ritz-Carlton Hotel in Boston, not just about science but about our children (her son was then a freshman at MIT; my daughter was seven). She was in town to receive another honorary degree, this one from "a famous university," she told me; she was forbidden to say the name. It turned out to be Harvard.

Blackburn studies telomeres—the very tips of our forty-six chromosomes, the threadlike structures nestled in the nucleus of every one of our one hundred trillion cells. Many of us have seen pictures of chromosomes: They are matched in twenty-three pairs (one from each biological parent), and together resemble an elongated X, two worms crossed at the middle, with our nearly twenty-five thousand genes—our DNA—as the spiraling, linear guts. Which genes are turned on in any particular cell determine that cell's identity and function. For example, skin genes are turned on in skin cells but not in liver cells, and vice versa. Telomeres (from the Greek words *telos* and *meros*, meaning "end" and "part") are the caps stuck on the ends of the chromosomes to protect our DNA—the chromosomal equivalent of the plastic tips on the ends of shoelaces that keep the lace ends from fraying. Each of our cells contains ninety-two of them, one on each end of the forty-six chromosomes tucked inside.

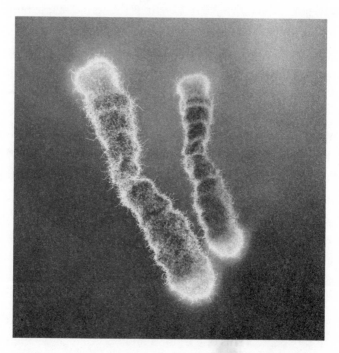

Figure 1. Tip-tops: Telomeres, on the ends of chromosomes, protect our DNA.

In the 1930s, geneticists Barbara McClintock, working with maize, and Hermann J. Müller, working with fruit flies, discovered telomeres at about the same time (Müller coined the name), each concluding that the structures' function was to prevent chromosomes from fusing end-to-end, which would be an unmitigated disaster for cells. But it wasn't until the 1970s, when Blackburn, as a postdoc at Yale in the lab of Joseph G. Gall, first sequenced telomere DNA from *Tetrahymena thermophila*—a one-cell creature that divides endlessly—that the molecular nature of telomeres was revealed.

Molecular biology has the uncanny ability to remind us simultaneously whence we came and how far we've come, and telomeres are a part of that memory jog. Telomeres, it turns out, are highly conserved in most eukaryotic cells or organisms (that is, ones with a distinct nucleus housing their DNA), from protozoa to people. In 1984, in collaboration with Blackburn, geneticist Jack W. Szostak, Ph.D., at what was then Boston's Sidney Farber Cancer Institute, found that the same telomere ends capped the chromosomes of the yeast *Saccharomyces cerevisiae*. And in 1988, geneticist Robert K. Moyzis, Ph.D., then at New Mexico's Los Alamos National Laboratory, identified the sequence of the human telomere. It was remarkably similar to that of Blackburn's lowly *Tetrahymena*.

Four chemical compounds, called bases—adenine, thymine, guanine, cytosine (dubbed A, T, G, C)—arranged in myriad permutations, make up all the DNA sitting on our chromosomes. Their arrangement is what determines our specific genetic inheritance. Telomeres, too, are made up of those bases, but they have a distinction: They are composed of just a single repeating sequence—TTAGGG—bound by proteins. The very end of the telomere hooks around and tucks back into the DNA, forming a loop like the noose at the end of a rope. The TTAGGG sequence—a kind of molecular thumbprint—along with the loop structure, acts as a harbinger: It tells surrounding cells that what they are looking at is the tip of a chromosome, a telomere, rather than a break in the genetic DNA. This is important, because DNA breaks set off alarm bells. They call forth DNA damage responses: enzymes (proteins causing chemical reactions) that rush in to "patch up" breaks by fusing the broken chromosome with another broken chromosome or capturing telomeres from neighboring cells.

"All cells abhor broken DNA," says cell biologist Judith Campisi, Ph.D., sitting across a round table from me in her small office at the Lawrence Berkeley Laboratory, in Berkeley, California. This is where she spends half her time; otherwise she's at the Buck Institute for Age Research, a soaring, meditative limestone-lined structure designed by I. M. Pei, in the dusty hills of Novato. Campisi is tiny and spry—just four-foot-eleven—with wavy auburn hair and a propensity to dress in all black. She has become famous in scientific circles for her discoveries regarding the evolutionary tradeoffs between cancer and aging, and the true nature of senescent, or arrested, cells. "A break in the middle of a chromosome is the most catastrophic lesion for a cell," she says. "The cell has to do something fast—fix that problem or die."

When the repair is perfect, the cell can return to business as usual. But imperfect, funky repairs can fuel mutations, vulnerability to additional breaks when the cell divides, and eventually genomic instability, wherein the chromosome becomes something of a molecular deck of cards, broken and shuffled and re-stacked. And mutations, says Campisi grimly, can cause cancer.

So telomeres are, in a sense, chromosome lifesavers, enabling the chromosomes to maintain their integrity, and working as a powerful cancer deterrent. Things get more complicated, though, when cells divide. Not all do, but immune and skin cells do, so they can multiply to repair or regenerate tissue or battle infections. Other dividing cells include adult stem cells and their first-degree offspring, progenitor cells, in organs ranging from intestines and bone marrow to—surprisingly—the brain. As explained in Chapter 1, cells that divide are known as mitotic cells. The end result of cell division is to produce an exact genetic replica of the mother cell. Cells that don't divide are called postmitotic cells. Among them are mature skeletal and heart muscle cells and mature brain cells (neurons).

The problem is, telomeres shorten with each cell division. Here's why: To produce daughter cells, the spiraling double-helix ladder of DNA on the chromosomes unzips so that enzymes can make a copy of each strand. But the enzymes that "read" the DNA strands to synthesize new copies run out of steam before they reach the ends of the telomeres. Which means that each time a cell divides, some of the telomere—the "unread" part (which amounts to some fifty to two hundred bases)—is lost. This is known in scientific circles as the "end replication problem." James D. Watson, Ph.D., of Watson and Crick double-helix fame, was the first to notice, in 1972, that daughter chromosomes were a smidgen shorter than their moms. At about the same time, Russian theoretical biologist Alexey Olovnikov, Ph.D., had an *aha!* moment regarding the phenomenon: He descended into a Moscow subway station, and the mechanism coalesced when he saw a train (the enzymes) chugging down but not yet reaching the end of the track (the DNA strands).

This erosion process is what makes telomere shortening a marker, to many scientists, of biological—or replicative—aging, a "molecular clock" ticking off the life span of the cell. Indeed, after about fifty to seventy doublings the telomeres have essentially eroded to nil, their loops gone and their protective function exhausted, and further division becomes impossible.

There are other biochemical processes at work as well, eating away at our DNA's tips. Chief among them are oxidation, caused by the release of reactive oxygen species (ROS), a type of free radical, and inflammation, the gathering of immune-system cells and fluids to an injury site, as described in Chapter 1.

During normal metabolism, our cells—specifically, their mitochondria—consume oxygen and nutrients to produce the fuel that powers them. Called ATP (adenosine triphosphate), this fuel enables cells to do everything from communicate with one another to metabolize glucose, their main source of nutrition. Mitochondria are oblong structures that sit in our cells' cytoplasm—the stuff (fluids, organelles) surrounding the nucleus and held in place by the cell membrane.

But as with any energy powerhouse, mitochondria have a downside. Just as car engines burning gasoline release carbon gases as a by-product, mitochondria converting oxygen and nutrients to ATP release free radicals as a by-product.

Free radicals are atoms (such as oxygen or nitrogen) or bunches of atoms (molecules) with one or more *unpaired* electrons. They race about, snatching electrons here from an atom, there from a molecule, in a frenzied attempt to regain equilibrium. In the process, they run roughshod over whatever's in their path, particularly DNA, proteins, and the lipids of cell membranes, leaving in their wake gene mutations, malfunctioning proteins, and leaky membranes. A chain reaction ensues as the newly robbed atoms go rogue themselves, attacking still other atoms to achieve coupled bliss.

When the free radicals involved have oxygen at their core, the process is called oxidation, or oxidative stress. (Hence the moniker "reactive oxygen species.") ROS are not all bad news: They're important for certain types of signaling between and within cells. Still, they can cause a great deal of damage.

Environmental factors such as pollution, ultraviolet light, and radiation can do the same damage, as can biological processes such as inflammation. The latter, as you'll recall from Chapter 1, begins as a *good* thing: Immune-system macrophages gobble up invaders to forestall infection. But while digesting their meal, they secrete ROS and pro-inflammatory cytokines into the tissue. As we age, not only does oxidative damage accumulate, but our mitochondria also operate less efficiently, releasing ever more ROS. In the mid-1950s, biochemist Denham Harman, M.D., Ph.D., captured the downward spiral in his free-radical theory of aging— that is, the idea that free-radical damage to cells leads to aging itself, as well as the degenerative diseases of aging (including cancer, heart disease, arthritis, cataracts, and cognitive problems such as memory loss and Alzheimer's).

"It's like rust on the Tin Man in *The Wizard of Oz*," says the University of South Florida's Paula C. Bickford, Ph.D., a specialist in the field of age-related changes in the central nervous system. "The Tin Man would freeze, and his arms and legs wouldn't work. A similar process happens in the cells of our body. When the proteins and the DNA and the lipids get oxidized, they don't function properly."

The body does have protection against ROS—internal antioxidants, including certain enzymes, vitamin E, and vitamin C, which neutralize the rogue atoms and molecules. Still, about 1 percent of ROS escape the antioxidant police daily. For years, we've been admonished to eat brightly colored fruits and vegetables, partly because they are rich in antioxidants: ascorbate, tocopherols, flavonoids, and carotenoids, to name a few. The thinking has been that perhaps what ROS our bodies can't sop up our diets can. But new research questions whether the amounts we consume can even make a dent. (For more on diet, see Chapter 4.)

New science reveals that oxidative stress does a number on telomeres, too. Cellular gerontologist Thomas von Zglinicki, Ph.D., at the UK's Newcastle University, has shown in the culture dish that oxidative stress accelerates telomere shortening, directly damaging the DNA in both human and animal cells, whether they're white blood cells (leukocytes) or neurons or muscle stem cells. "There's all the reason in the world to believe that it should occur in the body, too," says Calvin B. Harley, Ph.D., a pioneer in telomere biology and former chief scientific officer at biopharmaceutical company Geron, in Menlo Park, California. In fact, von Zglinicki reports that the higher the oxidative stress level, the faster the rate of telomere shortening.

Part of the problem lies in the chemical makeup of the telomeres themselves—their repeating TTAGGG sequence. "Telomeres are an easier target for oxidative stress," says UCSF's Jue Lin, Ph.D., who specializes in perfecting telomere and telomerase assays in Blackburn's lab. "They are G rich, and two or three Gs in a row are easier to oxidize. So the telomeres get degraded more easily than the rest of the chromosomes."

Cells such as leukocytes particularly suffer: They replicate to start with, thereby shortening their telomeres with each division, and are then whacked by scavenging ROS, which chew away at their ends. Throw in inflammation and those ROS-spewing macrophages, and you've got a triple threat.

The cells of the chronically stressed sit smack in the middle of this demolition derby. Studies have shown these folks to have increased levels of oxidative stress markers in their blood and urine, and decreased levels of antioxidant enzymes.

Where do postmitotic, or nondividing, cells such as mature brain and muscle cells fit into this? It may be that ROS alone erode their telomeres.

Geneticist Richard M. Cawthon, M.D., at the University of Utah, who performed many of the measurements for Blackburn and Epel's studies, speculates that it's oxidative stress to mitochondrial DNA in particular that may be doing the damage. Mitochondria contain their own brand of DNA—mitochondrial DNA (mtDNA), as opposed to nuclear DNA, which sits in the nucleus of our cells—as well as numerous enzymes, proteins, and fats important for cell metabolism. We inherit our mtDNA only from our mothers; it is shorter and circular, as opposed to elongated, as nuclear DNA is, and thus is much hardier. Indeed, it was mtDNA that enabled the identification of many 9/11 victims, as it was more likely to have survived the two-thousand-degree heat of the attacking planes' burning jet fuel.

"Telomeres don't shorten significantly with age in postmitotic cells," says Cawthon. "However, longer telomeres may protect postmitotic cells from oxidative stress better than shorter telomeres. Mitochondrial DNA damage accumulates with age in postmitotic tissues but not in rapidly turning over tissues. Perhaps telomere shortening contributes to cellular aging mainly in mitotic—replicating—cells, and mitochondrial DNA damage contributes to aging mainly in postmitotic cells."

Indeed, hair graying—that all-too-visible sign of aging—has been linked to ROS damage to stem cells called melanocytes: cells in the hair follicle that synthesize pigment, or melanin. One theory holds that the very process of producing the pigment lets loose ROS that erode melanocytes' telomeres and cause DNA damage, accelerating their demise.

Add to that the oxidizing effect of glucocorticoids from stress on telomeres and telomerase, and it's no wonder that President Obama is grayer than when he entered office.

All of this means, says Epel, "that telomere maintenance is important even in the cells that are not dividing. That the biochemical environment we live in might be affecting the health of that tissue as well."

At a certain point, the telomeres are shot and the cell can no longer divide. It then enters an arrested state known as senescence, or it commits a kind of molecular suicide known as apoptosis: programmed cell death for the good of the organism (see Chapter 1). After all, if the cell were to hang out with just the nub of a telomere or none at all, the DNA damage responses would kick into gear, fueling mutation-inducing fusions. "A cell that can't divide can never form a tumor," notes Campisi.

Senescence is bad news. For senescent cells are by no means dead and gone; they have, essentially, a life of their own. They pour all kinds of pro-inflammatory substances into the tissue and bloodstream, such as cytokines (including the interleukins and tumor necrosis factor-alpha), and enzymes called proteases that chew up proteins, particularly materials such as collagen and elastin, which hold together our organs (and yes, sadly, that includes our skin). Indeed, some scientists believe that it's the emissions from accumulating senescent cells that make our skin sag and our hair thin, and that set our immune systems on an inflammatory track linked with cardiovascular disease and cancer. "It's a toxic thing— a rotten apple spitting out bad stuff," says Blackburn.

Certainly, at the very least, tissues loaded with senescent cells, whether they're stem cells or differentiated cells, have a reduced ability to respond to illness and injury—that is, to repair and regenerate tissue in everything from kidneys to blood vessels to skin—a fundamental feature of aging. "Take a look in the mirror, and you know," laughs Campisi. "After the age of thirty you start: 'Oh no! What the hell is going on?'"

Nondividing cells not only emit stuff that degrades tissue and stimulates the activity of precancer cells, they also take up the valuable space of healthy ones.

Still, direct experimental evidence of senescent-cell buildup in people is hard to come by. Scientists such as Norman E. Sharpless, M.D., a cancer specialist at the University of North Carolina, have found that as mice age, indicators of senescent cells significantly increase; other studies have shown that cells with characteristics of senescence accumulate with age in multiple tissues in humans and primates. But actually *finding* large quantities of these fountains of anti-youth in human bodies (as opposed to in a culture dish) has proven more difficult. "It's guilt by association at this point," says UCLA's Rita B. Effros, Ph.D., who studies the cells of the immune system, particularly T cells and their telomeres, as they age. Effros has found that as cells age in a culture dish, they produce more of the pro-inflammatory cytokine interleukin-6 (IL-6), and that blood from frail old people has higher levels of IL-6. But careful scientist that she is, she won't draw a direct line from the dish to the body. "We can't *prove* that the IL-6 was specifically produced by senescent cells, even though the people may have senescent cells, because you can't see inside a person's body and follow what the cells are doing," she says. "It's still circumstantial evidence."

Campisi, who's credited with discovering senescent cells' propensity to spew out junk, is still the first to note that aging is not driven by an accumulation of senescent cells alone. "That's only one component," she says. "Aging is really quite complex. The only definition people in the aging field can agree on is: Aging is a process that turns a young, fit, healthy organism into an old, unfit, less healthy organism. Some people say it's telomeres, some people say it's senescent cells, some people say it's hormones. And you know what? I think they're all right."

~~~~~

In 1984, Blackburn and her graduate student Carol W. Greider, both then at the University of California, Berkeley, discovered a new twist to the telomere story while plumbing—again—the depths of the *Tetrahymena thermophila*. The breakthrough came on Christmas Day, after nine months of painstaking investigation.

What the two discovered was the enzyme telomerase, which synthesizes telomeric DNA, dabbing additional repeats of the TTAGGG sequence onto shortening telomere ends, making up for the ones that get lost during division or otherwise. It was this discovery, together with the understanding of how chromosome ends are protected, that jointly earned Blackburn, Greider, and Harvard's Jack Szostak the 2009 Nobel Prize in Physiology or Medicine.

Telomerase levels and telomere length, it turns out, may be a better predictor than cholesterol, glucose, or even C-reactive protein of overall health, susceptibility to disease risk, and where we fall on the aging spectrum. "Cholesterol tests just tell you about your lipid profile, glucose tests just tell you about blood sugar, and C-reactive protein just tells you about inflammation," Epel told the *Los Angeles Times* recently. "Telomere length is a more summative measure for multiple biochemical imbalances, a global marker of health status."

Do not be surprised if someday soon your doctor orders a telomere-length or telomerase-level test along with—or perhaps even in place of—the current blood tests run for your yearly physical.

Telomerase activity is very complex, but some generalities exist. In mammals, like us, it is high during embryonic and early fetal developmental stages, which makes sense, because cells are dividing at a rapid clip in order to form body parts and organs, differentiating kidneys from, say, noses. But the pace slows in later life. Indeed, most adult human cells have undetectable or very low levels of telomerase activity, with the exception of rapidly dividing cells such as skin cells and white blood cells and of course the "immortal" stem, progenitor, and reproductive (egg and sperm) cells. But just as size isn't everything, neither is amount: Even low levels of telomerase help forestall telomere shortening. Telomere pioneer Calvin Harley has shown in the lab that telomerase can extend the normal life span of human retinal pigment epithelial cells by at least twenty doublings—that is, the cells' life span would be extended by a robust 28 to 40 percent. Blackburn's lab has even detected low levels of telomerase in the progenitor cells of mature rat brains.

"It's like a little kid turning the [clock] hands back, because telomerase is there," says Blackburn. "It's not a whole lot; it gets turned down in adults in many cells—down but not off." Indeed, scientists are just now learning that telomerase might protect telomeres by just sitting on the things, even when it's not doing any elongating. Of course, in the end, the overall race is lost—but not for lack of trying.

Before you get too excited about the possibilities of telomerase as an antiaging elixir, stop and think for a minute about what a cellular Shangri-la might mean. What, after all, is another name for a cell that can divide and multiply ad infinitum—a cell with uncontrolled growth? Yes, a cancer cell. Indeed, cancer cells, despite their perpetually short telomeres, are telomerase rich, with "a hundredfold more telomerase" than normal cells, says Blackburn. Telomerase activity—though not the only factor in transforming a normal cell into a cancer cell—has been found in more than 90 percent of human cancers. That is the double-edged

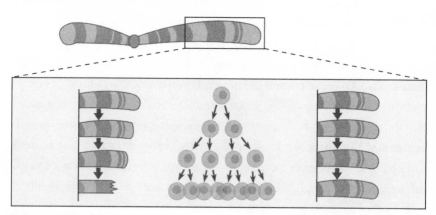

Figure 2. Without telomerase present, the chromosome is shortened each time the cell divides. Finally the telomere DNA is eroded and the chromosome is damaged. Telomerase maintains the telomeres at the ends of the DNA thread. This makes it possible to copy the entire chromosome to its very end each time the cell divides.   Illustration: Annika Röhl

sword that telomerase is—the "Dr. Jekyll and Mr. Hyde" of enzymes, as Blackburn puts it in a 1999 paper. Indeed, Harley's former employer, Geron, is running human clinical trials of so-called telomerase inhibitors and telomerase therapeutic vaccines to use as cancer treatments.

Telomerase, in other words, can give life but can also take it away. In a kind of supreme irony, it is cells' senescence program that keeps us alive.

About ten years ago, Campisi went out on a limb. She proposed in a paper an "evolutionary tradeoff": aging for cancer protection. We humans are kept relatively cancer-free for our first five decades (through our reproductive years), because our cells know when to stop dividing and call it quits. But the senescent cells that accumulate over those years increasingly degrade our organs and tissues. Cellular degradation is what aging is all about, says Campisi, and it's aging that sets us up for developing pathology. Campisi grabs a pencil and sketches out a seesaw as she speaks, writing "aging" on one end of the plank and "tumor suppression" on the other. "It's a very delicate balance to keep the organism cancer-free but not aging too fast," she says.

Over the past two decades, numerous cross-sectional studies of various types of leukocytes (cells that fight infection and are most readily available for assessing telomeres and telomerase) have shown that, in general, older people have shorter telomeres and lower levels of telomerase than younger ones. There are of course exceptions, such as centenarians (the "oldest old"), who fall into a class of their own, as well as more typical folks. "You can always find a relatively young person that doesn't do as well as a relatively old person," says Campisi, who counts herself among those who don't consider telomere length a reliable marker of aging.

Indeed, according to a study by von Zglinicki, telomere length doesn't correlate with survival in the oldest old, suggesting that other factors hold sway at that stage of life. Other research, including a 2008 paper by Boston University's Dellara F. Terry, M.D., suggests that when it comes to centenarians, not age but *wellness* correlates with telomere length: In her study, healthy centenarians ages 97 to 108 (we should all be so lucky) had significantly longer telomeres than their unhealthy matched counterparts.

Early on, telomere length is influenced by genetic factors, but later, environmental and lifestyle factors—smoking, exercise, diet, infections, and as Blackburn and Epel revealed, chronic stress—come into play. "By the time you're over seventy," says Blackburn, "that heredity similarity can be all but erased by everything else." Indeed, a study of identical twins age seventy-three to eighty-five, by Indiana University's David P. Gilley, Ph.D., found no evidence of heredity but much association of hypertension and cardiovascular disease, as well as shared environmental factors, on telomere length. Exercise figured prominently among those factors: In a 2008 study of 2,401 twins (2,152 of them women), Lynn F. Cherkas, Ph.D., at King's College London, showed that the most active subjects had telomeres that were two hundred bases longer than those of the least active subjects—the biological equivalent of ten years.

Other studies have linked short telomere length in white blood cells to increased mortality—from stroke, vascular dementia, heart disease, hypertension, atherosclerosis, osteoarthritis, Alzheimer's disease, and insulin resistance, a precursor of diabetes, among other diseases. In an elegant twenty-year study of 143 men and women age sixty-plus that was published in 2003, the University of Utah's Cawthon found that those with the shortest telomeres had a threefold higher mortality rate from heart disease and an alarming eightfold higher mortality rate from infectious diseases. Overall, the mortality rate of people with shorter telomeres was nearly double that of people with longer telomeres. In 2008, Elissa Epel's team pushed the association even further, showing for the first time that not just telomere length but the *rate* of telomere *change* predicts mortality from cardiovascular disease in elderly men. Those whose telomeres had the highest rate of change (shortening) over a period of 2.5 years were three times more likely to die from heart disease than those whose telomeres had the lowest rate of change.

This is not to say, of course, that telomere shortening *causes* these disorders. For serious scientists, the distance between an association, or a link, and cause-and-effect can be a chasm as vast as the Grand Canyon, and they're terrifically careful about limning the distinction between the two. And don't forget about all those nondividing, or postmitotic, cells. But the mounting piles of research papers drawing similar conclusions do indicate that telomere shortening has a remarkably suspicious relationship with certain diseases and with people dying from them.

Clearly, some kind of unholy alliance is at work.

~~~~~

Elissa Epel is an associate professor in the UCSF Department of Psychiatry, where she investigates chronic stress, tunneling down to a place where psychology, neurology, biology, and endocrinology meet. She is small boned and petite in all directions, very fashionable, and very, very smart. She studies how stress throws our hormones out of whack and how that chemical soup circulating throughout our bodies affects the way we eat, how much we weigh, where we carry our fat (bellies versus hips), and our susceptibility to diseases of aging, such as type 2 diabetes, depression, and heart disease. She works to unravel why some people are particularly vulnerable to stress and what traits or behaviors make others resilient.

She's also—rare in science—a natural synthesizer. In the early 2000s, as a postdoctoral fellow in health psychology at UCSF, she was dissatisfied with her field's standard of just linking stress to disease; she wanted to find a marker, a biological flag, that would permit her to measure not just how stress upsets our systems—say, the cardiovascular system to contribute to heart disease, or the immune system to contribute to infections—but how stress affects our very cells. "In my field, health psychology, there's a lot of research linking stress to systemic dysregulation—high blood pressure, high cholesterol, heart disease, diabetes, abdominal fat, that is, to disorders, or 'systemic-level markers'; they indicate disease processes," says Epel in her uncluttered office, her young son's tiny *Sesame Street* Bert finger puppet dangling from her whiteboard. But such systemic disorders reflect multiple factors at work: Type 2 diabetes, for example, reflects caloric input and output, glucose tolerance, insulin levels, fat buildup, and so on. Epel wanted a "clean" marker—one that could connect stress to cellular processes and thereby provide a window on to its direct biological effects. "I wanted to look at a marker that was unconfounded by disease, that we could measure in kids if we wanted to, or young adults who don't have disease. There really aren't many markers that fit that bill."

She scoured the scientific literature and was drawn to the work of molecular gerontologists—folks investigating molecular defects associated with aging, such as DNA damage and the mutations that can result from misguided repairs. "They are studying all of these reductionistic measures of aging," she says, "but—where is the biological clock? And what popped out from that literature so clearly was that if there is a clock on cell life, telomeres are the best candidate."

Epel knew from her research that Liz Blackburn was the telomere guru. She also knew that, fortuitously, Blackburn had been running a lab at UCSF since 1990. So she sent the senior scientist an e-mail—"as hundreds of people do every day," says Epel, hoping for but not counting on a response—asking Blackburn to collaborate with her on a study looking at how chronic stress might relate to telomere length in mothers who were the primary caregivers of a chronically ill child, a stressful circumstance if there ever was one. "Liz had to take a leap of faith, because I was suggesting that chronic stress affects all these bodily systems, so just maybe it affects telomeres as well," says Epel.

Blackburn was intrigued and impressed with Epel's rigorous study design, which "controlled" for as many variables as possible, from smoking to body mass index to sex to age, so that in the end she would be comparing only the endpoints that answered a specific question, such as "What is the relationship between telomere length and duration of stress?" Blackburn can afford to be picky. "If the study's not well designed, we're not going to lift a pipette for it," she says. Luck played a role, too. When Blackburn asked her lab group if anyone wanted to help answer this "wacky question," says Epel, it was the stressed mother of two young sons, postdoc Jue Lin, who raised her hand. Blackburn got back to Epel. "You know, nobody's ever looked at this," she recalls telling the young scientist. "Why don't we?"

For the study, Epel recruited a group of some sixty women ages twenty to fifty, more than half of whom—like Lia Spiliotes—were caring for a chronically ill child of their own. The women completed the Cohen Perceived Stress Scale, included at the start of this chapter, to rate their own stress—"stressful meaning out of control, meaning unpredictable, meaning 'I don't have the resources to cope, I'm overloaded,'" says Blackburn. The researchers then took blood and urine samples from the women to measure several biological markers: telomere length, telomerase activity, level of oxidative stress, and level of stress hormones (cortisol, chief among the glucocorticoids; and epinephrine and norepinephrine, the catecholamines). They also correlated, at the suggestion of coauthor Richard Cawthon, telomere length with how long the moms had been in the caregiving role (one to twelve years). "If there is no relationship with the duration of the stress," Cawthon scribbled to Epel on an early draft of the paper, "then the telomere-length differences you found might have existed even before the stress began." Epel didn't want to leave any stone unturned.

Epel and Blackburn's results sparked a twenty-first-century blaze among stress researchers. The caregiving moms who perceived themselves as being under the highest stress had telomeres that were, on average, shorter by the equivalent of at least ten years than those of the moms who perceived themselves as under low stress. In fact, the more years of caregiving, the shorter the telomere length, the lower the telomerase activity, and the greater the level of oxidative stress. Indeed, the mean telomerase activity for the high-stress group was a startling 48 percent lower than that of the low-stress group. Shorter telomeres were also associated with higher levels of stress hormones. Could it be that stress might play a role not only in fraying our cells but also in dampening the activity of the enzyme that could make them whole again?

Sapolsky, Effros, and Harley, among others, think so. In his *PNAS* commentary on the study, Sapolsky traces a speculative path of how chronic stress may do its dirty work: Stress, modified by our perceptions, leads to the release of stress hormones, including glucocorticoids. The released hormones increase oxidative stress to white blood cells, which in turn leads to oxidative damage to telomerase. That begets impaired telomerase function, which results in shortened telomeres and possible acceleration of cell senescence.

Indeed, several years later, UCLA's Effros traced the pathway in culture: She exposed T cells, a type of white blood cell, to cortisol and found that the cells' telomerase production dropped. The likely culprit? Oxidative stress.

"What really blew people away was the unexpected link—the report of 'stress accelerates telomere shortening,'" says Sapolsky, who has studied baboons in the national parks of Africa for years to learn the stress effects of social hierarchy on health. "The stress people all said, 'DNA! It's all the way down to the DNA level, stress screwing up something that a lot of people think of as a basic molecular mechanism for cell aging! Amazing.' And the molecular people said, 'Humans! They're going from human stress down to the level of telomeres? Amazing.'

"A remarkable number of people are now thinking about telomeres," adds Sapolsky, "including me."

In a follow-up study with the same group of women, this one published in 2006 in the journal *Psychoneuroendocrinology*, the Blackburn and Epel team found that the caregiving mothers with high stress and low telomerase activity also had higher blood pressure, cholesterol, and fasting glucose, and more belly fat—all cardiovascular risk factors—as well as elevated stress hormones. "It just blew me away," says Blackburn. "You just split the telomerase [for the high- and low-stress groups] and you said, 'Look at the curves for these folks. Look at these for the others. . . . They're like two different species!'" Could low telomerase be a red flag for disease risk, a marker of trouble even before telomeres shorten? "We can see things with telomerase that are just hard to see numerically speaking with telomere length," says Blackburn. Think of it as a neon sign flashing in the cellular dark.

Since the publication of the 2004 paper, a critical mass of studies has replicated Blackburn and Epel's findings regarding chronic stress and leukocyte telomere length—the official stamp of approval in the scientific world. Among the most prominent are these: a 2007 paper by Amanda K. Damjanovic, Ph.D., from Nan-ping Weng's lab at the National Institute on Aging, in collaboration with Janice Kiecolt-Glaser, Ph.D., and Ronald Glaser, Ph.D., at Ohio State University, that looked at the immune function and telomere length of caregivers of Alzheimer's patients, and a 2009 paper by the National Institutes of Health's Christine G. Parks, Ph.D., which considered perceived stress, stress hormones, and telomere length in 647 women ages thirty-five to seventy-four.

Interestingly, Damjanovic's group found a big bump in telomerase activity in its caregivers, indicating "an unsuccessful attempt of cells to compensate the excessive loss of telomeres," the authors write. And Parks found the most significant perceived-stress-related differences not across the board but among women ages fifty-five to sixty-five, those with the most epinephrine in their morning urine, and those who'd experienced a recent major stressor, such as premature death of a close relative. That may have been because the women in Parks's study were not caregivers, so their levels of perceived stress were much lower from the get-go. "We enrolled anybody who volunteered for the study and then controlled for variables analytically," says Parks. "We weren't representing the worst-off, very high-stress women. But even with our low stress scores, we saw differences."

On a shelf in front of me in Blackburn's lab is a DNA sandwich: two rectangular glass plates, upright on a stand, with a four-millimeter layer of burnt-yellowish gel mashed between them. Traces of blue and purple dye migrate downward, like hairline cracks accelerating in a sheet of ice. Each is a single strand of floating DNA representing double helixes that have drifted apart, or been "denatured" by a combination of radioactive chemicals and heat before being dropped in the wells at the top of the gel. The DNA is from the white blood cells of women in another Blackburn and Epel collaboration, and Jue Lin is measuring their levels of telomerase. A computer in another room will calculate the actual amount; the darker the images of the bands of radioactive DNA, the more telomerase present. While preparing the wells, Lin had put the tubes of denatured DNA on ice. "If you let them go back to room temperature, the strands gradually find each other," she'd told me. I'm charmed by their fidelity.

Lin painstakingly measures telomere lengths and telomerase levels in the Blackburn lab from eight thirty a.m. to five p.m. every day. As an accomplished postdoc, she could be designing her own studies somewhere—a decidedly more glamorous gig. But the regular hours enable her to see her young sons off to school and be home in time for dinner. Besides, her contribution to a follow-up study to the mom caregivers may just turn the field of stress and aging on its head.

For that study, Blackburn and Epel wanted to see if chronic stress affected telomere length not just in a moment in time, as it had with the mom caregivers, but over a period of one year. It was the first longitudinal study in humans—the gold standard in science—to investigate stress and telomere length. Abraham Aviv, M.D., a longevity researcher and hypertension expert at the University of Medicine and Dentistry of New Jersey, recently devoted an entire paper to calling for more longitudinal analyses, with large groups and long-term follow-up, to ascertain the credibility of links between leukocyte telomere length and aging. As this book goes to press, there are only a handful of longitudinal telomere studies out there.*

This time, Blackburn and Epel recruited older women, including both caregivers of spouses with dementia and low-stress controls matched on factors such as age, education, and BMI. They took telomere-length

---

* Among those studies are the Bogalusa Heart Study of Wei Chen, M.D., Ph.D., and Aviv; the Heart and Soul Study of Mary Whooley, M.D., and Ramin Farzaneh-Far, M.D.; a hypertension study by Zhiwei Yang, M.D, Ph.D.; Epel and colleagues' own elderly men study; and one from Sweden's Katarina Nordfjäll, Ph.D.

measurements and administered the Perceived Stress Scale to everyone at the start of the study, and then again twelve months later.

The results replicated those of Blackburn and Epel's earlier cross-sectional study with the caregiver moms: Those who *perceived* themselves as being under greater stress had shorter telomeres at the study's start than those who didn't—caregivers and controls alike. What blew the scientists' socks off (OK, their lab coats) was that after twelve months the telomeres actually *lengthened* in those caregivers whose stress levels had dropped. In just one short year of stressing less, their biological aging had not just slowed but had *reversed.*

"We'd thought that telomere length went in one direction, which is slowly shortening. But what we find is that actually when you look in short time periods, like a year apart, there are changes in all directions," says Epel. "There's this great new phenomenon, where shortening is reversible in a sense. In this one-year period of change, the women who showed decreases in stress were the ones who showed more lengthening. When I looked closely, what had happened to bring about these drops in stress? Some of the time it was an increase in nursing care, or a sad culmination of caregiving, in that the partner had died or had been placed in hospice." These women, whose stress levels had been sky-high at the outset, ended up showing a greater drop in stress than some of the controls. "So there's mourning, but there can also eventually be positive change as well—less of this burden and life feeling uncontrollable," she says. "It may be that short telomeres bounce back when they can, probably due to telomerase. When your mind takes a breather, your body can too."

The longitudinal spouse-caregiver study may be as close as we can get to "seeing" what's going on inside our cells as they go about their business deep within our bodies.

To actually observe such changes internally over time, of course, scientists must turn to animals—subjects whose stressors they can ethically manipulate long term. Yet the literature in animal models is stunningly slim when it comes to telomeres and stress; as this book goes to press, there is just one clinical controlled study out there, using wild house mice. It came out in 2007.

"The mouse study," says Epel, "is fantastic."

Over a period of six months, Alexander Kotrschal, a Ph.D. student at Switzerland's University of Bern, exposed female wild-caught house mice (whose telomeres are much closer to humans' than lab mice's are) to two forms of stress: crowding and amorous males (read: sexual aggression and perpetual birthing). At the end of the experiment, the stressed females had significantly shorter telomeres than the controls had; indeed, the controls' telomeres actually lengthened, just as they had in Blackburn and Epel's spouse caregivers.

"What we find is that it really does look causative," said Blackburn about what her and Epel's caregiver studies, taken together, reveal about the stress-aging relationship. She was speaking to Adam Smith, editor in chief of nobelprize.org, immediately following the announcement of her prize, on October 5, 2009. "Now, the question is, does [telomere shortening] cause the bad, clinical effects of stress, which have been well documented in the literature for years and years? It's a plausible model, actually. And I'm inclined to think it does. But you have to be very careful about what, exactly, is the complete mechanism by which these adverse effects of stress are mediated. Certainly we see the effects on telomere maintenance in the immune system, which is, it turns out, a very good window into what's happening in terms of disease risks in the body."

~~~~~

Blackburn and Epel's spouse-caregiver study constitutes a breakthrough— but still it's no panacea in the Talmudic world of science, where every finding is ripe for further hairsplitting.

For starters, a central question of aging research remains: Does cellular aging actually mean organismal aging?

Does the clock winding down on our cells mean it's winding down on the tautness of our muscles and the thumpability of our hearts, on our ability to conquer the treadmill and to remember why we've entered a room seconds after crossing the threshold? Does telomere attrition in those ubiquitous leukocytes reflect primarily a weakening immune system and increased inflammation (which scientists agree drives aging), or does it represent what's happening across all tissues? And don't forget those non-dividing cells in our brains and skeletal muscles—the ones whose telomeres aren't in the path of this molecular time bomb but age nonetheless.

Do shortening telomeres, when all is said and done, mean a shortening of our lives?

It's a hotly debated topic among scientists, and an important one for anyone growing older (you, me) to address in the quest for the truth (as opposed to a phony magic bullet) about what drives our own aging process. Only by grappling with the complexities of the causes of aging can we arrive at legitimate ways to hold those causes in check.

The best model of how cellular aging relates to organismal aging in humans may come from genetically engineered mice. Yes, of course there's still a vast divide between the two species. For starters, unengineered laboratory mice have very long telomeres, and at the end of their short life spans (two years and change), show little if any telomere attrition. "There's a saying in the field that humans are not a very good model for the mouse," notes Cal Harley wryly. Yet with enough molecular tinkering to make their systems more closely mimic human ones, mice can reveal some startling insights into our own internal mechanisms.

Scientists from labs around the world have manipulated lab-mouse genes so that in one scenario the critters produce excessive levels of telomerase *and* are cancer resistant (remember, telomerase is cancer's friend), and in another are telomerase deficient because one of the genes for telomerase has been knocked out.*

---

* The most prominent researchers genetically engineering such mice include Maria A. Blasco, Ph.D., Manuel Serrano, Ph.D., Antonia Tomás Loba, Ph.D., and Irene Siegl-Cachedenier, Ph.D., at the Spanish National Cancer Research Centre, in Madrid; Ronald A. DePinho, M.D., at the Dana-Farber Cancer Center, in Boston; Karl Lenhard Rudolph, M.D., formerly with DePinho in Boston and now at Germany's University of Ulm, and, of course, Carol W. Greider, Ph.D., at Johns Hopkins.

Mice pumped up on telomerase have superfit skin and intestines, and delayed aging—meaning less inflammation, atrophy, and susceptibility to type 2 diabetes, and higher levels of muscle-bulking insulin-like growth factor (IGF-1). They also have longer median and maximum life spans. Their telomeres are significantly longer than those of controls, and their DNA breaks are decreased. Indeed, in some studies, there has been a 9 to 26 percent increase in overall life span and a 40.2 percent increase in median life span; 42 percent of the engineered mice have lived to extreme old age (three years), compared to just 8 percent of controls.

The telomerase-deficient mice, on the other hand, have a very bad time of it. They turn gray (some at as young as six months) and go bald. Indeed, the more gray hair they have, the shorter their telomeres. They are fatter than controls, their nails atrophy, and their skin ages prematurely, meaning poor wound healing, skin lesions from superficial trauma, and difficulty in recovering from surgery and chemotherapy. Clearly, the organs that depend on high cell turnover, including skin and bone marrow, are running out of reinforcements. These poor mice also have more malignant tumors than controls, as cancer is a disease of aging, and die earlier.

The nail-atrophy part of the mice's fate made me wonder: Could the reverse—rapid nail *growth* in humans—be a marker of robust telomeres and longevity? I had a personal interest at stake: My nails are soft and grow like weeds. Even now as I type, they're curling over my fingertips, clattering on the keyboard. The thought that their sproutability might be a good thing, rather than just a source of embarrassment, made my eyes light up. And indeed, some scientists, including Anne C. Hofer, as an undergrad, and Marc S. Lewis, Ph.D., at the University of Texas at Austin, posited just that: The velocity at which our fingernails grow may indicate not only how fit our telomeres are but also how long we may live. In a 2005 paper, Hofer and Lewis cite research showing that nail-growth velocity in people, beagles, and pigtailed macaques (go figure) slows with age, as well as a ten-plus-year longitudinal study on rhesus monkeys that posits nail-growth velocity as a "surprisingly good predictor [of longevity], correlating significantly with both years of survival and age at death."

Further evidence for how cellular aging relates to aging of our entire selves comes from research into accelerated-aging syndromes and pulmonary fibrosis, which occur in humans. Genetically based, the rare progeroid syndromes—including dyskeratosis congenita (DC), Hutchinson-Gilford progeria syndrome, and Werner syndrome—leave patients devastatingly old before their time. Their hair and skin thin, they go bald, their nails atrophy, they have high levels of pro-inflammatory cytokines in their blood, and they may get osteoporosis, atherosclerosis, type 2 diabetes, cataracts, and increased infections. Twelve-year-olds can look forty-five; forty-year-olds can look ninety-five. The telomeres of these patients, it turns out, are alarmingly short. Indeed, white blood cells of patients with Werner syndrome, says David Kipling, Ph.D., D.Phil., a pathology professor at the UK's Cardiff University who specializes in the disease, may divide in the culture dish perhaps just ten times, compared to the fifty divisions of normal cells. "They behave as if they've already used up their number of cell divisions," he says. He uses a car metaphor to bring the point home: In these patients, he says, "the petrol tank is a lot smaller from the beginning than that in most cars. You can't even get off of the local block, let alone go into the next city."

Short telomeres and/or telomerase deficiencies are often the culprit in these diseases. Patients with DC, for example, have a mutation in the gene that codes for an essential component of telomerase. The mutation leaves sufferers with just half the usual amount of telomerase. Most eventually die of failure of the bone marrow—an organ involved in producing new blood—after the telomeres of bone-marrow stem cells erode away and the cells senesce. Johns Hopkins oncologist Mary Y. Armanios, M.D., who's worked with Carol W. Greider, Ph.D., recently found that patients suffering from idiopathic pulmonary fibrosis—pulmonary fibrosis with no known cause, such as smoking—also had short telomeres in their white blood cells and in the tiny air sacs in their lungs, leading to limited tissue-renewal ability in the lung; some also had a mutation in the gene encoding for telomerase.

Still, telomeres and telomerase are not the be-all and end-all of organismal aging. Far from it. Blackburn and Epel, of course, know that well. Those engineered mice, for example, showed only *some* of the aging symptoms that beset us humans: Where, for instance, was the cardiovascular disease, the osteoporosis? "Something else in the aging organism cooperates with telomere dysfunction to compromise fitness," noted Ronald A. DePinho, M.D., of the Dana-Farber Cancer Institute, when his 1999 study of aging telomerase-deficient mice came out. Furthermore, the brains of Werner syndrome patients remain top notch; only the rapidly proliferating tissues and organs (bone marrow, skin) deteriorate. "You've got a body that looks like a 110-year-old, but the brain of a thirty-five-year-old," says Kipling.

Buttressing Richard Cawthon's theory that perhaps telomere shortening contributes mainly to cellular aging in replicating cells and mtDNA damage contributes to aging mainly in postmitotic cells is a study by Jan Karlseder, Ph.D., and Andrew Dillin, Ph.D., at the Salk Institute for Biological Studies. They note that telomere length in worms (*C. elegans*), which as adults have no dividing cells, doesn't matter a jot when it comes to life span. Worms with long telomeres can die early, while ones with mere telomeric nubs can have lots of time in the sun (OK, in a petri dish). "For successful aging you have to control both— aging in your dividing cells, which hinges on telomere maintenance, but also aging in your nondividing cells," said Dillin when the study came out in 2005. "We thought that telomeres might play a role in the latter, but that's clearly not the case."

Cal Harley and Abraham Aviv, among others, would add a big caveat to that view: vascular aging. The vascular system—that web of veins and arteries that carries blood and nutrients to and from all parts of our bodies—is lined with a layer of what are called endothelial cells, as are the inside surfaces of body cavities such as the heart. "And all tissues," whether replicative or not, says Harley, "are impacted by the aging of endothelial cells." Harley's lab was the first to show, in the nineties, that endothelial cells in areas of chronic physical stress—say, a spot in an artery with turbulent blood flow—divide and turn over rapidly in an effort to keep up with the necessary tissue repairs. As they replicate, their telomeres shorten, eventually leading to senescence. Loaded with underperforming and senescent cells, the vessels are then less able to feed organs made up of nonreplicative cells, such as heart and skeletal muscles and the brain. Think of vascular aging as a rubber hose that's sprung leaks: Flowers (organs such as the heart and brain) don't need rubber (dividing endothelial cells) to survive, but it's the rubber that permits the water to flow onto the petunias. "That's the link in how shortened telomeres impact essentially all tissues in the body even if the tissue itself is not showing significant telomere loss," says Harley.

Judith Campisi, for one, remains cheerfully skeptical about the role of telomere attrition per se in *both* cellular and organismal aging. "There is no evidence that before cells become actually senescent there's anything wrong with them," she says. "You see that the telomeres can go from ten kilobase to five kilobase and still be perfectly functional.* To equate a change in telomere length to a change in age is a huge leap based on the assumption that this path to senescence is a continuum. And so far as we know, it is not; it's a step function. We have cells in the lab: They're fine, they're fine, they're fine, they're fine, the telomere fails, boom, they're senescent. It's not like they're young, and then they're middle aged, and then . . ." her voice trails off. "But the literature is loaded with those kinds of words, which sets up this prejudicial idea that it's a continuum, and it's not."

Still, a gathering storm of new evidence makes it harder and harder to discount the argument that telomere length is a reliable biomarker of aging, even in the qualifier-rich world of science.

Consider this study, released in November 2009, which focused on a

---

* Telomeres are measured in kilobase. One kilobase is one thousand base pairs of DNA.

unique group of subjects: eighty-six Ashkenazi Jewish centenarians (average age ninety-seven), 175 of their offspring, and ninety-three age- and gender-matched controls whose parents had lived a typical life span of eighty-five or fewer years. The average age of the centenarian offspring and controls was a sprightly seventy. Because the centenarians came from a population that was both culturally and genetically homogeneous, the scientists got a rare glimpse into the source of their longevity.

The research team, led by Gil Atzmon, Ph.D., and Yousin Suh, Ph.D., at the Albert Einstein College of Medicine, had two primary questions: Do those who live exceptionally long lives have longer telomeres? (They guessed yes.) And do variations in the genes that code for the enzyme telomerase account for that length?

They analyzed all participants' leukocyte telomere length and levels of telomerase and got these fascinating results: Not only did the centenarians and their offspring have longer telomeres than the controls, but their genes coding for telomerase had similar mutations that revved up the enzyme's action.

"Telomeres are one piece of the puzzle that accounts for why some people can live so long," said Atzmon when the study came out. Added Suh: "We found that they owe their longevity, at least in part, to advantageous variants of genes involved in telomere maintenance."

CHAPTER 3

Your Brain on Stress

I felt a Cleaving in my Mind—
As if my Brain had split—
I tried to match it—Seam by Seam—
But could not make them fit.

—Emily Dickinson, from poem 937, 1864

Anne Erni is a terrifically put-together lady, from her smart navy slacks to her white-tipped French-manicured nails and alligator-trimmed belt. As a high-powered businesswoman in financial services on Wall Street, she built the diversity department at the once-towering Lehman Brothers from scratch, overseeing employees in New York City, where she was based, and in offices around the world. Among her proudest achievements was establishing Women's Initiatives Leading Lehman (WILL), a network committed to supporting women in their professional development. "Men run in packs, women don't," Joe Gregory, then Lehman's chief administrative officer and later president, told her. "Go create your pack." WILL included a strong recruiting arm to move Lehman from being a self-perpetuating "old boy place," says Anne, to a cohesive organization with the best talent. "And the best talent doesn't just come in a male package," she says.

Anne was an eleven-year Lehman veteran when the place crashed. She'd started as a salesperson on the equities trading floor, where she was one of the first women to go from full time to a four-day week, the better to care for her two children. "I loved this firm, and I mean this," she says. "When Lehman died, I cried."

She experienced the most intense stress, she says, over the six months before the firm actually declared bankruptcy—when day by day everyone's future hung in the balance.

Over that time, Lehman's stock had plummeted from about fifty-one dollars a share to about forty, and by the end was trading at a ludicrous fifteen cents. For senior management, like Anne, 40 percent of compensation came in the form of company stock options, pieces of paper that didn't hold their full value for five years. "Over the last six months, you saw five years of your top earnings literally losing money, losing money," says Anne. "And there was nothing you could do about it."

Her personal currency at the office teetered, too. "When you're hemorrhaging money, when you're not doing deals, when clients are unwilling to trade with you, when your credit lines are being pulled, everything becomes about survival," she says. "If you're doing things to make the corporate culture a better place, to make meritocracy a reality, when you are attracting, retaining, and advancing the best talent—all of a sudden that doesn't mean anything. We had to constantly reinvent ourselves."

Reinvention didn't only mean finding new projects. It meant severely downsizing. Between March and October 2008, Anne's team suffered three rounds of layoffs, with Anne having to decide who stayed and who went. The numbers of heads that would have to roll kept changing. "I had to face people every day knowing 'You're on the list, you're on the list, you're on the list.' But the list could change the next day: Now they needed dollars; now they didn't. So people went on the list and off the list, on the list and off the list."

To enable as many people as possible to keep working, Anne and other managers "brokered deals," parsing employees to each other's departments. Her job, she says, "became saving souls." Her own group diminished to seven, including herself. Budgets were slashed—hers from many millions to a piddling fifty thousand dollars by year's end.

On September 14, 2008, the night Bank of America was to rescue

Lehman through a merger, Anne had her parents over for dinner: grilled pork, Israeli salad with crunchy noodles, and grilled vegetables. She remembers every detail in Technicolor. "We had the TV on, and all of a sudden my mom looks up and she goes, 'Oh my God. That's Lehman Brothers!' I go, 'Yeah?' She goes, 'Why are people carrying boxes?' And I was like, 'What?'

"And I remember seeing people walking through the revolving doors with boxes. The announcer said that the deal with Bank of America had fallen through and that Merrill Lynch and BOA were merging. And I remember I said to my mom, 'They ran off with our bride.' And then I kept thinking, 'What does that mean for us?'"

Through it all, Anne remained remarkably clearheaded; she was in survival mode. Indeed, her office became a respite for not just her team but for the others left standing. "My office was like Lucy's, 'The doctor is in,'" she says, recalling the beloved *Peanuts* character. "Everyone was waiting outside my office to just talk." That sense of purpose helped pull *her* through.

Still, she paid a physical—and a cognitive—price. Her eyebrows went suddenly and totally gray (she dyes them now). "It was the strangest freaking thing," she says. "My right eye started to tic. And it was unbelievable how bad my short-term memory became during this time. Someone would tell me something and if I didn't write it down, I couldn't remember it." She started recording everything in small notebooks, as if compacting—reminding herself—who she was.

"It was really intense," she says.

Rating Your Memory

Stress does a number on our memory, leaving many of us searching for words—and various items (glasses, car keys, our pants)—before our time. The following test can help you quantify how far you believe your memory has slipped. It doesn't measure your memory per se (something only a clinician can do), but how you see your memory now compared to when you were younger. Regardless of your score, don't despair: This book can help you recall your recall to that earlier place.

Answer the following questions on a scale of 1 to 5:

As compared to when you were in high school or college, how would you describe your ability to perform the following tasks involving your memory?

Much better now (1)	Somewhat better now (2)	About the same (3)	Somewhat poorer now (4)	Much poorer now (5)

1. Remembering the name of a person just introduced to you

2. Recalling telephone numbers or zip codes that you use on a daily or weekly basis

3. Recalling where you have put objects (such as keys) in your home or office

4. Remembering specific facts from a newspaper or magazine article you have just finished reading

5. Remembering the item(s) you intended to buy when you arrive at the grocery store or pharmacy

Answer the following question on a scale of 2 to 10

Much better now (2)	Somewhat better now (4)	About the same (6)	Somewhat poorer now (8)	Much poorer now (10)

6. In general, how would you describe your memory as compared to when you were in high school?

Calculating your score:

Add together all of your scores. Total scores will range from 7 to 35. Higher scores indicate perception of greater memory decline.

Interpreting your score the *Stress Less* way*:

 7–14: See memory *improvement* over the years
15–21: See no memory decline
22–27: See slight to moderate memory decline
28–35: See significant memory decline

———~~~———

We've all been there: Something horrible happens, and the experience burns itself—as a fragment of a picture—into our brains. I was twenty-one, looking for volunteer social-service work in Chicago, when a young man I'd met pushed me into a stairwell and lunged at me. Today, a quarter of a century later, I can still see his thin face leering above me, but I have no recollection of where I'd met him—on the train? on the street?—or what I did after I pushed past him. I do vaguely remember taking him to task for scaring me, driven as I was by the chutzpah of youth and pumping epinephrine. But that's it. I've no idea where I went next (did I have an interview with an agency?), or how I got back to my apartment in Evanston.

That's a "flashbulb" memory, formed during extreme acute stress: The salient images sear, but the surrounding, more neutral details evaporate into thin air.

We've also, like Anne Erni, experienced the opposite: We're stressed for weeks or months on end and find that nearly every detail seems to slip our minds. *Ach! Forgot to pay the Visa bill and now I have a penalty. Gah! Turned on the stove to hard-boil an egg, then got lost in researching assisted-living facilities for my mother—until the thing burst (gross).* I was the victim of both lapses, and much more, during the time my mother lay fully conscious but on a ventilator in a hospital for more than a year. And the forgetting gets worse as we age, extending from our short- to long-term memories for verbal and visual (but not emotional) information: "Where did I leave my glasses?" morphs into mentally misplacing

* The *Stress Less* interpretation was developed by the author, not the scientists.

phone numbers we've known for years and even, shockingly, ourselves, as we forget to show up for doctor's appointments, dinner dates, or, most recently for me, telephone interviews.

No, we're not suffering from early Alzheimer's, as often as that fear flits across our minds. But we are experiencing the effects of stress on not just the function but the very structure of our brains. It's not a happy circumstance—but the good news is it can be reversed. The ability to do so lies within us: By altering our perceptions via the strategies in this book, we can change the very substance of our minds.

Snap!: Acute Stress Can Enhance Memory

Behavioral neurobiologist David M. Diamond, Ph.D., is warm and funny, and loves to talk about his work. He made a bit of a media splash recently when he showed that rats that ate a typical American diet (high in sugar and partially hydrogenated fat) were plumper and more stressed than those who chowed down on Atkins fare (high in animal and vegetable fat, low in sugar) or low-fat, low-sugar foods. Diamond was surprised—and pleased—by the results: He personally loves to eat large pieces of red meat, and based on his research he believes that a ketogenic diet, such as Atkins, is neuroprotective. But I, an anti-Atkins acolyte, argue that the real test would be to compare the Atkins diet to a low-fat, low-sugar one to learn the long-term effects on overall health—variables other than stress and weight gain.

Diamond is ambidextrous in more than just his food choices. Professionally, he swings between Tampa's University of South Florida, where he studies the effects of stress on memory in rats, and the nearby veterans hospital, where he investigates ways to improve the treatment outcomes of combat veterans suffering from post-traumatic stress disorder (PTSD).

The former informs the latter via a rat model of PTSD that Diamond devised: He exposed a rat to a predatory cat for two one-hour sessions, ten days apart. (The animals were separated by a transparent

Plexiglas barrier to prevent the rat from becoming an actual meal.) He also stressed the traumatized rat by housing it with a new cage mate every day, to ensure that it didn't form attachments (social isolation exacerbates PTSD). At the end of the "treatment," the behavior of the traumatized rat reflected that of a traumatized veteran: It had horrible anxiety, its heart raced, and its memory was impaired. From the way Diamond tells it, I wouldn't be surprised if images of snarling cat teeth flashed across its mind as well.

When we experience an acute stressor, a cocktail of hormones and neurotransmitters—including epinephrine, norepinephrine, and the terrifically excitatory amino acid glutamate—shoot into two interconnected brain regions, the hippocampus and the amygdala (see figure 3). Both are part of the brain's limbic system, which helps regulate the expression of emotion and emotional memory. Glutamate, which relays

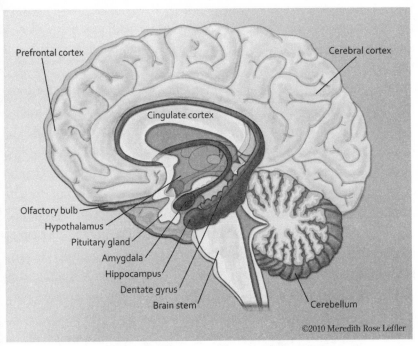

©2010 Meredith Rose Leffler

Figure 3. Brain drain: Parts of the brain affected by stress.

messages between brain cells (neurons), is crucial for what's known as long-term potentiation (LTP), simply put, a strengthening of the communication network between neurons that relates to learning and long-term memory (see Chapter 5 for more detail). Heart rate and blood pressure soar, which increases blood flow, and hence glucose—a necessary ingredient for the energy-intensive work of memory retrieval and storage—to the brain.

The hippocampus (from the Latin word for *seahorse*, though if you ask me it looks more like a banana) is the seat of memory consolidation and retrieval (see Chapter 8 for more on how memories are made). It provides the context for our memories: the who, what, when, where, and how (it's the brain's journalist, in a way). It reigns supreme for declarative memories—memories of an experience, event, or fact—that is, things you can "declare" and that you're conscious of knowing. The amygdala, nestled near the tip of the hippocampus, registers the emotional content of our memories, particularly fear. Together they craft the particular type of declarative memory known as an episodic memory, a memory comprising, logically, episodes, such as walking down the aisle and saying "I do."

Simplistically speaking, memories, once made, are moved for long-term storage from the hippocampus to the cerebral cortex, that folding blanket of gray matter overlaying the brain. (Our brains are made up of two kinds of matter—gray and white. The gray matter is the billions of neurons themselves, which process information. The white matter consists largely of bundled nerve fibers coated with myelin, a fatty substance that aids in transmission of messages.) "The hippocampus is telling you exactly what's getting you stressed," says Diamond. "It's helping you remember the details. And the amygdala is working with the hippocampus to add the emotional flavor. When you have a simultaneous activation of the amygdala and the hippocampus, you make a very powerful memory."

Meanwhile, the prefrontal cortex (PFC) takes a bit of a nap. It's the seat of executive function, which includes working memory; for example, I read a scientific paper and can explain the contents, recognizing consequences, scheduling, and planning. When you're stressed, these functions aren't primary; after all, it's silly to plan tomorrow's breakfast when you might be a giant cat's dinner right now.

"When an animal's life is threatened, all of its attentional and sensory resources, including its memory-storage processes, focus on the threat," says Diamond, explaining the evolutionary roots of the process. The animal needs to reach back into its memory stores to see how it has coped with similar threats before, and store the current experience so it can save its skin in the future.

So the hippocampus and amygdala are all hyped up, compacting both the event and its emotional punch. But why do the events following the trauma fade to a blur?

Consider again that huge burst of glutamate shooting into the hippocampus at the stressor's onset. It activates receptors on the hippocampal neurons to let calcium rush into the cells. And it is the calcium, says Diamond, that, through a process called phosphorylation, causes the neuron membranes to change enough so memories can imprint. "Getting calcium into the cells is the real trigger mechanism to make memories," he says. The problem is, calcium can be toxic: Too much inside a cell will kill it. "If you put hippocampal neurons in a dish and you increase the calcium concentration, they will die," he says. "So just the right amount of calcium must come in to make the memory. The more intense the memory, and the more often the emotional memories are formed, the more likely it is these cells are getting closer and closer to dying, because they're taking in more and more calcium."

To protect themselves once the calcium deluge has passed, the hippocampal neurons close their doors to the stuff. "The receptors are actually inhibited from permitting calcium to come into the cells," says Diamond. Short on calcium, the neurons can't imprint subsequent events. And so we—and that traumatized rat—are left with frozen, fragmented images. As I saw it that day in Chicago, the city faded away and only the man's leering face, Cheshire cat–like, remained.

Blur: Chronic Stress Can Impair Memory

Stanford's Robert Sapolsky penned the commentary on Blackburn and
Epel's groundbreaking paper about stress and cellular aging for good reason: He and Bruce McEwen, working with animals, have made fundamental contributions to the science of stress, including learning how
excessive glucocorticoids can damage the hippocampus. Indeed, it was
McEwen who discovered, in the 1960s, that the hippocampus is chock-
full of glucocorticoid receptors, making it a magnet for the hormone to
ensure that stressful events are recorded. And it was Salpolsky, in the
1980s, who revealed that high levels of glucocorticoids accelerate aging
of the hippocampus. We *need* glucocorticoids to make memories. But too
much of a good thing backfires.

One reason is that the hippocampus has two types of receptors that
glucocorticoids can attach to: mineralocorticoid and glucocorticoid receptors. Glucocorticoids bind much better and faster to mineralocorticoid receptors than to glucocorticoid receptors, and so that's where they
head when they initially increase, at the onset of a stressor. That's a good
thing, because mineralocorticoid binding enhances memory formation.
Recall those flashbulbs that go off with acute stressors? The mineralocorticoid receptors have come into play. But with a major stressor, the
glucocorticoid levels go through the roof, which means the hormone
needs additional receptors to attach to. That's when the glucocorticoid
receptors start filling up, too. That's a bad thing, because glucocorticoids
exerting their influence long term through glucocorticoid receptors disrupts memory formation.

Sapolsky's team has conducted untold numbers of experiments with
rats to uncover those and other mechanisms underlying the impact of
stress on the brain. A visit to his lab at Stanford makes it easy to understand why students and postdocs gravitate to the place. It's not just
for Sapolsky's genius (he's the winner of a MacArthur "Genius" Grant),
but also for his wry wit, colorful mien, and creative flair with both words

and experimental design. His fans have even set up two Facebook pages in honor of him—or rather, parts of him: Robert Sapolsky's Beard and Robert Sapolsky's Hair.

Abutting Sapolsky's lab proper is a worn "chill out" room, complete with upright piano and Gibson acoustic guitar, a couch made up as a bed with sheets and coverlet, another couch as couch, and a big poster of Einstein punctuated by the words "I want to know God's thoughts . . . the rest are details." A well-doodled whiteboard reveals that lab denizen Nate carries a "man-sac" and Shawn prefers "free or expired food." Who wouldn't want to work here?

Dozens of researchers such as Nate and Shawn have, under Sapolsky's guidance, tested the stress basics and then pushed the envelope. Some basics for you and me:

Neurons form vast networks—patterns of electrical excitation that bring to mind constellations flickering against the night sky. Extending from one end of a neuron is a fiber-like projection through which it sends messages to other neurons. That's the axon. Extending from its other end is a shorter, bushier projection through which the neuron receives messages from other neurons. That's the dendrite. As mentioned earlier, neurons talk to each other through chemical messengers called neurotransmitters, and in the hippocampus and the cerebral cortex, glutamate is the big man on campus. As their name implies, neurotransmitters *transmit* the electrical charges that signal thoughts or needs.

A minuscule gap separates the axon of neuron A and the dendrite of neuron B (after all, a neuron's got to have its integrity). It's called the synaptic gap. Now, picture neuron A conversing rapidly with neuron B after that menacing cat has bared his teeth. Neuron A sends a message (*Incisors!*) through its axon via glutamate to the dendrite reaching out from neuron B. *Zinggg!* A point of connection, or synapse, across which impulses can pass, has been made. As the electrical message passes from axon to dendrite to axon to dendrite, a neuronal circuit is essentially etched into the brain. This is the establishment of long-term potentiation, which, as described previously, is the strengthening of the communication network between neurons for learning and long-term memory.

This process is why you hear the phrase "use it or lose it" so often regarding aging and the brain. Learning stimulates the brain both to form new synapses, which expands electrical networks, and to make existing ones stronger, carving experiences into our gray matter. This is the positive side of adaptive plasticity—the brain's ability to reconfigure itself, structurally and functionally, as it adapts to outside stimuli. Amazingly, learning can also spark the birth of new neurons, a process called neurogenesis (more on that later).

Repeated or chronic stress does the opposite of learning, as the brain tries to protect itself from the hormonal onslaught. Neurons in the hippocampus are particularly vulnerable to physical insults, including glucocorticoids and reactive oxygen species, the latter of which are released during normal cell metabolism (see Chapter 2). "The hippocampus is a part of the brain that's very expensive," says Sapolsky. "Virtually by definition, fancy neurons are expensive ones, and expensive neurons are vulnerable ones."

Bruce McEwen has shown in rats that after just a few weeks of stress or exposure to excess glucocorticoids, dendrites in the hippocampus actually retract: They shrink up like a child cowering from a ghost, their limbs withering. In the process, connections from neuron to neuron are lost; the circuit is broken, and information transmission stalls. David Diamond thinks that the dendrites retract, at least in part, to limit the amount of calcium entering the cell. (Recall that the glutamate released into the hippocampus during stress opens up the cell to calcium, and too much calcium can kill the cell.) "The neurons have to protect themselves because all that calcium coming into the dendrites is threatening their lives," he says.

Meanwhile, Sapolsky's and other teams have shown that in neurons in the amygdala—that bastion of fear conditioning—stress induces the very opposite reaction. There the dendrites expand, multiplying their branches and synaptic connections. What was several trees becomes a forest; anxiety soars.

In Sapolsky's lab, researchers led by Rupshi Mitra, Ph.D., gave rats either a single injection of glucocorticoids, producing a hormone level comparable to that of several hours of stress, or ten daily doses of the stuff, producing a level comparable to that of a major chronic stressor. They measured anxiety levels in the rats by watching their reactions in a raised maze with both closed and open arms (anxious rats huddle in the closed ones), and twelve days later, they dissected their brains to measure changes in amygdala neurons. The amygdala dendrites, they found, had expanded by a whopping 54 percent in length and 23 percent in branching points with the single glucocorticoid dose, which was comparable to the overgrowth in the multiple-dose group.

Acute stress (several hours' worth) had had a similar effect on the amygdala as chronic stress. No wonder we set ourselves up for trouble if we freak out over every little thing.

You'd think the prefrontal cortex, particularly the middle part (the medial prefrontal cortex), whose job it is to bring the amygdala back to its senses, might intervene to save the day. But no. McEwen's lab has shown, again in rats, that repeated stress makes the PFC's dendrites recoil, too, severing "voice of reason" connections. The physiological changes manifested themselves in the rats' behavior: The PFC facilitates shifts in attention, but these rats were unable to redirect theirs.

This is the negative side of adaptive plasticity, at least when a sharp memory is what you're after; the brain, of course, reacts this way to protect itself from further damage. Yet dreadful as the process sounds, all is not lost: These dendrite changes can reverse after the stressor passes. They stretch their limbs and reform connections with neighboring axons. "In the rodent models, there is spontaneous recovery when you end the stress," says McEwen.

What no one really knows is if there's a tipping point—a point at which the stress has gone on for so long that the dendrites can no longer regain their earlier glory. What is known is that there may be no turning back if major depression, compounded or even sparked by stress, becomes part of the dynamic. Indeed, autopsies on people who've had major depression show no reduction in the number of neuron cells in the hippocampus and prefrontal cortex, but there is a loss of the support cells—the glial ("glue") cells—that fill the spaces between the dendrite branches to provide nourishment to the neurons and mop up excess chemicals. The neurons themselves are smaller, too. And it's "very likely," says McEwen, that the dendrites have atrophied as well.

What do these rat studies tell us about humans? In a rare kind of scientific synchrony, Conor Liston, M.D., Ph.D., while in McEwen's lab, translated McEwen's attention-shifting study of rats to an analogous trial for humans. He recruited twenty of his fellow medical students who, for a month, had been stressed to the hilt studying for their board exams. He had them fill out the Cohen Perceived Stress Scale, described in Chapter 2, to assess their stress levels. Then, with a colleague at Cornell Medical College, he put them in an fMRI machine and scanned their brains while they performed an attention-shifting task that relied heavily on the prefrontal cortex (pressing a button when a particular target appeared, while ignoring competing images). Functional magnetic resonance imaging (fMRI) looks at the brain in slices, front to back, like a loaf of bread, and tracks blood flow to its various parts. One month later, after the students had recovered from the stress of the medical boards, he scanned the subjects again as they performed the same attention-shifting task. He compared the results of the before and after scans to those from twenty controls, a group of low-stressed folks that matched the subjects for age, sex, and sleep habits.

The results? The higher the perceived stress score, the poorer the attentional control, indicating disrupted functional connectivity in a brain network of the PFC devoted to attentional shifts. Just as in rats, the situation righted itself here, too. Given a month of reduced stress after the boards, the same subjects showed no significant difference on their fMRIs from the controls. "Conor could not, of course, look into the human brain and see if there were a loss or shrinkage of dendrites and a loss of synaptic connections," says McEwen. "But the functional connectivity certainly says that this circuit is not working as efficiently, and it's consistent with what we had found in the rodent."

~~~~~

What happens to memory during all this Alice in Wonderland shrinkage and expansion? Does it, too, under the influence of stress, fall down the rabbit hole?

Unfortunately, the answer is yes. During repeated or chronic stress, memory—specifically declarative memory—declines. And retrieval suffers most. The memories are still there; they're just harder to access. This was certainly no news to me, as, stressed under deadlines, I struggled to remember while talking with a friend: Who was that guy who told Dan Quayle he was "no Jack Kennedy"? Wait. John Kerry? No, wrong job. Gary Hart? No, no, no. Hart was the guy on the boat with the girl (who wasn't his wife) on his lap. Ah, in a flash: Lloyd Bentsen. Whatever happened to him? Is he even still alive?

Part of what's going on is that when a stressor doesn't let up, hippocampal neurons get hungry, and therefore can't function at their peak. "They're not starving, but a little bit queasy," says Sapolsky. That's because glucose levels in the hippocampus drop to some 25 percent below normal. Recall that when a stressor first strikes, stored glucose in fat cells is released and ferries to the brain—the hunter-gatherer from Chapter 1 needs razor-sharp attention. But soon after, any extra glucose rations are shoveled to the parts of the body that, from an evolutionary standpoint, need them most: thigh muscles and diaphragm, for instance, so the hunter-gatherer can flee.

"What parts of your brain are saving your life while you're running?" asks Sapolsky. "It's brain stem reflexes; you want to have your diaphragm working fast enough to get you oxygen. The parts of the brain that do calculus and your taxes and all of that, they're not pertinent at that point. The hippocampus is a superfluous fancy area that can be triaged. So you're shifting glucose uptake and utilization from hippocampus-fancy-frontal-cortical areas to your reptilian-keep-your-heart-beating-at-the-right-speed area."

Generally, the somewhat energy-deprived hippocampal neurons

can recover fine. But if they've been compromised in any way, by, say, a stroke or even low blood sugar, they could be in big trouble.

"While there is evidence that glucocorticoids by themselves do not necessarily cause cell death, that doesn't mean they're not an important player," says Arizona State University's Cheryl D. Conrad, Ph.D. "If a person is exposed to many stressors in their life, that increases the likelihood that any one of them might coincide with some type of challenge to their brain. The challenge to the brain could be very benign by itself, and so, too, stressors by themselves could have no noticeable impact in the brain. But when the stressor and the challenge coincide, then you have a very exasperating synergistic negative outcome on the brain. For example, a benign metabolic challenge to the brain could be hypoglycemia—someone who has very low blood sugar and is not regulating it well. That by itself could be easily corrected. But a person who experiences that often and is under high stress—those two variables combined could lead to minute damage to the brain. And once you have a little bit of damage to the brain—and the hippocampus is hugely susceptible to this—then it is less likely to regulate glucocorticoids." And so the cycle continues, until eventually hippocampal cells might become so damaged they die.

As we age, our glucocorticoid levels rise, and yes, sadly, our hippocampus shrinks—at least that's what imaging scans tell us. In men, hippocampal volume starts to decrease in their twenties, while in women it doesn't start until around age forty, possibly because estrogen has protective effects. In 1986, Sapolsky proposed the glucocorticoid cascade hypothesis to help explain the stress-aging phenomenon: As rising glucocorticoid levels take their toll on the hippocampus, the hippocampus itself becomes less proficient at helping to shut off the hypothalamus-pituitary-adrenal axis, which in turn kicks off the secretion of even more glucocorticoids, which do an even bigger number on the hippocampus, which . . . It's another self-perpetuating cycle.

Past imaging studies have shown that animals subjected to extreme stress and people suffering from PTSD, prolonged major depression, and

Cushing's syndrome, a tumor disorder that leads to hyper-glucocorticoid secretion, have smaller hippocampi. Psychophysiologist Peter J. Gianaros, Ph.D., at the University of Pittsburgh, wanted to know if chronic stress in folks *without* a psychiatric or medical diagnosis had the same result. "Bruce McEwen and Robert Sapolsky made some very seminal observations showing that chronic stress in rats and primates leads to changes in the gray matter of the hippocampus," Gianaros tells me. "What we tried to do is translate those findings to see whether chronic stress in humans is also related to gray matter changes in the brain."

His team was already investigating the relationship of stress to cardiovascular disease in women, following forty-eight healthy women for twenty years and rating them on the Cohen Perceived Stress Scale every one to three years. At the start of the study, the women were forty-two to fifty years old. Then, twenty years later, in 2005 and 2006, when their mean age was sixty-eight, he scanned their brains using structural MRI. Lo and behold, those with higher perceived stress scores over the twenty years had less gray matter in their hippocampi. The differences persisted after accounting for numerous variables, including age, time since menopause, and use of hormone-replacement therapy. The scientists speculated that the women with the smaller hippocampi were more vulnerable to memory and psychiatric problems.

The study had limitations: It was cross-sectional rather than longitudinal—a snapshot in time rather than the more rigorous tracking of changes over the months or years—so there was no way of knowing if those with smaller hippocampal volume had started out that way. But the results still sound a warning bell: These women didn't report horrific, wildly fluctuating stress but "modest levels of life stress," which remained "relatively stable."

What does that mean for you and me?

The Cycle Can Be Broken

Sonia J. Lupien, Ph.D., is at once supersmart and outrageously collo-quial—as well as breezily fashionable in white linen pants and a denim jacket. The scientific director of the University of Montreal's Mental Health Research Centre, Lupien talks a mile a minute, flipping between English with me and French with her preteen daughter, who occupies herself with a handheld Nintendo game in a San Francisco café as Lu-pien and I talk. "I always do seventeen thousand things at the same time," Lupien says briskly. "Parallel worlds."

Lupien works with people to learn where neurological aging and stress meet. She initially worked with healthy elderly people at McGill University but has circled back to study children, with whom she now believes the stress-and-cognitive-function story begins.

At McGill, Lupien followed people ages sixty-five to seventy at the trial's start, testing their glucocorticoid levels over a period of twenty years. In year nine, she began testing their memories as well, asking them to re-call lists of words and navigate a virtual maze, and later added a follow-up MRI scan of their brains to see how their hippocampal volume had fared. By the study's end, she had about sixty-five subjects whose glucocorticoid levels she'd collected for ten years and who'd taken the memory tests and been scanned. She found that those with high levels of stress hormones had poorer memories and hippocampi that were about 14 percent smaller than those whose glucocorticoid levels had remained stable or sunk.

In other studies, in which she either administered synthetic cor-tisol (hydrocortisol) to participants or stressed them by having them deliver a speech to a frozen-faced panel and then do mental arithme-tic, she confirmed the results: While small increases of glucocorticoids increased memory acuity, larger increases—whether synthetic or self-manufactured—decreased memory performance.

And so for much of her career, Lupien ascribed to the so-called neu-rotoxicity theory of stress—that, in general, prolonged exposure to glucocorticoids makes neurons more vulnerable to damage by challenges, metabolic or otherwise, and the hippocampus atrophies accordingly. And then she heard about the twins study.

In 2002, a team led by Harvard's Mark W. Gilbertson, Ph.D., and Roger K. Pitman, M.D., published a paper looking at identical twins, one of whom had PTSD after serving in the Vietnam War, the other of whom had stayed home. Earlier research, you'll recall, had shown that the hippocampal volume of people with PTSD is smaller than that of people without the disorder. But here the scientists found a surprise: Yes, the hippocampal volume of the veterans with PTSD was smaller than the norm, but so was the hippocampal volume of their identical twins, who had *not* been exposed to the trauma of combat. Did the egg, perhaps, come before the chicken?

The authors of the paper think so. "These data indicate that smaller hippocampi in PTSD represent a preexisting familial vulnerability factor rather than the neurotoxic product of trauma exposure *per se*," they write. They nail the lid on the coffin of the neurotoxicity hypothesis of stress thus: "In light of the current findings, reference to hippocampal 'atrophy' in PTSD may be a misnomer." And they introduce a new theory: The vulnerability hypothesis of stress—that is, that a smaller hippocampus, whether due to genes or early exposure to stress—can *predispose* you to the damaging effects of stress, rendering you more vulnerable to age-related memory loss and disorders such as PTSD.

Lupien's scientific world flipped upside down. Might it be that because different brain regions develop at different points in time, her observations in her older stressed subjects weren't so much atrophy as a window on to their pasts?

"So I was out walking the dog," she begins, a preamble to many of her insights, "and I said, 'Yeah, that's it! Exposure to adversity early in life will delay the development of the hippocampus, rendering you more vulnerable.' I'm not saying that there is no degeneration that happens with chronic stress in my older adults, but I think that their sensitivity to stress may have been driven much earlier in life."

And so Lupien designed her own very elegant hypothesis, which she calls the "life-cycle model of stress," to reconcile the neurotoxicity hypothesis with the vulnerability hypothesis.

The hippocampus develops very early in life, between birth and two years of age. The amygdala develops much more slowly, starting at birth and continuing until the late twenties. And the front part of the cerebral cortex does most of its growing between the ages of eight and fourteen. "What we think is that if you are exposed to different adversity at different times of your life, this will impact on the development of the structure through a neurotoxic process, rendering it smaller, increasing your vulnerability to develop different types of disorders," says Lupien. "So when I measure it later, for sure it's smaller, not because of atrophy but because it never developed in the first place. The life-cycle model goes along with data that has always had discrepancies. What it implies is if you had adverse experiences between ages zero and two, it would delay the development of the hippocampus. But if the adversity persists after two, it would have an impact on other structures like the amygdala or the frontal cortex. So at the end, the reduced volume you see would not be a good reflection of the type of trauma you had but more a reflection of the *time* that you were exposed to the trauma. For example, women who report physical and emotional abuse before the age of twelve have a hippocampal atrophy, whereas those women who report abuse after twelve have a frontal atrophy."

How would those different women fare functionally? Broadly, those with hippocampal atrophy would have a poorer memory, while those with frontal atrophy would have impaired reasoning and less impulse control.

An update of the Vietnam-vet PTSD study, led by the University of Tokyo's Kiyoto Kasai, M.D., Ph.D., and Harvard's Roger Pitman, supports Lupien's theory, showing that both vulnerability and neurotoxicity play a role in hippocampal shrinkage. Looking at the same Vietnam vets and their twins, the scientists used sophisticated technology to examine exactly *where* in the hippocampus the gray matter had shrunk. And indeed, the combat-exposed twins with PTSD had lower density in one region—the anterior cingulate cortex (ACC)—than their unexposed twin. Yes, they'd started out with a smaller hippocampus, but the trauma of war had injured it even further.

At first glance, the revelation may seem damning, but in fact it provides new hope. McGill University's Michael J. Meaney, Ph.D., working with rats, pioneered studies showing how early life experiences—say, a mother who nurtures her pups by licking and grooming—shape not just stress responses into adulthood but the expression of the very genes that control those responses (the burgeoning field of epigenetics). Meaney's licked and groomed rats were less emotionally reactive and more adventurous, lived longer, and had better memories than the ignored ones. They, in turn, passed those traits along to their offspring.

As Lupien sees it, her research opens the door wide to timed, early interventions. "If the brain is so plastic to adversity," she says, "then it means it could be plastic to intervention." Indeed, Meaney and others have shown that placing rats not so fortunate in the licking and grooming department in an enriched environment—toys, running wheel, and so on—can reverse the negative effects.

"I do research for one reason," says Lupien firmly. "To change social policies—to give politicians a very convincing argument that they cannot push away."

New Brain Cells Can Be Born

Neuroscientists shunned the idea of neurogenesis—the birth of new cells in the postmitotic world of the adult brain—until the end of the twentieth century. But then, in the late nineties, scientists including Fred H. Gage, Ph.D., at the Salk Institute, and Elizabeth Gould, Ph.D., now at Princeton, rattled the mature-brain cage: They showed, independently, that new neurons are born in one part of the hippocampus, the dentate gyrus. Gould showed the birth of new neurons in adult rats and primates, and Gage showed it in humans, using brain cells of people who had died of cancer. Later research showed that the brain's olfactory bulb, which processes smell, generates new neurons, too. Ever wonder why pregnant women start heaving when they smell, say, broccoli or brussels sprouts? In another evolutionary hangover, pregnancy spurs neurogenesis in the olfactory bulb, ensuring survival of the species—albeit generally for the nonhuman among us, for whom sniffing equals surveillance.

Not surprisingly, chronic stress decreases neurogenesis. When Gould's team removed rats' adrenal glands, the source of glucocorticoids, they watched new neurons sprout in the dentate gyrus. Conversely, when they injected those rats with glucocorticoids, the flowering stopped. External stressors had the same effect in a variety of animals: rats exposed to the scent of a fox, tree shrews exposed to same-sex shrews (apparently shrews are homophobes), and marmoset monkeys housed with already settled-in monkeys. Gould also showed, in young to middle-aged marmosets, that—also not surprisingly—neurogenesis in the hippocampus decreases linearly with age.

But, as it does repeatedly regarding stress, other research suggests that we have some control over that process.

An enriched environment and voluntary exercise (see Chapter 5 for more on exercise) boost neurogenesis, as do antidepressants and estrogen. (This is not a recommendation to take either but a subject worth investigating. Estrogen, by the way, has also been shown to increase telomerase levels in lab studies. All of this has led Sapolsky to develop a chimeric gene, for gene therapy, that would convert the bad effects of glucocorticoids in the brain into the good effects of estrogen—an amazingly nifty trick.) In one study, Gage showed that the hippocampi of rats raised in an enriched environment upped new-cell production by 15 percent and also increased dendritic branching and synaptic connections. And Gould reported at a recent neuroscience conference that—yes!—sex increases hippocampal neurogenesis in mature rats, particularly in the area regulating anxiety, and also increases dendritic growth, despite the fact that it raises stress hormones.

The scientists believe that the hormone oxytocin may play a role in the phenomenon.

"It's uniquely important work showing that glucocorticoids are context dependent," says McEwen about Gould's promiscuous rats. "They don't have a unitary effect—they depend on other factors."

Here, briefly, is how those new brain cells are born.

Embryonic stem cells—the stem cells there's such a political ruckus over—form soon after fertilization and can divide indefinitely, producing either new versions of themselves or differentiating into various types of cells: blood, muscle, gastrointestinal, neurons, you name it. Their first-degree offspring are called progenitor cells. These can divide only a limited number of times, and differentiate into limited types of cells. In other words, their fate is predetermined.

The new cells generated in the dentate gyrus of the hippocampus arise not from true-blue stem cells but from progenitor cells, here also called neural stem cells, that can only become neurons. The progenitor cells live in the subgranular zone, a layer deep inside the hippocampus, and their progeny will eventually wander to the higher-up granule-cell layer and become mature neurons, complete with dendrites and axons. The growth factor BDNF (brain-derived neurotrophic factor) is crucial for this process. Growth factors, or neurotrophins, are chemicals in the brain that regulate the growth, proliferation, and survival of certain neurons. (Glucocorticoids, research shows, dampen the flow of BDNF, hence contributing to stress's decreasing neurogenesis.) Thousands of new cells are generated in the dentate gyrus each day, but only a small percentage of them go on to become mature neurons. Learning new things, notes Rutgers University's Tracey J. Shors, Ph.D., in a recent paper on neurogenesis in animals, can make a huge difference.

"Indeed, between about 1 and 2 weeks after their birth, as many as 60 percent perish," writes Shors about the nascent neurons, citing the work of Elizabeth Gould, adding that "with learning, however, the percentage of cells that survive is increased." Shors explains further: "That is, if animals are trained when the cells are approximately one week of age, more of the newly born population survive. Therefore, the cells are essentially rescued from death by learning."

"Rescued from death by learning." I love that. And numerous other studies support the contention. In one, led by Gerd Kempermann, M.D., now at the Center for Regenerative Therapies Dresden, old mice "educated" for ten months by playing with novel toys, rearrangeable plastic tubes, and a running wheel showed a fivefold increase in the birth of new neurons, compared to mice housed in their usual humdrum quarters.

If you're thinking mice are not us, consider this: Bogdan Draganski, M.D., at University College London, conducted a similar "real-life" learning intervention with people. He did MRI scans of the brains of German medical students while they were studying for a dreadful exam called the Physikum, which comprises new information about subjects from biochemistry to physics and the social sciences. Because it takes three months for newly generated neural cells to differentiate into mature neurons, the researchers scanned the cramming students at three points in time: three months before the test, one or two days after the test, and three months later.

The students' brains were fairly bursting with new growth. Gray matter in the hippocampus expanded "continuously through the three time points," the scientists write. Another region, the posterior parietal cortex—known for manipulating mental images and integrating sensory and motor portions of the brain—increased between the first scan and the second, and was still in its heftier state three months later.

All learning, though, is not equal. Leading scientists remain wary, for example, about computerized "cognitive training" programs. A panel of experts associated with the Stanford Center on Longevity recently issued a consensus statement noting that while such programs may help, the scientific evidence is just not there yet to know for sure.* "Consumers need to consider hidden costs beyond dollars and cents," the panel

---

* For the full statement, see www.longevity.stanford.edu/mymind/cognitiveaging statement.

notes, adding that "every hour spent doing solo software drills is an hour not spent hiking, learning Italian, making a new recipe, or playing with your grandchildren."

Stress, Telomeres, and Our Aging Brains

To say that the study of telomeres and the brain is in its infancy is an understatement. It's essentially—if not literally—*prenatal* at this point. Neural stems cells, described earlier, are the only brain cells that divide, and are therefore the only ones with telomeres at risk for shortening through mitosis. Still, as noted in Chapter 2, reactive oxygen species can do a number on the telomeres of mature brain cells, given the particularly vulnerable makeup of the DNA tips. Could there be other drivers for telomere erosion as well?

A team led by Sacfi R. Ferrón, Ph.D., of Spain's Universidad de Valencia, found that telomerase plays a role. In a paper just out in November 2009, they showed that some neural stem cells of mice engineered to be deficient in telomerase had "critically short" telomeres, which led to fewer new neurons being produced and stubby dendrites in the ones that did make it. Fewer new neurons, the scientists wrote, "suggest that age-related deficits could be caused partly by dysfunctional telomeres . . ."

And a study just released this year speaks even more directly to those of us worried about the effects of worrying on the rate at which our brain cells age.

Susanna Wolf, Ph.D., a former postdoc in Robert Sapolsky's lab who's now at the University of Zurich, subjected twenty pregnant mice to five days of chronic but mild stress: Each day, for a set period of time, she tilted their cages, inverted their water bottles so drinking would be a struggle, removed their food, and exposed them to "predator odor," that is, a cotton ball soaked in bobcat urine. The stressed mice were matched with pregnant control mice, who were hanging out, enjoying their days in the sun.

All the mice's pups were born after twenty-one days, the normal mouse gestation time, and raised by their biological mothers. Then came the guillotine ("sacrifice by decapitation," in scientific parlance) at designated time points: On day one, three subjects and three controls lost their heads. On day two, three of each did. And so on up to day ten. Wolf then assessed the telomere length and telomerase levels of the neural stem cells in the slain pups' hippocampi.

Amazingly, the baby mice of the stressed mothers had shorter telomeres and lower levels of telomerase than those whose moms had twenty-one days on easy street. And this was from stress before they were even born. Who knew stress could be so potent? Had those mice lived, says Wolf, "they would have had lower levels of neurogenesis"—older brains from the get-go. Why? With shorter telomeres, their neural stem cells had fewer divisions left in them, which meant fewer new neurons would be born, and an earlier demise of the neural stem cell itself.

Wolf's is a cautionary tale if there ever was one. And it's buttressed by a few earlier studies tying poorer cognition or psychiatric disorders to the more standard telomere measure: that of white blood cells or leukocytes. (Keep in mind that since the field is so new, the evidence is just surfacing.)

Ana M. Valdes, Ph.D., at King's College London, found in 382 healthy women ages nineteen to seventy-eight that the worse the women's memory, the shorter their leukocyte telomeres and the worse their ability to learn, even after adjusting for age and prior intellectual ability. Telomere length, the authors write, therefore might be "a biomarker of cognitive aging in women before the onset of dementia." Harvard's Naomi M. Simon, M.D., found that the leukocyte telomere lengths of people with psychiatric disorders (major depression to bipolar disorder) were shorter than those of matched controls by as much as ten years. Citing oxidative damage to cells as a mechanism, the combination, she writes, "results in accelerated organismal aging."

How can we apply these revelations to revitalizing our memories and keeping them sharp?

That's exactly what the rest of this book is about: The chapters that follow lay out the latest interventions, along with their action-inspiring underpinnings, for slowing and even reversing the aging process of your brain and your body. Exercise is a biggie. So is learning—specifically, thinking outside your usual box and opening your mind to new perspectives (even taking a new route home challenges brain circuits!). Diet and frame of mind can help rejuvenate your mental and physical well-being, too. As Elizabeth Blackburn and Elissa Epel revealed in their research, perception is key in how stress affects our aging processes. Keep reading to learn how you can change the way *you* see the world.

CHAPTER 4

Stress and Diet

What determines human life is the mind, which is the master of the body. If the body is at ease and in harmony with its environment, the mind will be able to deal with all changes in life. Thus it is important to keep the body in good repair and maintenance, the essence of which is to keep the golden mean. This is not to be deficient in nutrition and not to indulge in excesses. Use the five tastes [saltiness, sweetness, sourness, bitterness, pungency] to temper the five vital organs. If these are at peace, the vital fluid in us will flow smoothly, then our mind will find its equilibrium, and the whole person will find himself in a state of supreme well-being.

—Hu Sihui, *Principles of Correct Diet*, 1330

It's three a.m. and Debbie Meyer can't sleep. Again.

She tosses off the covers, takes a peek at Carl, her husband of thirty-three years, to make sure he's still snoring, and steals downstairs to the kitchen of their home in Brockton, Massachusetts.

It's time to eat.

Debbie is, by her own account, a "middle of the night nosher"—a very specific type of stress eater. A scoop of peanut butter here, a handful of popcorn there—anything salty and crunchy that she hasn't labeled "forbidden" and banished to her husband's backyard shed will do in the dark of night. Sometimes she's hungry. Sometimes she's not. Always, these days, she's stressed.

Debbie laughs easily and talks with gusto, but her good cheer belies an excruciating year and a half. Her mother, who resides in an independent-living facility, has a serious heart condition and has been showing signs of dementia. She can no longer manage her own finances or medications, so every week, in addition to transporting her to doctor's appointments, Debbie, the oldest daughter, pays her mom's bills and doles out the eighteen pills a day a nurse's aide will give her.

Her stress threshold dipped precariously two months ago, when she lost her father to end-stage dementia. He'd been in a nursing home for five years, virtually immobile, his hips and knees shot, a colostomy bag poking up on his belly, a bladder bag dangling low to the floor. Recently, her support structure caved some, too. Maureen, her best friend since they were both twelve and the smartest kid in junior high, was shipped to Iraq to serve as a medical commander outside the Baghdad airport. No more picking up the phone on impulse to vent: "You're not going to believe what my sister did with my mother today!"

Work used to be her escape. A thirty-year veteran of Gillette, she'd risen from secretary to senior planner through sheer will and night classes. "If I had a pretty low-key day, I could just sit and deal with numbers and not have to deal with anybody," she says.

But Gillette moved out of town after Procter & Gamble bought it, and Debbie switched careers—to pastoral ministry, a dream of hers for years. Today she does elder outreach for Catholic Charities USA, counseling low-income elders and caregivers of chronically ill relatives, and facilitating bereavement groups. She loves the work, but it's exhausting. The stress has added inches to her waistline and battered her immune system: She gets frequent colds and stomach bugs, and recently had her first bout of bronchitis in fifteen years. "I've been neglectful of my own health," she says. "I feel like I don't have any downtime."

Does Stress Drive You to Eat?

For most of us, stress and eating are inextricably linked. This test will help you determine your drive-to-eat baseline—and thus how likely you are to make a beeline for the snack cabinet when the going gets tough.

Please indicate the extent to which you agree that the following items describe you.

Use the following 1 to 5 scale for your responses:

1 Don't agree at all
2 Agree a little
3 Agree somewhat
4 Agree
5 Strongly agree

1. I find myself thinking about food even when I'm not physically hungry. _____

2. I get more pleasure from eating than I do from almost anything else. _____

3. If I see or smell a food I like, I get a powerful urge to have some. _____

4. When I'm around a fattening food I love, it's hard to stop myself from at least tasting it. _____

5. It's scary to think of the power that food has over me. _____

6. When I know a delicious food is available, I can't help myself from thinking about having some. _____

7. I love the taste of certain foods so much that I can't avoid eating them even if they're bad for me. _____

8. Just before I taste a favorite food, I feel intense anticipation. _____

9. When I eat delicious food I focus a lot on how good it tastes. _____

10. Sometimes, when I'm doing everyday activities, I get an urge to eat "out of the blue" (for no apparent reason). _____

11. I think I enjoy eating a lot more than most other people. _____

12. Hearing someone describe a great meal makes me really want to have something to eat. _____

13. It seems like I have food on my mind a lot._____

14. It's very important to me that the foods I eat are as delicious as possible. _____

15. Before I eat a favorite food my mouth tends to flood with saliva. _____

Calculating your score:

Add up your scores from the 15 items. Scores will range from 15 to 75. The higher your score, the more likely you are to reach for the goodies.

Interpreting your score the *Stress Less* way*:

15–25: Unlikely to be driven to eat
26–41: Somewhat likely to be driven to eat
42–59: Moderately likely to be driven to eat
60–75: Highly likely to be driven to eat

How Stress Manages Your Eating

Why is it that when we're really stressed we reach, like Debbie, for the sweet, salty, fatty stuff? The simple carbs, the saturated and trans fats, the greasy crunch? It's almost as if there's something in our *blood* that cries out for fries or doughnuts or buttered popcorn—and that calms down once we've downed a fistful of them. After all, they can't be called "comfort foods" for nothing.

Research shows that when stressed, about two-thirds of people (and

* The *Stress Less* interpretation was developed by the author, not the scientists.

lab rats, for that matter) reach for food, primarily of the sweet, starchy, fatty variety. (The remaining one-third *lose* their appetite). To top off the bad news: When we eat fatty stuff when stressed, the fat goes straight to our bellies—the worst place for it to be.

Intra-abdominal fat, as belly fat is technically called, because it lies between the organs in the abdomen, leaves us with an "apple" as opposed to a "pear" shape. It is a known risk factor for conditions ranging from hypertension to heart disease to type 2 diabetes. "Apples" have waists that are bigger than their hips (a waist-to-hip ratio, or WHR, larger than 1.0). "Pears" have hips that are bigger than their waists (a WHR less than 1.0). Sure, there's a genetic component, but lifestyle plays a huge role, too. And talk about aging: The 2003 National Health and Nutrition Examination Survey linked an apple shape with reduced life span, as well.

Yet it's not the stress response itself that drives this overindulgence and the subsequent packing on of heft but the repeated and chronic *turning on* of that response.

As explained in the introduction, challenge stress (you're waiting in the wings to debut as Rosalind in *As You Like It*) sparks fight-or-flight, the first stage of the stress response, when epinephrine floods the bloodstream and digestion shuts down. The corticotropin-releasing hormone burst and glucocorticoid boost that follow are short-lived. You're fine holding off eating until the cast party, several hours later.

But threat stress (you're Debbie Meyer, juggling crises intermittently all day long) keeps CRH spurting and glucocorticoids constantly elevated. Each time CRH clears (it takes just minutes), your body believes recovery has begun. Digestion restarts; appetite shoots up: Gotta replace the glucose burned during the most recent crisis! And those elevated glucocorticoids? Unlike CRH, they stick around for *hours*, and they don't just stimulate appetite—they make you preferentially yearn for junk.

Here's why.

Stress and Drugs and R & R

That we eat when we're stressed is an evolutionary necessity, wired into our brains to ensure our survival as a species. But these days, with food so accessible and stress so constant, the circuit has gone haywire.

Since at least the mid-1970s, scientists have been showing, through animal and human studies, that glucocorticoids activate the same reward system in the brain as cocaine, heroin, and other drugs of abuse. Indeed, in one of her papers Elissa Epel refers to the system as the "neural circuitry of addiction."

True, the *degree* of activation is different, but the process is the same. Both glucocorticoids and addictive drugs stimulate neurons in a part of the brain called the ventral tegmental area, which sits atop the brain stem, to release the neurotransmitter dopamine (see figure 3, page 69). The dopamine then zips via nerve fibers over to the nucleus accumbens, a.k.a. the pleasure center of the brain. The information, *ahh, pleasure*, is then relayed to the prefrontal cortex, where it makes its way into consciousness.

Mind you, the dopamine itself is not the reward. Rather, it sparks the motivation to do the work to *get* the reward. The good feelings are ones of delicious anticipation and mastery: "Yes we can!" chanted Obama volunteers, their dopamine flowing, knowing in their hearts that the presidency was within reach. This dopamine-inspired drive exists for a reason: to keep us alive. When we're hungry or thirsty, it drives us to seek food and water. When it's time to reproduce, it drives us to seek sex. *Good job!* the reward circuit tells us when we've located the watering hole or a mate, thereby reinforcing the behavior. We beam. Glucocorticoids pump up that drive, making the water appear even more sparkling and the mate even hunkier. They supercharge the *wanting*.

What we want during stress, scientists say, depends on context. The reward just has to be palatable, a natural reinforcer—something veggies are not. Studies have shown that if a rat is stressed and a hunk of pork fat and regular chow are both within reach, it'll make a beeline for the pork fat. If cocaine is available at the push of a lever, it'll go for that. If a running wheel is the only game in town, it'll exercise its little legs off.

The food-as-drug comparison goes even further. Sweet, high-fat foods increase the release of endogenous opioids, or endorphins—naturally occurring brain chemicals that also activate the brain's reward system, increasing the release of dopamine into the nucleus accumbens. Drugs such as morphine and heroin, known as opiates, mimic these effects, though of course to a heightened degree. The release of opioids as a result of eating these foods, in turn, leads to the intake of more sweet, high-fat foods, which then increases the release of opioids, which . . . It's a cycle remarkably similar to that of drug addiction.

Opioids exist in part to decrease activity in the hypothalamus-pituitary-adrenal axis, thereby helping to end the stress response and permit recovery—the replenishing of energy stores—to begin. Indeed, when people (or rats) in research studies are given opiate blockers, their interest in sweet, high-fat foods diminishes.

Mary F. Dallman, Ph.D., professor emeritus at UCSF, may be the grande dame of comfort food research. Now in her seventies, she has been studying stress physiology since 1959, and was the first to describe "fast glucocorticoid feedback"—how rising glucocorticoid levels can, when everything's working right, inhibit further glucocorticoid release within seconds.

I speak with her in her box of an office at UCSF Parnassus, pictures of her grandchildren and a "much loved" yellow lab tacked on the wall, paper clasps tumbling out of the desk drawer. They're remnants of her nearly forty years in the space, which she's now packing up to leave. Dallman is feisty and irreverent, partly, I'd imagine, because she came of academic age at a time when being a woman in science was a grueling uphill battle. Back then, an engagement ring was enough for the president of the Rockefeller Institute for Medical Research (now the Rockefeller University) to deny her admission as a graduate student. "I knew it was a mistake to interview a woman," he sniffed upon spying the stone when she entered the room.

Dallman and her colleagues conduct elegant experiments with rats: stressing them (using cold or restraint), putting palatable rewards nearby (lard, sugar water, exercise wheels), manipulating and measuring their hormone levels, then chopping off their little heads in a tiny operating theater and examining slides of their brains under a microscope.

She has shown that while normal rats run miles each night on their wheels, those whose adrenal glands have been removed and therefore can't produce glucocorticoids snooze the night through. When she implanted glucocorticoids in the brains of the rats without adrenals, the rats once more became night runners—but ran strictly in proportion to the amount of glucocorticoids they'd received. She got the same result when she substituted saccharin water or lard for the running wheels: As the dose of glucocorticoids rose, so did the intake of the goodies.

"The more glucocorticoids, the more dopamine," she says flatly. "The more the dopamine, the more this pleasure center stuff turns on—the wanting, the salience."

In other experiments, in which she's dissected the rats after the protocol, she's found that the intake of lard and sugar water following a stressor actually *cuts down* on the secretion of the crucial stress hormones: CRH, adrenocorticotropin hormone, glucocorticoids, and catecholamines. The opposite is also true: Rats that eat comfort food *before* being restrained secrete lower levels of the stress hormones. Comfort foods act, in essence, as a natural tranquilizer. "The results suggest strongly that ingestion of highly palatable foods reduces activity in the central stress response network," Dallman concludes in a 2009 paper. She makes the leap to humans in another one: "Do the effects of chronic stress and glucocorticoids apply to humans?" she and her colleagues write. "We believe the answer to this question is a resounding 'yes!'"

No wonder we're snarfing up the sweet, fatty stuff.

UCSF's Elissa Epel, among others, has done experiments with people that back up Dallman's *yes!*—and they describe the same reward-system relationship: Glucocorticoids set off the dopamine rush over the nucleus accumbens in proportion to the amount of glucocorticoids released. The dopamine in turn drives our wanting for that natural tranquilizer: comfort food.

In one study, Epel and her colleagues exposed fifty-nine women ages thirty to forty-five to a stress session: They had to do puzzles, subtract prime numbers serially, and deliver a speech to evaluators behind a one-way mirror, all in a ridiculously short period of time. At several intervals, the researchers took saliva and measured levels of cortisol, the glucocorticoid that plays the leading role in the stress response in humans (the rat version, recall from Chapter 1, is called corticosterone). After the grueling session, the women received a basket of snacks: high-fat, sweet, and salty treats (chocolate granola bars, potato chips), and low-fat salty ones (sweetened rice cakes, pretzels). On another day, they followed the same protocol but without the stress session.

Guess who downed more calories and more sweet and fatty foods? Yup, the women whose cortisol shot through the roof during the stress session: On average, they consumed 216 calories, compared with 137 for those whose cortisol remained lower.

Eating because of stress makes perfect evolutionary sense. After all, the primary role of glucocorticoids, as the *gluco* in their name suggests, is to ensure that there's plenty of accessible energy (read: calories) available to save our skins, and to replenish the stores once the stressor has passed (read: time to eat again). Glucose, the simplest sugar, released from the liver and muscles, provides just that. Indeed, research has shown that the more glucocorticoids you release in response to a stressor, the hungrier you will be *after* the stressor.

"Sweet things and things high in carbohydrates replenish energy sources quickly," says Health Canada's Samir Khan, Ph.D., waving away waiters offering trays of Kobe burgers (not sweet, not carbs) at the July 2009 International Society of Psychoneuroendocrinology (ISPNE) conference in San Francisco. Kahn is here to present new research that attempts to separate any psychological drives to eat from the purely biological ones.

To do that, Kahn and his colleagues began by giving fourteen subjects IV injections of either placebo or ovine CRH. The CRH would do its usual job of stimulating cortisol, without psychological stress coming into the picture, so the scientists could separate the effects of *cortisol* itself on the subjects' food choices from any *psychological* reasons for those choices. They took blood samples both before and after the injections, then delivered food (sweetened rice cakes, chips, and pretzels) and followed up by measuring in calories and grams how much each subject ate. Not surprisingly, the subjects who got the CRH injections—and thus had the cortisol-loaded blood—ate significantly more, in terms of both calories and grams.

Is it any wonder, then, that with our stressing these days over everything from job security to our kids' education to our aging parents' health, we're scrambling for the Ben & Jerry's hidden behind the frozen spinach?

～～～～

When the glucocorticoid flow never lets up, the reward circuit can backfire, as it does with drug addiction—and with depression, which is often the endpoint of chronic stress. The dopamine receptors just conk out, and the ability to experience pleasure diminishes.

"We believe that the addictive property of drugs is due to the fact that they can increase the concentration of dopamine in the brain," explains Nora D. Volkow, M.D., director of the National Institute on Drug Abuse. If the dopamine release goes on long enough, she says, eventually "the number of receptors starts to decrease."

Think about it: Nerve cells, or neurons, talk to each other through chemical messengers such as dopamine. As their name implies, the neurotransmitters *transmit* the electrical charges that signal thoughts or needs. Say that the thought *I'm hungry!* lights up neuron 1 in your nucleus accumbens. Neuron 1 releases dopamine carrying the message *I'm hungry!* into the receptor of neuron 2 through the tiny junction, or synapse, between them. Once attached, the dopamine transmits *I'm hungry!* into the body of the neuron. Neuron 2 then takes up the charge, passing the signal to neuron 3, and so on. It's like a game of telephone, without the garbled-message part. Neuron 1's dopamine then detaches from neuron 2's receptors and slips back into neuron 1 to be reused, or it dissolves in the synapse.

Now imagine glucocorticoids raining down on the neurons thick and fast. Neuron 1 is spewing out buckets of dopamine. Because of the onslaught, nothing is detaching or dissolving in the synapse. The receptors on neuron 2 are aghast. To save themselves they mount defenses, becoming less sensitive. They may even reduce their numbers.

What to do? Eat even *more* palatable food, in an attempt to get that same bump of calm. Pretty soon, you're eating not to elicit calm but just to maintain the status quo.

Control Through Willpower? Fat Chance.

It sounds like a bad dream: We eat sweet, fatty foods when stressed, and the fat goes straight to our bellies.

But it gets worse, becoming more like a recurring nightmare. Large fat deposits inside our bellies make us more susceptible to stress and to secreting even *more* glucocorticoids. That in turn jacks up our craving for sweets and fat. We indulge, and the fat again lands in our bellies, which . . . You get the picture.

Why ever were we built this way? And can the cycle be broken?

Epel and colleagues wanted to know. They are one of the few groups to explore how the many animal studies of Mary Dallman and others showing the stress–belly fat connection relate to humans.

Over the course of four days, the researchers subjected a group of women ages thirty to forty-six—half apple shaped, half pear shaped—to three stress sessions (serial math, puzzles, and speech tasks) and one rest session. They measured cortisol in saliva and administered psychological tests. And true to form—literally—the belly phenomenon stuck: Faced with a new stressor, the women who were apple shaped reported higher levels of stress and secreted significantly more cortisol than the women who were pear shaped.*

And the belly-fat indictment went even further. The scientists also compared the lean women with big bellies (colloquially "lean apples") to the overweight women with big bellies, and found that the lean apples reported higher levels of stress: They felt out of control, gave up coping with the stressful tasks, and most strikingly, never *habituated* to the tasks. Physiologically this meant that while the overweight women stopped secreting excess cortisol after the first task go-round, the lean apples continued pouring out the stuff even on round three.

The correlation between glucocorticoids and belly fat is not arbitrary; it exists for a reason. Cortisol's job, remember, is to make sure that fast fuel keeps coming so the brain and body have the energy to respond to—and then recover from—a challenge or a threat. One way to ensure adequate supplies is to instruct the body to move stored fat from the periphery (say, the hips) to a place where it's readily available to the liver to be converted into fuel. The liver, of course, lies in the abdomen. What better spot for future rations? At the same time, cortisol inhibits the production of hormones that would only get in the way during an emergency, including growth hormone (don't want to waste energy reaching six feet now) and sex steroids (certainly not time to reproduce)—hormones that in better times help break down and *eliminate* fat. It also inhibits the production of insulin, another key player in the stress and aging story.

---

* Epidemiological studies show the same stress–belly fat relationship. Among one of the most cited is the twenty-year Whitehall II prospective study that came out in 2007. It showed that those with poor social support, little job control, and high job strain—in other words, those exceptionally stressed—had increased BMI and abdominal obesity. The study, which followed more than ten thousand British civil servants ages thirty-five to fifty-five, was established by University College London's Sir Michael Marmot in 1985 to investigate the role of social class, psychosocial factors, and lifestyle in disease.

The Stress, Aging, and Insulin Connection

Insulin, which is produced by the pancreas, is a major player in the stress-aging story. It's what permits the nutrients produced by the liver and released through digestion to enter target cells so they can do their job of providing energy. Think of insulin as the doorman controlling passage into a fancy Manhattan co-op building. Without it, no one gets in. Insulin permits fat cells to take up fatty acids, muscle cells to take up amino acids, cells all over to take up glucose. When we eat a big meal or sweet snacks, the level of glucose in our blood soars. The high glucose sparks the pancreas to release buckets of insulin, to open the doors to the cells so they can be nourished.

Except when stress is in the picture. Remember, in the midst of a stressor, glucocorticoids work to keep nutrients (glucose, fatty acids, glycerol) in the bloodstream, ensuring they'll be available for the cells that need them most and, later, for recovery, when depleted stores must be replenished. So glucocorticoids initially *inhibit* insulin secretion from the pancreas and put a vise on the insulin that might be floating around. They're particularly vigilant about keeping the doors shut to the fat, liver, and muscle cells.

This is all fine and good in the short term. But if the stress is chronic or repeated, the glucose and other rations in the bloodstream just build and build—buttressed, of course, by all that comfort food we've eaten to soothe ourselves. The sky-high glucose again sparks the pancreas to pour out insulin. By now the glucocorticoids, raised for so long, have lost their ability to inhibit insulin release from the pancreas. So insulin floods the bloodstream. However, the glucocorticoids *continue* to keep the insulin from opening the cell doors. The pattern repeats, and the insulin levels in the blood climb and climb.

This is type 2 diabetes, also known as insulin-resistant diabetes.

Experiments that artificially raise glucocorticoid levels have replicated the process: In a study in which overweight people were given a synthetic glucocorticoid called dexamethasone, their levels of insulin in the blood shot up by a whopping 83 percent. And insulin wasn't the only hormone to go wacko in that study. The subjects' levels of leptin soared by 80 percent. Leptin is an appetite-suppressing hormone secreted by fat tissue; its job is to tell the brain when we're full. Glucocorticoids make brain cells less sensitive to leptin, so in the presence of chronic stress, leptin, like insulin, never makes it past the cells' doormen, and its levels in the bloodstream rocket. The message *You're full!* never penetrates our brain; we keep chomping away.

"All the stress hormones—epinephrine, norepinephrine, cortisol— are acutely anti-insulin," says C. Ronald Kahn, M.D., head of the Obesity and Hormone Research section at the Joslin Diabetes Center, in Boston. Kahn and his colleagues are known for, among other things, development of the FIRKO (Fat Insulin Receptor Knockout) mouse, a creature genetically engineered to have no insulin receptors on its fat cells, which means no doors on the fat cells can open to let fatty acids and other nutrients inside. FIRKO mice can gorge to their hearts' content and still remain thin and in good health. "When there's a need for an acute stress response, your body doesn't care if your sugar goes up," says Kahn. "It may *want* your sugar to go up, because it may need more fuel. It may *want* to shut down storage of fat and say, 'Use all that extra energy you've got. Don't store it away in fat cells; use it. To run, to fight, to do whatever it's going to take to survive your stress.'"

Not only stress but excess fat, particularly belly fat, contributes to the development of type 2 diabetes. Why? Fat cells don't just store calories; they also secrete stuff, including pro-inflammatory proteins such as cytokines, leptin, adiponectin, and resistin—the last of which is especially concentrated in belly fat. These proteins, too, can impair insulin signaling.

Of course, genetics plays a role in developing type 2 diabetes as well—but not as large a role as you'd expect. If you have two parents with the disease, your chance of developing it by age fifty, says Kahn, is "something like ten times that in the general population." But if through lifestyle interventions you can maintain a normal body weight, he says, "you can lower your risk to the same as the general population—about 5 percent or so." Indeed, the genes for type 2 diabetes are very common—most of us have some, says Kahn.

Excess insulin on its own is bad enough for our health. But couple it with excess glucocorticoids and you've got a particularly lethal brew. While glucocorticoids heighten "wanting," says Mary Dallman, the excess insulin in the bloodstream during stress determines *liking*—that is, which foods are most enticing. Insulin, it turns out, shapes the drive for fat.

To prove this, Dallman and her colleagues took rats that had been rendered both diabetic (without insulin) and without glucocorticoids (their adrenal glands had been removed) and infused them with synthetic glucocorticoids. As expected, the rats' appetites increased and they ate more standard rat chow. But when they gave the same rats doses of insulin along with the glucocorticoids, those rats passed up the chow and dug into available lard; indeed, the amount of lard the rats ate was directly proportional to the level of insulin in their bloodstream.

Perhaps even more concerning, when Dallman dissected other rats sans adrenals, she found that in the presence of high synthetic glucocorticoids and high insulin, fat stored in peripheral sites in the rats' bodies—say, their thighs—left its home base and migrated to the abdomen, the worst place for it to be.

The converse is true, too: Researchers led by Nir Barzilai, M.D., at the Albert Einstein College of Medicine, found that when they removed the belly fat of five-month-old rats, insulin's ability to open cell doors shot up, insulin levels in the blood dramatically decreased, and the rats lived longer.

Intra-abdominal fat cells, scientists have learned, have more glucocorticoid and insulin receptors than peripheral fat cells do, which means that when we're stressed, we pack on more fat precisely where it hurts us most. Here's an additional way that belly-bulking happens: Another job of glucocorticoids is to activate the enzymes in fat cells that enable the

storage of fat after a stressor is over. The more receptors, the more glucocorticoid and insulin activity; the more glucocorticoid and insulin activity, the more active the fat-packing enzyme will be and the more doors
that will be opened for the circulating fat to find its way inside the cell.

Belly fat has another, more insidious role: It provides a feedback signal to the brain to inhibit catecholamines in the brain stem and CRH
from the hypothalamus. The reduction of CRH cuts down on the release of ACTH from the pituitary, which then cuts down on the release
of glucocorticoids from the adrenals. *Ahhh. Calm.* Activity in both the
sympathetic-adrenal-medullary and the HPA axes has been dampened—
all because of that spare tire in and of itself, even without food in the
picture.

"Belly fat reduces the stress output," says Dallman bluntly. "It's very
tough to break the cycle. Plus my recent realization is that habit has got
be hugely important to all this. What's also driving you to eat comfort
foods is the memory that you felt better the last time."

Stress = Belly Fat: The Reason Y?

Zofia Zukowska, M.D., Ph.D., gets so excited talking about stress and
diet and fat in the belly that you swear she's going to hurtle through
the phone from her lab in Washington, D.C., and land at your feet.
Zukowska is chair of Georgetown University's Department of Physiology
and Biophysics, and with her colleagues there she's been studying how
one small peptide may be driving comfort food straight to our bellies.

A peptide is similar to a protein, but it's smaller; both are made up of
chains of amino acids, yet peptides have only fifty amino acids or fewer
(a typical protein contains about four hundred). Zukowska's passion is
a peptide dubbed neuropeptide Y (NPY), whose release is triggered by
the activation of the sympathetic nervous system and by glucocorticoids
during prolonged or intense stress.

Discovered in the 1970s, NPY stimulates appetite and decreases anxiety when released in the brain. Recent research has shown that it's released from the nerve endings of the sympathetic nervous system shortly after the norepinephrine of fight-or-flight fame squirts out, and it makes its way into the body, including blood vessels and fat tissue. One of NPY's jobs in the body is to continue and enhance the blood-vessel constriction that norepinephrine starts, so if we're injured as we flee, we won't bleed to death. "I compare the action of norepinephrine to starting a fire with twigs, and NPY is adding the logs and keeping the fire going," says Zukowska.

Keeping the fire going is a good thing—in the short term. But Zukowska's team has shown that if NPY is around for too long, it causes the cells forming the smooth muscle of blood vessels to thicken. "This is exactly what can lead to hypertension," she says. "It's like a cuff around the tube; it can even completely close the vessel when it contracts." NPY, secreted during stress, can also stimulate inflammation in the vessel wall, accelerating the formation of plaques.

Over a period of four years, Lydia Kuo, an M.D./Ph.D., candidate in Zukowska's lab, and other researchers ran a series of experiments with mice to learn how NPY and certain of its receptors on fat cells (Y2Rs) interact to bulk up belly fat and lead endothelial cells—which form the slippery, innermost lining of blood vessels—to proliferate.

In one experiment the scientists injected NPY directly into the intra-abdominal fat of mice and watched their bellies bloom. In another, using mice engineered to be massively obese, they injected a nontoxic chemical that blocks NPY receptors to see if they could "melt the fat." Indeed, the fat disappeared. It was like liposuction without the vacuum. Should these actions translate to humans, NPY and Y2R blockers could be every woman's dream: a nonsurgical way to add fat to plump up wrinkles and to remove fat in chunky areas.

Moreover, the Y2R blocker also reduced fat in the animals' livers, and helped control insulin resistance, blood pressure, inflammation in blood vessels, and glucose intolerance.

The researchers went on to stress mice directly and intensely, trying to mimic the kinds of stress people experience. They stood them in a puddle of cold water daily for an hour for at least two weeks, "simulating what we experience when we stand in winter slush waiting for a late bus," says Zukowska. Or they would let an aggressor mouse have at them for ten minutes, "inducing a surprise encounter with an angry boss." Broken into groups, the mice ate either standard chow or sweet, fatty comfort food—the latter a sure glucocorticoid booster. Within just two weeks, NPY levels in the belly fat of the junk-food junkies soared, as did the number of NPY receptors. The belly fat itself increased by 50 percent—twice as much as the researchers had anticipated, given the number of calories their charges were downing. After three months, the stressed junk-food eaters had the mouse equivalent of metabolic syndrome, exhibiting these symptoms: abdominal obesity, inflammation, excess insulin, glucose intolerance, hypertension, and fat in their livers and muscles. "Their whole system just exploded," says Zukowska. Meanwhile, the junk-food eaters that were not stressed and the chow-eaters that were stressed pretty much maintained the status quo.

"The high-fat diet by itself increases glucocorticoids," explains Zukowska. "If you add stress, you not only get more glucocorticoids on top of those stimulated by the high-fat diet, but you get them in the wrong place." That is, you get excess glucocorticoids in the fat itself—specifically, the intra-abdominal fat. Once there, the glucocorticoids, as already noted, activate the enzymes that allow even *more* fat to be packed in.

To learn how this happens, Zukowska's team stuck NPY in a petri dish with the cells that give rise to fat cells, called fat precursor cells or preadipocytes, and the endothelial cells that line blood vessels. The NPY triggered both types of cells to proliferate and the preadipocytes to mature into actual fat cells capable of storing fatty acids. Voilà: more fat cells in the belly and more vessels formed from existing ones to provide them with nourishing blood.

Zukowska's lab has also found that NPY from human fat operates similarly to that in rats. "My collaborator, Steve Baker, from plastic surgery, would give me all kinds of fat," Zukowska says enthusiastically. "Buckets!" They put the fat into mice engineered not to reject transplants. "When we had NPY on board, that fat nicely grew and stayed there," she says. "So we know that NPY in humans can work in the same way as stress-induced NPY worked in mice."

NPY, Zukowska believes, could be used as a diagnostic marker in the future, with high levels indicating the person was at risk for metabolic syndrome even before symptoms appeared.

Belly Fat and Cellular Aging

At UCSF, Ramin Farzaneh-Far, with the team of Mary Whooley, have uncovered what may be the strongest incentive yet to unpack that belly fat and keep it off. "Abdominal fat," he says, "is accelerating cellular aging."

Farzaneh-Far and colleagues were the first to show that folks who are fat in the belly actually have shorter telomeres. The findings sprang from a large trial of Whooley's called the Heart and Soul Study, one of the few longitudinal studies looking at risk factors for telomere attrition, mentioned in Chapter 2.

In this study, Farzaneh-Far's team measured the leukocyte telomere lengths of 608 outpatients with stable coronary artery disease when the patients joined up (between 2000 and 2002), and again five years later. At five years out, the average age of the participants was sixty-five, and 80 percent were male. The scientists also measured body mass index to assess whole-body obesity and abdominal obesity, using the waist-hip ratio (WHR).

What they found was astonishing: BMI was "not related at all" to telomere length, says Farzaneh-Far, but WHR absolutely was. "The people who were more abdominally obese had more telomere shortening, after adjusting for everything," he says. "Which says that *only* abdominal obesity—not total body obesity—is an independent cause of accelerated cellular aging."

The mechanism, he says, might be a combination of oxidative stress and inflammation, but the bottom line matters most: The accumulation of belly fat during chronic stress could be cutting our days short.

Eating to Manage Stress

Given those physiological realities, what can we do?

Are there diets or particular foods that are simultaneously good for us *and* counteract the effects of stress, permitting us to slow down the aging process as we soothe our souls? Can we put the kibosh on those stress-induced cravings for sweet and fatty foods? And what about the *way* we eat: on the run, mindfully, counting calories and/or carbs? Does that alter our stress-aging profile?

The answer to all those questions is an enthusiastic yes. Here's a look at how to eat to dampen the stress that drives our aging all the way down to the telomeres inside our cells.

The Stress of Dieting Itself

A. Janet Tomiyama is just twenty-nine, but she has the clear, steady voice and refined gestures of a seasoned speaker as she clicks through her slides at the July 2009 ISPNE Conference. As part of her thesis for her Ph.D. in social and health psychology from UCLA, Tomiyama has been studying why dieting fails over the long term. She's come up with a straightforward answer: Dieting is not just psychologically but *biologically* stressful.

For the study she's presenting on this chilly summer day, Tomiyama and her team divided 121 young women into four groups to see how the main components of dieting—tracking and restricting calories—affected stress levels. For three weeks each group either restricted calories to twelve hundred a day and diligently tracked them, just tracked them without restricting them, just restricted them (this group got prepared meals of twelve hundred calories daily), or neither tracked nor restricted them (the control group). The women assessed their stress levels with the Cohen Perceived Stress Scale (see Chapter 2) and had their saliva tested for cortisol levels.

The result? Those tracking calories increased their levels of perceived stress, but only those actually *restricting* calories raised their cortisol levels. The very process of restricting what they ate kicked the stress response into gear. Why might that be? "It could be that the restrictors needed more glucose," says Tomiyama.

Recall that cortisol's primary function is to ensure that there's enough glucose available in the bloodstream during a stressor, which it does by releasing stored energy from the liver and muscles. If we're eating what our bodies demand, we're providing glucose from the outside. But if we cut down on calories, we cut down on that external supply. So cortisol may kick in to release the stored glucose, leaving us hungrier than ever.

Tomiyama's work backs up the epidemiological studies showing that folks trying to diet are significantly more likely than nondieters to eat when stressed—and to choose high-fat/high-sugar foods when they do. One study reported that an alarming 71 percent of dieters ate more when stressed. Psychological factors, of course, play a part, too: We may reach for the cookies as a way to be nice to ourselves during a rough time or even as an act of defiance. The end result? Weight gain rather than weight loss.

The stress from chronically struggling with dieting may eat away at our telomeres, too, aging our cells. A UCSF team led by Amy K. Kiefer, Ph.D., and Elissa Epel looked at thirty-six premenopausal women ages twenty to fifty, and twenty postmenopausal women ages fifty-three to sixty-nine. All were perpetual dieters but not participating in a controlled program such as, say, Weight Watchers. The scientists assessed leukocyte telomere length with a simple blood test, and dieting attempts with a standard eating-behavior questionnaire. In both groups of women, the more rigid the dieting attempts, the shorter the telomere length, regardless of age, BMI, and smoking.

"Dietary restraint," the authors note in their 2009 paper, may relate to "accelerated aging of the immune system." Wildly fluctuating glucose and insulin levels from skipped meals and compensatory overeating, they speculate, may be a direct cause.

How Can We Eat to Reduce Stress?

We struggle to limit our eating so we can be healthy and live longer, and it turns out that all that rigorous effort may actually be aging us—down to our cells. Are there *any* diet approaches out there that have the opposite effect?

Regain control, not pounds

Numerous studies and reviews spanning decades compare types of diets—low carbohydrate, low fat, high protein, and various permutations of these macronutrients—to see which are best for health and weight loss. I've synthesized their results, and here's the bottom line:

What matters most is *not* the mix of macronutrients but that you *cut calories* so that output (what you burn) exceeds input (what you eat) in a way that is sustainable for you.

That means finding a way to eat that reduces, rather than exacerbates, stress by putting *you*—not a self-appointed diet guru or some rigid program—in control of your food choices and eating habits. The new Healthy Eating Pyramid, developed by Walter C. Willett, M.D., and colleagues at the Harvard School of Public Health (HSPH), is the best guide yet to doing that.

Based on forty years of research at Harvard and around the globe, the new Healthy Eating Pyramid is, notes Willett, "not actually a diet" but a distillation of broad, healthful *choices*—just what the doctors (stress ones, that is) ordered for reducing stress. It suggests a total way of eating—not a list of dos and don'ts regarding particular foods—that nixes nothing completely except those dastardly trans fats.

"I like to believe that our Healthy Eating Pyramid way of eating will bring enjoyment along with health in a way that is stress reducing and empowering," Willett tells me in an e-mail. "It will provide a good metabolic and physiological state, and lead to lower risks of heart disease and type 2 diabetes—stress-reducing factors in themselves."

Willett points to a study led by David S. Ludwig, M.D., Ph.D., of

THE HEALTHY EATING PYRAMID

Department of Nutrition, Harvard School of Public Health

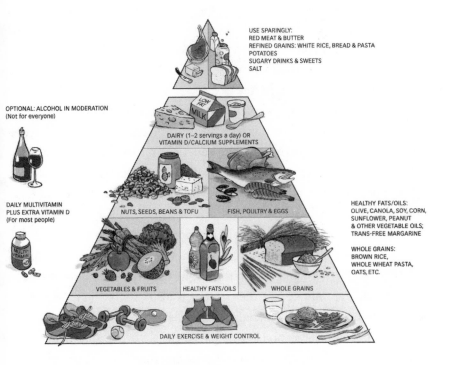

USE SPARINGLY:
RED MEAT & BUTTER
REFINED GRAINS: WHITE RICE, BREAD & PASTA
POTATOES
SUGARY DRINKS & SWEETS
SALT

OPTIONAL: ALCOHOL IN MODERATION
(Not for everyone)

DAIRY (1–2 servings a day) OR
VITAMIN D/CALCIUM SUPPLEMENTS

DAILY MULTIVITAMIN
PLUS EXTRA VITAMIN D
(For most people)

NUTS, SEEDS, BEANS & TOFU   FISH, POULTRY & EGGS

HEALTHY FATS/OILS:
OLIVE, CANOLA, SOY, CORN,
SUNFLOWER, PEANUT
& OTHER VEGETABLE OILS;
TRANS-FREE MARGARINE

WHOLE GRAINS:
BROWN RICE,
WHOLE WHEAT PASTA,
OATS, ETC.

VEGETABLES & FRUITS   HEALTHY FATS/OILS   WHOLE GRAINS

DAILY EXERCISE & WEIGHT CONTROL

For more information about the Healthy Eating Pyramid:

WWW.THE NUTRITION SOURCE.ORG

Eat, Drink, and Be Healthy
by Walter C. Willett, M.D. and Patrick J. Skerrett (2005)
Free Press/Simon & Schuster Inc.

Figure 4. Stress less over diet: The pyramid doesn't prescribe specific amounts of food to eat, but instead relies on this simple guideline: Ground your approach in daily exercise and weight control, and choose more foods from the base of the pyramid than from the higher levels. Mix up a blend of fresh, whole foods from all the categories listed below the "Use Sparingly" tip, and you'll get the nutrients you need while putting control back in your own hands.

Children's Hospital Boston, showing that high-carbohydrate diets, in particular, induce stress responses. The researchers measured food intake using glycemic index (GI)—a ranking of carbohydrates on a scale from one to one hundred based on how much each carb raises blood-sugar levels after it's eaten. Carbs that are rapidly digested, converted into glucose, and absorbed into the muscles and liver, such as refined grain products and potatoes, have a high GI. Those that break down and release glucose slowly, in a sustained way—such as fruits and veggies—have a low GI. In general, low is better.*

On three occasions, Ludwig and his colleagues fed twelve obese teenage boys breakfast and lunch with either a low, medium, or high GI. After breakfast they took blood to measure various hormones and energy indicators, including epinephrine (of fight-or-flight), insulin, glucose, and fatty acids. For five hours after lunch, the boys had access to platters of food loaded with bread, bagels, cold cuts, cream cheese, cookies, and fruit.

Not only did the boys gobble up more goodies after the high-GI meals, but their epinephrine levels had shot up, no doubt in an effort to counterbalance the rapid absorption of glucose from the high-GI foods.

One of the most recent diet studies is also one of the most telling regarding the best way to manage what we eat, because of its long duration (two years), large number of participants (811), and diversity of diet types (four diets, each with different emphases on fat, protein, and carbs). Led by Frank M. Sacks, M.D., of HSPH, the study appeared in 2009 in the *New England Journal of Medicine*. It is also the study in which Debbie Meyer—the night eater who introduces this chapter—lost fifty-one pounds from her five-foot-plus frame three years before we spoke, dropping from 179 to 128 pounds. And despite her continuing yet fewer forays to the kitchen—which drove her into the study in the first place—she's maintained a svelte 133.

All the diets followed heart-healthy principles, replacing saturated fat with unsaturated fat, and were high in whole grains, fruits, and veg-

---

* For a full list of foods' GI levels, visit www.ajcn.org/cgi/content/full/76/1/5; for a searchable database of GI visit www.glycemicindex.com.

gies and low in cholesterol—just as Willett's Healthy Eating Pyramid is. Participants were encouraged to cut 750 calories a day from their regular diet, though not to go below twelve hundred calories, to exercise moderately for ninety minutes a week, to keep a food diary, and to attend individual and group counseling sessions.

All four groups showed similar losses in weight and waist size: An average of thirteen pounds after six months, a bit of regain by the end of the year, and a final loss of an average of nine pounds after two years. Waists shrank an average of two inches. Even the regain was modest: about 20 percent of the average in previous diet studies. Heart-disease risk markers changed, too: Good cholesterol (HDL) rose and bad cholesterol (LDL),* triglycerides, blood pressure, and insulin dropped. Interestingly, the participants who attended the most counseling sessions lost the most weight: an average of twenty-two pounds.

CALMM the fat away

Creating a sustainable eating plan is one way to reduce stress and therefore slow aging. But Elissa Epel and her team wanted to find an approach that put something besides food at its core.

Enter CALMM (Craving and Lifestyle Management through Mindfulness), led by Jennifer J. Daubenmier, Ph.D., assistant professor at UCSF's Osher Center for Integrative Medicine. CALMM is not a diet but a stress-reduction program that concentrates on mindful eating, yoga, and meditation to reverse the packing on of belly fat and the aging processes it sparks. Its pilot trial, presented at the 2008 American Psychosomatic Society conference, did just that.

The scientists broke forty-seven overweight and obese women into

---

* Cholesterol is a lipid, a fatty substance found in our cell membranes and blood that's manufactured and removed from the blood stream by the liver; it also comes from the food we eat. HDL, or high-density lipoprotein, is mostly protein with little cholesterol. It removes cholesterol particles from the cells and shunts them back to the liver to be recycled. LDL, or low-density lipoprotein, comprises a moderate amount of protein with lots of cholesterol that's just waiting to attach to an artery wall and contribute to an atherosclerotic plaque.

two groups: Half spent four months in the CALMM stress-reduction program; half did not (the controls). The program included meditation CDs, gentle yoga classes, and mindfulness-based eating strategies such as "surfing the urge"—pausing before, say, grabbing that chocolate—to analyze your motivation (is it impulse? real desire? habit? boredom?) and permit the sensation to pass. These strategies also included concentrating attention on the texture, shape, flavor, and smell of every bite.

Among other measures, the researchers assessed the participants' body fat before, during, and after the intervention, noting the amount of fat in their bellies and thighs, their morning cortisol levels, and their levels of perceived stress. At the end, they found that the more the women practiced the mindful techniques, the greater the shift of fat away from their bellies, the lower the rise in morning cortisol, and the greater their weight loss—even though no one was actually dieting.

The results were the opposite of Tomiyama's, which showed that restricting calories through dieting was biologically stressful.

"Many weight-loss programs provide a one-size-fits-all prescription of what foods to eat or avoid," says Daubenmier. "While this type of 'outer wisdom' information can be valuable, people can also learn to pay attention to 'inner wisdom,' that is, the body's signals that tell us when to start and stop eating, and what foods we truly enjoy and can eat without guilt in moderate amounts. By slowing down and paying attention to the actual experience of eating, people can gain insight into their eating patterns and discover new ways of relating to food."

What Can We Eat to Reduce Stress, for the Long Term and Slow Aging?

As Mary Dallman's studies with mice have taught us, sweet, fatty foods do, initially, dampen the stress response. But in the long term they send us into a dreadful frenzied spiral: increased belly fat; greater sensitivity to stress; higher cortisol; more guzzling of chips, fries, ice cream; even *more* belly fat; and on and on.

And as our guts expand, our health deteriorates, our hair grays, and our skin sags off our bones.

Has research uncovered any *healthful* comfort foods—foods that will reduce stress *and* slow aging? Or is "healthful comfort food," in fact, an oxymoron?

The stress and telomere experts are just starting to investigate the nutrients that influence that place where stress and aging meet. And UCSF's Ramin Farzaneh-Far is at the forefront.

In analyzing the telomere data from the Heart and Soul Study, Farzaneh-Far noted that about a quarter of his subjects actually showed telomere *lengthening* over the five years. Recall that Epel, too, found telomere lengthening in her cohort of elderly men, and the Bogalusa Heart Study found it in its midlife men and women. "We think that's a real biological phenomenon, that telomeres can lengthen in vivo," says Farzaneh-Far, referring to lengthening inside the body as opposed to in a petri dish (in vitro). But the young cardiologist wanted to push beyond the observation to the source: What was behind this lengthening? Could there be something that *reversed* the cellular aging that came with chronic stress?

Initially Farzaneh-Far thought the antidote might be a cardiac medication, such as a statin, given that all of his subjects had stable coronary-artery disease. So he did an exhaustive analysis of possible drivers, everything from vitamins and aspirin to education and physical activity. He was stunned by what he found: The only factor associated with telomere lengthening was the level of omega-3 fatty acids in the blood. "Omega-3 fatty acids are actually associated with telomeres' *lengthening*, not just with their not shortening," he says over the phone from San Francisco.

I put him on hold when I hear this so I can run upstairs and take a double dose of the fish oil.

Of course, numerous studies in both animals and humans have shown that omega-3 fatty acids, DHA (docosahexaenoic acid), and EPA (eicosapentaenoic acid)—found naturally in fatty fish such as salmon and sardines, and in supplements available everywhere—are important for normal cognitive function and brain plasticity, as well as cardiovascular health and inhibiting age-related macular degeneration. DHA, for example, is a crucial component of neuronal membranes, and since the human body is not great at synthesizing DHA, we need to get it from our diet. Other studies over the past decade have linked deficiencies of omega-3 fatty acids with clinical depression and everyday despair. But no one has ever linked omega-3 fatty acid deficiencies to cellular aging—from chronic stress or any other source—let alone suggested that these fatty acids might reverse such aging. Until now.

"It's very preliminary, but it's exciting because it suggests there may be a way you can manipulate cellular aging with simple supplements," says Farzaneh-Far.

Omega-3 fatty acids may not be the only nutrient that can make a difference regarding stress and telomere length.

In March 2009, scientists at the NIH's National Institute of Environmental Health Sciences released a cross-sectional epidemiological study showing that, on average, women who took daily multivitamins had longer telomeres than those who didn't.

Led by Qun Xu, Ph.D., the researchers analyzed leukocyte telomere length in blood samples from 586 healthy women ages thirty-five to seventy-four and crunched the numbers on 146-item questionnaires about diet. Telomeres on average were 5.1 percent longer in those who took daily multivitamins compared to those who did not. Higher intake of antioxidant vitamins C and E from food was also associated with longer telomeres, even after adjusting for multivitamin use.

Could it be that those who take multivitamins just have healthier lifestyles all around, and that the results might be reflecting that? The authors addressed that possibility, taking extra caution in their analyses by adjusting for factors that could affect telomere length, such as age, smoking status, BMI, socioeconomic status, and lifestyle choices. The results remained the same: A multivitamin a day may help keep cellular aging at bay.

Food, Glorious Food

Taking multivitamins is a smart way to help alleviate the ravaging effects of stress. But as Walter Willett explains in *Eat, Drink, and Be Healthy*, his best-selling book based on HSPH's Healthy Eating Pyramid, multivitamins are "insurance," not a replacement for getting nutrients the natural way.

"A multivitamin can't in any way replace healthy eating," he writes. "It gives you barely a scintilla of the vast array of healthful nutrients found in food. It doesn't deliver any fiber . . . The only thing it can do is offer a nutritional backup or fill in the nutrient holes that can plague even the most conscientious eaters."

The implication: Eye with caution any diet that advocates numerous supplements as the "answer."

Obviously, we cannot live—or extend our lives—by supplements alone, as exciting as the Omega-3 and multivitamin findings may be. Which raises the question: Are there any healthful *whole* foods that science has shown can dampen our stress response and thus slow aging?

One food that some self-help books and Web sites hawk turns out to be more legend than fact. We've all heard about turkey and tryptophan—an amino acid that's a precursor to the neurotransmitter serotonin and rumored to make you drowsy. Our bodies can't synthesize tryptophan, so it must come from the proteins we eat. The last time I plugged *turkey* and *tryptophan* and *calm* into Google, I got 17,500 hits. But science has given the lie to that tale. Our drowsiness after the Thanksgiving feast doesn't come from tryptophan. Rather, it comes from the rush and subsequent crash of glucose after the meal, our body's focus on digestion, and the activation of the parasympathetic nervous system, which slows other systems down to promote growth and energy storage. The claim that carbohydrates kick off serotonin release itself, and therefore calm us down, doesn't fare any better under scientific scrutiny.

While scientifically sound research on healthful antistress foods is alarmingly slim, there's a virtual (in all senses of the word) library of material on "brain foods"—foods associated with improving cognition as we age, partly through influencing signaling between brain cells. These foods are rich in everything from vitamins B, D, and E to choline and antioxidants. Might there be a revolutionary place where antistress and antiaging foods meet?

Two areas of research come close: that of scientists investigating pistachios at Pennsylvania State University, and that of teams in the United States and abroad burrowing past the all-too-familiar territory of oxidation and antioxidants to the land of hormesis.

The Nutty Professor

Penn State's Sarah K. Gebauer, Ph.D., is fascinated by pistachios. As a postdoc in the lab of Sheila G. West, Ph.D., Gebauer had seen plenty of evidence regarding how stress and diet affect vascular function—in particular, the innermost, slippery lining of our blood vessels known as the vascular endothelium. But most of the diet experiments in the lab focused on nuts at the top of the chain: walnuts and almonds, for instance. Gebauer wanted to look at a nut less traveled: pistachios—the nut with the highest level of plant sterols, compounds that have been shown to significantly reduce "bad" cholesterol (LDL). So she designed and ran a vigilantly controlled eighteen-week soup-to-nuts trial on diet for her dissertation.

"Each nut has a unique nutrient profile," says Gebauer. "Pistachios are low in saturated fat and rich in mono- and polyunsaturated fats, the good fats. They're also rich in numerous vitamins and minerals, and contain more lutein, beta-carotene, and gamma-tocopherol than other nuts." The latter two are precursors to antioxidant vitamins A and E, respectively.

As Chapter 1 explains, chronic stress can lead to lesions in the blood-vessel walls—sticky sites that act like magnets for immune cells, platelets, and fats. Gobs of these gather to form atherosclerotic plaques, which narrow and harden our arteries and put us at higher risk for hypertension and other cardiovascular diseases. West's lab had made its name showing that diet could alter the force with which blood surged through those vessels during stress and thus increase or lower the risk for disease. Foods high in saturated fat, for instance, pumped up the heart's output, intensifying the risk of lesions; those high in unsaturated fats did the opposite.

For her study, Gebauer took ten men and eighteen women ages thirty to seventy and fed them four different diets:

- A typical American diet, relatively high in saturated fat (for base-line measurements of factors such as cholesterol and inflammatory markers)
- A standard healthy diet with 25 percent total fat and 8 percent saturated fat
- A diet with 30 percent total fat and 8 percent saturated fat that included 1.5 ounces of pistachios
- A diet with 34 percent total fat and 8 percent saturated fat that included 3 ounces of pistachios

The twenty-eight subjects ate the pistachios in various forms: roasted, salted and roasted, unsalted, by the handful as snacks, and in recipes such as pistachio muffins, granola, and pesto.

The researchers weighed the participants every day and made adjustments in their portions if they showed any added or lost pounds. "We wanted to be sure the effects were due to the pistachios and not weight loss," says Gebauer.

They then subjected them to two stressors: mental stress, in the form of a math test; and physical stress, in the form of plunging a subject's foot into ice water for 2.5 minutes. During each stressor the researchers measured participants' blood pressure and how resistant their blood vessels were to blood flow, an indicator of vessel elasticity. Finally, they compared those results to the participants' blood pressure and blood-vessel resistance at rest.

The numbers don't lie: Pistachios reduced the vascular stress response.

During both pistachio diets, blood pressure dropped, and LDL fell in a dose-dependent manner (12 percent with the 3-ounce dose and 9 percent with the 1.5-ounce dose). "So we were able to see that the results were directly due to the amount of pistachios in the diet," says Gebauer.

Triglycerides dropped, too, with the higher dose, compared to the standard healthy diet. And on both pistachio diets, IL-1, a marker of inflammation and thus of heart-disease risk, dropped by 15 percent compared to the fatty American diet.

Interestingly, the lower pistachio dose lowered blood pressure more than the higher-pistachio dose, which sounds counterintuitive but in fact is not. Given pistachios' ability to relax blood vessels, the larger dose sent the vessels fairly swooning (a good thing in the long term), which made the heart rate drop. To compensate and maintain equilibrium for the moment, the heart pumped harder to protect against the blood pressure's plunging. "This pattern of change would be beneficial if it is maintained in the long term," West said when the results came out. "It is possible that other foods that are high in unsaturated fat and antioxidants would have a similar effect."

Cellular Resistance Training

Remember the concept of hormesis, from the introduction? We discussed how challenges to the system, or "stressors," in small doses, can actually benefit us, while in large doses they can do us in. Certain foods, it turns out, have hormetic properties as well—possibly helping to slow the aging process.

When cells are hit with mild, intermittent stressors—chemicals, temperature, radiation, exercise, and so on—they emit various molecules to protect themselves. The cells are rattled but then regroup, facing their enemies with even stronger defenses. As I phrased it earlier, metaphorically, they thicken their skins. The molecules emitted include heat-shock proteins (also called stress proteins), growth factors such as insulin-like growth factor and brain-derived neurotrophic factor, and antioxidant enzymes such as superoxide dismutases (SOD). Mind you, the last are not antioxidants; they're the enzymes that kick natural, internal antioxidants into action. The cell may become resistant not just to the particular stressor that raised its hackles, but to any number of stressors. Hormesis may partly explain why mild stressors such as exercise (see Chapter 5) and caloric restriction* have not just one but a myriad of health benefits

"The definition of hormesis is that if we deliberately challenge—or stress—the system, it will try to match it up, and as a result, there is an overshoot in the defense mechanism and you get beneficial effects," says Aarhus University's Suresh Rattan, Ph.D., D.Sc., an exuberant man with a full belly laugh who spends his days feeding various types of cells nutritional hormetics to witness hormesis in action. Among the compounds he's found to elicit the effects are curcumin (turmeric is the active compound), ginger, garlic, onion, and zinc.

For years we've been reading about the antioxidant properties of brightly colored fruits and vegetables—blueberries, Concord grapes, broccoli, spinach, you know the drill. Plants, the antioxidant story goes, are rich in phytochemicals—substances they manufacture to cope with environmental challenges such as solar radiation, pests, and infectious agents. These protective molecules contribute to the plants' color, flavor, smell, and texture. Scientists, and the mass media on their coattails, have been falling all over themselves singing the praises of these phytochemicals' antioxidant properties—that is, their ability to neutralize those nasty electron-scavenging free radicals resulting from normal metabolism that damage cells in their quest to balance out their orbits.

But the latest research by scientists such as Rattan, Mark P. Mattson, Ph.D., at the National Institute on Aging, and Robert Krikorian, Ph.D.,

* In numerous studies, caloric restriction—reducing caloric intake by 30 to 40 percent while maintaining proper nutrition—has been shown to extend life span in animals ranging from rats and mice to dogs and, just a year ago, rhesus monkeys. It's also been shown to delay diseases of aging such as cancer, cardiovascular disease, brain atrophy, and type 2 diabetes.

at the University of Cincinnati, suggests that something else entirely—something stress related, in fact—is what gives fruits and veggies their antiaging punch.

The quantity of antioxidants we consume in fruits and vegetables is just not enough to make a difference, say hormesis proponents. And so the benefits of phytochemicals come not from their ability to neutralize reactive oxygen species (ROS, a form of free radical) but from their ability to kick hormesis into gear. "[I]t is unclear, and in most cases unlikely, that humans ingest the fruits and vegetables that contain these phytochemicals in amounts sufficient to achieve the high . . . concentrations of the phytochemicals required to scavenge free radicals," writes Mattson in a 2008 review paper in *Aging Research Reviews*.

Hormesis requires not mass quantities of those foods to achieve antiaging benefits, but human-size portions. Moreover, hormesis acts as a prophylactic, preventing aging rather than attempting to treat it. If the nomenclature catches up with the science, perhaps someday we'll be calling such foods hormetics (Rattan's word) rather than antioxidants.

Large epidemiological studies on foods touted as antioxidants have shown that people who eat mounds of berries, spinach, and broccoli—or take supplements such as vitamin E—have less heart disease, and that these foods are associated with a reduced risk for cancer, inflammatory diseases, and cognitive disorders such as Alzheimer's and Parkinson's.

And clinical trials with rats have backed up those observations: Many studies have shown that rats fed such diets—of spinach, spirulina, and blueberries, for example—improve their memories and even reverse brain impairment. A particularly striking study led by University of South Florida's Paula Bickford found that rats fed a formulation of blueberries, green tea, carnosine, amino acid, and vitamin D for two weeks before a surgical stroke (yes, she zapped their brains) had 75 percent less brain damage than the animals not eating the formula pre-stroke.

But when the research moved up the evolutionary ladder—both scientifically and species-wise—to randomized human trials using supplements, the positive associations dwindled. In fact, two large trials of smokers and/or workers exposed to asbestos resulted in a slight *increased* risk of lung cancer among those taking beta-carotene supplements for four to eight years.

"The problem is, it gets harder as you go from animal models to humans and then to clinical trials; the evidence gets weaker and weaker," says the Joslin Diabetes Center's C. Ronald Kahn. Indeed, the participants in almost all epidemiological studies looking at so-called antioxidants have other healthful behaviors, too. "And in the clinical trials that have been done, it's not clear about the dosages or whether there were enough events to see an effect," says Kahn.

Many scientists blame the discrepancies on comparing whole foods to supplements; the synergistic effect of antioxidant activity, other nutrients, and fiber in whole foods gets lost, they say. And indeed, various studies have found that eating whole-food fruits and nuts—tart cherry juice, cactus pear, almonds, mixed-berry juice, among others—does lower markers for oxidative stress in adults.

But they haven't gone the additional step: showing that foods labeled "antioxidants" have the ability to improve cognitive function in humans. That may be, say those on the cutting edge, because the biochemical action making the antiaging difference is hormesis.

"Antioxidant effects of phytochemicals may be just the tip of the iceberg," says Krikorian. "There may be other benefits that are more potent. The basic neuroscience studies have shown antioxidant effects of berry fruits and other vegetables and fruits but also anti-inflammatory effects, direct effects on neuronal signaling—the talk between neurons—particularly in areas of the brain that mediate memory function. Cellular studies have shown that the presence of anthocyanins, phytochemicals that give some fruits their red or purple color, improves resistance of neurons to different sorts of stressors like toxins and radiation. But there's another category of potential benefit that may underlie all this stuff that may be more fundamental than anything else: hormetic effects—that is, a low dose of a toxin that the body responds to in a beneficial way or in multiple beneficial ways."

Among the hormetic phytochemicals scientists have found are: ferulic acid, or FA (in sweet corn and tomatoes); epigallocatechin-3-gallate, or EGCG (in green tea); phenethyl isothiocyanate, or PEITC (in Chinese cabbage, turnips, rutabagas, watercress, and radishes); res-everatrol (in red grapes and wine); and polyphenolic compounds, most prominently anthocyanins (in blueberries, strawberries, and spinach), curcumin (in turmeric), sulforaphane (in broccoli and other cruciferous vegetables), and flavonoid polyphenols (in Concord grapes).

Indeed, Ying Xu, M.D., Ph.D., at the University of Florida, Gainesville, and colleagues found curcumin to reverse hippocampal damage in chronically stressed rats—in a way that was similar to the tricyclic antidepressant imipramine. The curcumin also prevented a typical stress-induced decrease in serotonin and brain-derived neurotrophic factor—brain molecules involved in hippocampal neurogenesis.

Why does it matter whether the hero here is antioxidants or hormesis, as long as we eat our greens (and reds and blues)? Because knowing *what* our food does inside us to slow and perhaps even reverse the aging of our brain and other cells may be just the push we need to grab that glass of Concord grape juice instead of water, orange juice, or soda to quench our thirst.

When I started researching this book, in 2007, I could find *no* randomized clinical trials with people showing that eating fruits and veggies improves cognitive ability—regardless of whether it was antioxidant action or hormesis that was bringing about the effect. There were human clinical studies linking Concord grape juice with lowered inflammation and blood pressure, and plenty of evidence that rats' memories improved after eating a variety of berries (they were better at finding their way out of mazes). But with no evidence in people, even rooms full of scientists at aging conferences weren't reaching for the fruits—except for the ones putting the rodents through the mazes in the first place.

Now, three years later, I've unearthed just two small preliminary studies, very likely the first randomized controlled trials in older people—those most likely to suffer from memory problems—that examine the benefits of Concord grape and wild blueberry juices on cognition.

Robert Krikorian and his team recruited twelve healthy adults ages sixty-eight to seventy-two with "mild memory decline," that is, very early memory changes such as forgetfulness. They randomized the participants into three groups: For twelve weeks, five of the subjects drank Concord grape juice, seven drank a placebo drink (the controls), and nine drank wild blueberry juice. Neither subjects nor researchers knew who got the grape juice or placebo (a double-blind controlled model, the gold standard), but the researchers did know who got the blueberry juice (a single-blind controlled model). (Don't try to add these numbers—it will stress you out! The researchers were short on funding, and so conducted both studies simultaneously, using the same subjects.) Before and after the trial, all the subjects took neuropsychiatric tests to assess their memory and mood. The subjects drank between fifteen and twenty-one ounces of their drink a day, based on weight.

At the end of the trial, those drinking both the wild blueberry juice and the Concord grape juice had significantly improved their memories compared to the controls. The folks downing the blueberry juice improved their performance by a whopping 45 percent compared to those drinking the placebo. And those drinking the Concord grape juice showed a 41 percent improvement in their performance compared to before the intervention.

"These were preliminary studies just to see if we could get a signal, so to speak—a positive indication—and that's what we got," says Krikorian.

Where do telomeres fit into all this? Since one mechanism behind telomere attrition may be oxidative stress (as described in Chapter 2), would increasing our intake of foods rich in antioxidants perhaps slow the cellular aging associated with chronic stress? The hormesis folks would say no, that it's unlikely we eat antioxidant-rich foods in quantities large enough to scavenge those pesky ROS. But then, hormesis-inducing foods may be just what we need.

As this book goes to press, there are no studies showing the effects of hormesis on telomere length. But Suresh Rattan may be getting close. He found that repeated mild heat shock to human skin fibroblasts, endothelial cells, and bone-marrow stem cells in a petri dish increased the replicative life span of the cells by 10 to 15 percent by boosting levels of emitted heat shock proteins and other cellular processes. That is, the cells were able to live, and thus divide, longer than cells not subjected to the mild stressor. When you recall that cell division is one way telomeres shorten, you can't help but wonder if hormesis-inducing foods might actually *slow* the rate at which our telomeres erode, thus increasing the life span of our cells.

As Rattan puts it on his Web site: "The long-term aim of these studies is to find effective hormetic treatments for delaying the onset and/or the prevention of age-related diseases related to replicative senescence, such as thinning of the skin, neurodegenerative diseases, immune deficiency, and muscle loss leading to sarcopenia."

Think of the trajectory this way: If chronic stress works to shorten the number of times our cells can divide—in other words, if it shortens their life span—eating foods that increase cells' replicative life span may counteract or even prevent that effect, putting our cells back at baseline. Even nondividing cells, such as mature brain cells, could benefit, given that their progenitor cells divide, too (see Chapter 3). Might such foods help our skin perk up and our immune systems revive? It certainly can't hurt to try.

Put that in your curcumin-spiced wild salmon and smoke it.

To Reduce Stress and Slow the Cellular Clock Using Diet

Eschew rigid diets and use Walter Willett's new Healthy Eating Pyramid as your guide to reducing belly fat.

There is no magic bullet for reducing belly fat, despite what outfits such as RealAge say in e-mails that promise "Foods That Fight Belly Fat." The notice I received in my own in-box, for instance, promising to trim my middle, referred to a 2008 study led by Maastricht University's Laura A. E. Hughes, M.D., showing that women who consumed more flavonoids (phytochemicals found in fruits, veggies, tea, seeds, herbs, spices, and whole grains, among other foods) had less of an increase in BMI over a fourteen-year period than those who didn't. This is good news; however, it relates to one's height-weight ratio, *not* waist-hip ratio, which is the measurement relevant to belly fat.

Instead of dieting, put yourself back in control of your eating by making your *own* choices based on the Pyramid, which avoids simple carbs and uses whole grain foods, plant oils (rich in unsaturated fats), fruits, veggies, and nuts as its base.

Try eating mindfully.

Indiana State University's Jean. L. Kristeller, Ph.D., cofounded an entire center to educate people about mindful eating.* The site includes everything from "Principles for Mindful Eating" to downloadable MP3s of presentations on topics such as "Unintentional Eating" and "Different Types of Hunger." With Kristeller's method, explains Elissa Epel, people first rate their level of hunger and fullness when they're ready to eat. Epel is describing strategies used in the CALMM study to shift away from the automatic eating so many of us do. "They then savor the food for part of the meal, which slows down eating in a manageable way, and increases enjoyment," she says. "You can't enjoy food—or notice how it's affecting your fullness—if you aren't aware that you're eating it! Even a few moments of being fully aware can change the quality—and the size!—of a meal."

A simple exercise to get you started: Jon Kabat-Zinn, Ph.D., founder of the Stress Reduction Clinic at the University of Massachusetts Medical Center, began his clinic sessions by asking clients to eat three raisins, one at a time, "mindfully, with awareness." I've adapted the exercise, which follows, from his influential book *Full Catastrophe Living*. You might roll your eyes at the start of the exercise, but stick with it. I know a woman who lost several inches in her belly by extending the raisin exercise to everything she ate.

* Access the Center for Mindful Eating at www.tcme.org.

Take your time. Allow the examination and eating of the raisins to take about ten minutes.

Pick up a single raisin, not your usual handful. Lay it in the center of your palm and look at it, as if you "had never seen one before," instructs Kabat-Zinn in *Full Catastrophe Living*. Roll it between your fingers. Smell it. Examine its folds and creases, hills and valleys. Become aware of any thoughts about raisins or food that come to mind. Now, with awareness, slowly bring it to your mouth, tracking the distance it travels and how its color and texture shift as it moves closer. Breathe deeply and slowly as you go through every motion, moment to moment. Notice how your salivary glands begin to secrete saliva as the raisin rises to your mouth. Open your mouth and place the raisin on your tongue. What does it feel like? What does it feel like after you close your lips? What does it taste like, just lying there? Roll it around on your tongue. What's your saliva doing now? When you feel ready, begin to chew it, slowly. Move the raisin around with your tongue to different teeth. How does its texture and taste change as you chew? Recognize how your throat begins to constrict as you become ready to swallow. Feel the raisin slide down your throat. "We even imagine, or 'sense,' that now our bodies are one raisin heavier," writes Kabat-Zinn.

"Since many of us use food for emotional comfort, especially when we feel anxious or depressed, this little exercise in slowing things down and paying careful attention to what we are doing illustrates how powerful and uncontrolled many of our impulses are when it comes to food, and how simple and satisfying it can be and how much more in control we can feel when we bring awareness to what we are actually doing while we are doing it," he writes. "By paying attention, you literally become more awake."

Take omega-3s daily.

The brand I prefer is OmegaBrite* because I trust its history and purity, but others are fine, too; just research your choices. Dosage will be on the box or bottle.

---

* Access the site at www.omegabrite.com.

Take a multivitamin daily.

Eat pistachios.

In Gebauer's study, participants ate 1.5 to 3 ounces a day.

Drink Concord grape juice or wild blueberry juice.

Participants in Krikorian's studies drank 6 to 8 milliliters per kilogram of their weight. Use this formula to figure out your dosage:

1 milliliter = 0.03 ounces
1 pound = 0.45 kilograms

Convert your weight from pounds to kilograms by multiplying it by 0.45. Then multiply your weight in kilograms by either 6 or 8 to find out how many milliliters of juice you should drink. Take that product and multiply it by 0.03 to determine how many ounces of juice you should drink.

Sever the stressed-digest connection.

As Mary Dallman puts it: "Partly what's driving you to reach for that brownie when you're stressed is the memory that the brownie made you feel better last time. It's habit."

So develop a *new* association—to something that makes you feel better *and* is good for you. Remember, you'll be activating the exact same reward circuit the fatty, starchy food activates. In his book *Spark*, John J. Ratey, M.D., asked one client who enjoys jumping rope to "start jumping rope every time she felt the stress coming on." The woman's choice of de-stressor had been a glass of chardonnay, but after embarking on the plan, she told Ratey that she "had jump ropes stashed on different floors of the house."

What will work for you?

CHAPTER 5

Stress and Exercise

Exercise ferments the Humours, casts them into their proper Channels, throws off Redundancies, and helps Nature in those secret Distributions, without which the Body cannot subsist in its Vigour, nor the Soul act with Chearfulness.

—Joseph Addison, *The Spectator*, 1711

Tragedy struck for Janet Noonan, a retired pharmacist from Hamilton, Ontario, just weeks before she was to begin participating in an exercise study for older adults at McMaster University. Little did she know when she signed on how grateful she'd be not just for the distraction but for the sense of solidity—mental and physical—that she gained from those interminable leg presses, crunches, and lateral pull-downs.

It was Christmas 2003, and the Noonans' four children had traveled from England and all over Canada to their parents' condo to celebrate the holiday and throw a party for Janet and Jack's twenty-fourth wedding anniversary, the next day. But late on December 26, Jack developed a gastric bleed, and Janet had to race him to the emergency room. On arrival, according to the triage nurse, his blood pressure was "hardly existent."

Thankfully, by eleven p.m., Jack was stable, and Janet went home to get some sleep. The phone woke her at two a.m. on December 27.

"Have you discussed with your husband what he wants to do when he dies?" asked the doctor. Stunned, Janet dressed and stumbled to the car. "It was a cold, dark, and wintry night," she says. "I cried all the way there. 'He's not going to die; it's not going to happen this way.'"

Her husband was in the ER when she arrived. The sequence of events over the next four days remains fuzzy, but Janet recalls being told that Jack had had a minor heart attack during the surgery to stop the bleeding, and that he'd developed a massive intestinal infection after being moved to a room.

"I realized that he was not going to get better," she says. "There was too much going on in his body. He had very bad chronic psoriasis, so his immune system was affected; it couldn't fight things."

By December 31, Jack was on a ventilator. The ER chief minced no words. "His life is over," he told Janet. "That really hit home," she says. "It implied to me: 'The sooner you disconnect the ventilator the better.'"

It was early evening, and everything around town was closing for New Year's Eve. Janet, with her son and daughter, went looking for an open coffee shop. "We made the decision to unhook the ventilator that night," she says. "The timing was not good—Jack would have wanted me to wait till January first for tax reasons. But it was what had to be done."

The exercise study was set to start a short week later and, to say the least, was not exactly a priority. But Janet had already taken the preliminary tests and knew the benefits of working out; she plays golf and walks frequently in good weather, and during the winter she takes daily aerobics classes at her condo's clubhouse. She decided that exercise sessions three times a week over the next six months would be good for her.

They were. "It was a huge effort. It took my mind off everything," she says now. "It was therapy for me as well as my exercise. I could almost feel myself getting stronger." The facilitators, graduate students at the university, pushed their charges: "Is that the absolute best you can do?" they'd ask. "Here I am, four times their age, and they're telling me, 'Harder, harder.' Holy cow," says Janet.

The students' badgering paid off. At the start of the study, Janet pumped 140 pounds in the seated leg press; by the end of the six months, she was up to 210. Other measures soared, too: Her biceps-curl heft jumped from 40 to 65 pounds, her leg extension from 80 to 125, and her seated chest press from 70 to 90.

The DEXA scan, which uses a radioactive beam to analyze fat, muscle, and bone density, showed a drop in her body fat from 32.5 percent to 31.5 percent. "I came out pretty good at the start," she says, "but after the resistance exercise, I came out even better!"

"The study came at a good time," she says. "It settled me, calmed me, cleared my head."

What's Your Exercise Confidence Level?

Many of us design an exercise program for ourselves but too often end up being patrons of our gym or club rather than actual members (we pay the monthly fee but rarely go!). See how you measure up to your resolutions.

How sure are you that you can do these things?

Circle the number on a scale from 1 to 10 that best describes you:

I know I can   **Maybe I can**   **I know I cannot**

1. Get up early, even on weekends, to exercise.

   1   2   3   4   5   6   7   8   9   10

2. Stick to your exercise program after a long, tiring day at work.

   1   2   3   4   5   6   7   8   9   10

3. Exercise even though you are feeling depressed.

   1   2   3   4   5   6   7   8   9   10

4. Stick to your exercise program when undergoing a stressful life change (e.g. divorce, death in the family, moving).

   1   2   3   4   5   6   7   8   9   10

5. Stick to your exercise program when you have household chores to attend to.

    1   2   3   4   5   6   7   8   9   10

6. Stick to your exercise program even when you have excessive demands at work.

    1   2   3   4   5   6   7   8   9   10

7. Stick to your exercise program when social obligations are very time consuming.

    1   2   3   4   5   6   7   8   9   10

8. Read or study less to exercise more.

    1   2   3   4   5   6   7   8   9   10

Calculating your score:

Simply add together the eight numbers you circled above. Scores will range from 8 to 80. The lower your score, the more likely it is that you'll stick to a regular exercise program.

Interpreting your score the *Stress Less* way*:

8–25: Highly likely to stick to an exercise program
26–39: Moderately likely to stick to an exercise program
40–65: Fairly likely to stick to an exercise program
66–80: Not at all likely to stick to an exercise program

For eons, it seems, we've been hammered with the drill (even if we haven't heeded it): Exercise is good for our health.

It reduces allostatic load—the hormonal and systemic imbalance brought about by chronic stress that Bruce McEwen began writing about more than a decade ago (as described in Chapter 1). Indeed, say research-

* The *Stress Less* interpretation was developed by the author, not the scientists.

ers, many of exercise's benefits arise from its ability to counteract—and build resistance to—stress. Countless scientific studies have shown that exercise fortifies our hearts and vascular systems, our brains, our muscles, our bones, our immune systems, and our psychological selves. Lack of it predisposes us to age-related diseases that run the gamut from cardiovascular disease to type 2 diabetes, hypertension to osteoporosis. A recent Harvard School of Public Health review of thirty-eight studies on exercise and mortality covering more than 630,000 women found that, on average, the most fit women were 34 percent less likely to die than the couch potatoes over the course of the studies, who ranged from five to twenty-nine years.

Indeed, if we could put one health intervention into pill form and swallow it, the experts say, exercise would be it.

But can it actually slow aging? New research suggests that it can, and then some: It can actually *reverse* the aging process. And the studies point to the types of exercise that are particularly effective at doing so.

"Exercise is the only equivalent of a fountain of youth that exists today," declares S. Jay Olshansky, Ph.D., professor at the University of Illinois at Chicago, first author of *The Quest for Immorality: Science at the Frontiers of Aging* and a longtime runner himself. He notes that people are selling "every conceivable" antiaging product out there, and their claims are all-encompassing. Marketers vow, for example, that growth hormone can increase muscle mass, reduce bone loss, sharpen mental acuity, restore skin elasticity, and more. "Yet all these claims—benefits you can get in theory—have been documented in the scientific literature as benefits of exercise," says Olshansky. "And with exercise they are instantaneous. You immediately feel better."

John Ratey, in his book *Spark*, highlights how reducing stress drives the process: "Exercise is one of the few ways to counter the process of aging," he writes, "because it slows down the natural decline of the stress threshold."

Run (or Walk) for Your Life:
Turning Back the Cellular Clock

Behavior geneticist Lynn Cherkas, at King's College London, is a specialist on studies with adult twins—and coincidentally (or maybe not) a twin herself. Studies on twins can provide particularly telling evidence for how lifestyle variables affect health. After all, identical twins share 100 percent of their genes, and fraternal twins share 50 percent of theirs, and unless twins of either type are separated, they share the same environment growing up.

Knock genes and environment out of the picture, and the biological effect of lifestyle choices rises up like oil on water. Maybe one twin thrives on fries and burgers while the other eats tofu and greens, or one smokes and the other wouldn't consider inhaling. Their different biological markers—cholesterol levels, say, or blood pressure—can thus be clearly linked to their behaviors.

Scientists are just now learning that the same holds true for telomere length. The length of twins' telomeres would be identical or similar at birth, and so telomere changes in adulthood would result from lifestyle choices. Cherkas and her team wanted to see how aerobic exercise in particular might affect leukocyte, or white blood cell, telomere length, and turned to the UK Adult Twin Registry for subjects. "If you use twins, especially identical twins, you're controlling for the genetic variability of telomere lengths, so you're getting a much purer assessment of the influence of exercise on their telomeres," says Cherkas.

In 2008, Cherkas and her colleagues published the first scientific evidence that exercise not only protects us against age-related diseases but actually slows the aging of our cells. The results, the scientists write, "show that adults who partake in regular physical activity are biologically younger than sedentary individuals." Moreover, the length of the subjects' telomeres corresponded with how much exercise they did; the more they exercised, the longer their telomeres, even after the scientists adjusted for such variables as age, sex, socioeconomic status, smoking, and BMI. Like the pill we conjured up earlier, telomere length was dose dependent.

Here's how the researchers reached their conclusion: They asked 2,152 women and 249 men ages 18 to 81 to fill out questionnaires on their physical-activity level over the previous 12 months—that is, whether they had been inactive (exercised about 16 minutes per week) or had engaged in light (at least 36 minutes), moderate (102 minutes), or heavy (199 minutes) physical activity. They also recorded the lifestyle factors and physical variables mentioned earlier. Then they drew blood, analyzed telomere length, and related the exercise levels to the telomere results.

The findings rang a bell. "Overall, the difference in telomere length between the most active subjects and the inactive subjects corresponds to around ten years of aging," says Cherkas over the phone from London.

Ten years. It's the same shocking figure that Epel and Blackburn showed among their caregiving moms: Chronic stress, they reported, may speed up the rate at which our cells age by ten years or more.

The déjà vu makes sense: One theory as to why exercise is so beneficial is that it reduces psychological stress, says Cherkas. Reduce the level of stress people perceive, and longer telomeres should follow suit.

Next, to confirm their results, Cherkas sliced out of the group sixty-seven pairs of twins who were raised together but exercised different amounts, in order to zero in even more precisely on the behavioral piece. Fifteen of those pairs were identical twins. Voilà: similar findings. The conclusion? It isn't primarily genes or environment that drive our biological aging but how often we hit the gym.

Months later, a team led by Andrew T. Ludlow, Ph.D., at the University of Maryland's School of Public Health, delved deeper into the effects of aerobic exercise. Rather than looking at just the amount of exercise as it related to telomere length in white blood cells, the scientists meticulously interviewed each of their sixty-nine subjects—healthy men and women ages fifty to seventy—to learn their exercise history from age thirty on, how much time they'd spent in various physical activities over the past month, how intense each of those activities had been, and the number of hours per week spent in what they called "five distinct physical dimensions": vigorous activity, leisurely walking, moving, standing, and sitting. The nomenclature recalls time travel more than treadmill travel, which, as you'll see, may be fitting, given the relationship of those dimensions to turning back the clock.

The researchers then crunched the numbers to come up with each subject's weekly exercise energy expenditure (EEE). EEE is the rate at which your body consumes oxygen during exercise minus the rate at which it consumes oxygen when you're at rest. For example, if you burn 200 calories per hour while biking and 65 calories an hour while at rest, your EEE for biking will be 135 calories per hour (200 minus 65).

After completing the analysis, researchers divided the subjects into four categories based on their EEEs: 1) those who did little or no exercise; 2) those who did moderate exercise; 3) those who did moderate-plus exercise; and 4) those who were highly active, including competitive master athletes.

The findings replicated Cherkas's, with a twist. Those in the second and third groups, the moderate and moderate-plus exercisers, had significantly longer telomeres than those in both the first group (little or no activity) and, surprisingly, the fourth group (highly active). Men and women fared similarly.

Interestingly, the dose-dependent relationship Cherkas had found appeared here, too, but only in the two moderate-exercise categories. Moreover, the telomeres of the heavy-duty exercisers in the fourth group not only were shorter than those of their less-driven colleagues, but they were remarkably similar in length to those of the *lowest* activity group. Overdoing it long term, it seems, may affect telomeres similarly to doing nothing at all.

What might be going on here? No one knows for sure just *how* exercise affects our DNA tips and the aging of our cells; we'd have to shrink to microscopic size and tunnel through the fit folks' blood vessels to see the mechanism in action. But researchers have some good theories.

Ludlow speculates that the highly active group overtrained at some point in their lives, chronically increasing inflammation and thus sparking high turnover of white blood cells as well as increased oxidative stress or dampened antioxidant activity, all of which erode telomeres (see Chapter 2 for a telomere-oxidation refresher). Studies on endurance exercise and the immune response have shown that to be the case, with moderate levels of exercise—an acute stressor—*boosting* immune function, while inactivity and very high levels have done the opposite (see Chapter 1, "Your Immune System on Stress"). Yes, exercise briefly increases the release of reactive oxygen species, because we consume more oxygen while we're pedaling away. But it also boosts antioxidant-enzyme activity to the point that the balance tips in our favor—that is, oxidative stress overall *decreases*.

"The bottom line is that oxidative stress and other changes in cellular metabolism are signals to the cells to adapt," says Mark A. Tarnopolsky, M.D., Ph.D., a muscle metabolism and neuromuscular disease specialist at McMaster University Medical Centre, where Janet Noonan did her training. Tarnopolsky has shown that even in the resting state, people ages twenty to fifty who've had endurance training have lower oxidative stress and higher antioxidant-enzyme activity than the untrained do. "The fundamental principle of physiology is that you have a metabolic alteration and then the body responds in a strategic physiologic fashion to counter that so that the next time it encounters that stress, it's less of a metabolic perturbation to the system," he says. "There are infinite numbers of examples where you provide a stimulus and if that stimulus is pulsatile or intermittent, as exercise is, the body has a period of time to adapt and respond." But if you have chronic stress—say, some fanatic goes out and runs for forty-eight hours—you don't allow for adaptation. "That's when you cross from physiologic adaptation into pathology," he says.

The heat shock, or "stress," proteins described in Chapter 4 are one example of how acute stressors spur cells to build up their defenses and become not just more stress resistant but better at their jobs. Generally sequestered inside innate immune cells, heat shock protein 72 (HSP72), for instance, slips outside those cells during exercise and primes them, making them better bacteria killers, notes the University of Colorado's Monika R. Fleshner, Ph.D., who studies HSP72 in rats. "It's a very conserved feature of the acute stress response," she says, referring to the fact that it exists in species from worms to people, "and its primary function is to facilitate innate immune responses."

So now we know: From the inside out, moderate levels of aerobic exercise reduce stress and result in slower cellular aging. A study just out brings the chronic stress–cell aging link into sharp focus. Led by Eli Puterman, Ph.D., of the UCSF Blackburn and Epel team, the study showed that greater perceived stress corresponded to shorter telomeres *only* in sedentary subjects. Hence not only does exercise correlate with longer telomeres, it protects telomeres from stress as well.

The crucial question, then, for those of us struggling to keep the crepe out of our necks and our butts lifted off our knees, is: What constitutes moderate aerobic exercise? What should we be doing to reap the maximum benefits?

Ludlow's coauthor Stephen M. Roth, Ph.D., notes that his team didn't ask participants for specifics, but did know that the subjects engaged in an aerobic mix: jogging, biking, elliptical training, walking, and so on. Yet given the results, it doesn't really matter, because what divided the longer telomeres from their abbreviated brethren was the subjects' *level* of activity and their exercise history, not the type of activity. And he points to a way to put the findings into practice.

According to Roth, the 2008 Centers for Disease Control and Prevention (CDC) guidelines for aerobic activity, which are spelled out at the end of this chapter, match the activity level of his study's moderate exercisers. Wonderful news! Those in this second EEE group, he says, very likely meet the CDC's basic requirements, and those in the third, moderate-plus EEE group likely match the CDC's "For Even Greater Benefits" requirements. Excellent as well! "From a big-picture perspective, doing nothing or doing very high amounts of exercise—that is, beyond the higher CDC standard—appears to be detrimental for telomere length in our subjects," says Roth.

The CDC guidelines are straightforward and memorable—no complicated regimen here—and they're flexible enough for you to design your own program. That sense of control may be nearly as important as your regimen itself, not just for reducing stress, but for deriving the benefits of exercise at all, as the work of Monika Fleshner will make clear later. The American College of Sports Medicine (ACSM) and the U.S. Department of Health and Human Services endorse the CDC guidelines as well.

Roth's team also found a relationship between the *number* of years subjects had been exercising and their telomere length. Those who exhibited what the researchers call exercise's "protective effect" had been exercising consistently for five years or more. That indicates that what matters most is not when you start working out but that you keep going. Remember, telomeres neither shorten nor lengthen overnight—both actions take time. "The adoption of exercise at any age, even if you're elderly, is beneficial," says Olshansky.*

Stress-Proof Your Brain

Exercise's effect on the brain may be the most well-studied exercise intervention next to its effect on the cardiovascular system. Most of the research revolves around how exercise can boost cognitive function, but new science is emerging that investigates the place where stress, exercise, and brain function meet. It's about time: As you saw in Chapter 3, stress plays a big role in brain degeneration. Exercise is a prime way to ameliorate the damage—and slow neurological aging to boot.

---

* Olshansky cites the research of Maria Fiatarone Singh, M.D., now at the University of Sydney, in Australia, as the catalyst for the research that led to this finding.

I Exercise, Therefore I Think

Monika Fleshner spends her days designing experiments that let rats run at night to show how exercise makes the brain more resistant to stress. *Voluntary* exercise, that is.

Night is rats' natural time to run. They snooze all day and take to the wheel at night. I know. At age five, my daughter had two pet rats—a bribe to get her to fork over her pacifiers. At bedtime, we'd have to move Tom and Jerry, the fattest rats in history (my foodie husband fed them a gourmet diet), to the basement to keep their *thwump, thwump, thwump*-ing from constantly rattling us awake.

Recall that the brain, as Bruce McEwen puts it, is the key organ of stress; it decides what's stressful and how our bodies will respond to those stressors. Hence, anything that will make the brain more stress resistant, that ups its stress threshold, will lead to fewer destructive reverberations chipping away at our organs, muscles, and cells.

Voluntary aerobic exercise, a mild stressor, protects the brain by making it hardier. That is, by temporarily boosting glucocorticoids, it enables the HPA axis, various neurons, and connections between those neurons to adapt to a tiny assault and become stronger. Heat shock proteins are a case in point. But the words *voluntary* and *temporarily* are key: Forced exercise, Fleshner and others report, does the opposite. When researchers drop rats onto motorized wheels or treadmills and control the time, intensity, and duration of their runs, the animals' glucocorticoids (corticosterone, in rats) skyrocket and stay there, leaving the rats worse off than before they hit the turf.

"Voluntary exercise increases corticosterone, but then the levels go down—the rat becomes habituated," says UCLA's Grace S. Griesbach, Ph.D. Griesbach studies healthy and brain-injured rats to understand the effects of exercise on traumatic brain injury. She has directly compared the stress-hormone levels of rats that voluntarily run on wheels to those of rats forced onto motorized ones. "But with forced exercise, the corticosterone levels shoot up even higher at the beginning and do *not* decrease with time. The forced exercise acts as a chronic stressor."

People are likely no different. Which raises an important issue: Sure, you go to the gym—you're nothing if not responsible, and you *make* yourself go. You even have a personal trainer whom you suspect was a drill sergeant in a former life. But if you're consistently forcing yourself to exercise—by that I mean dreading it and counting the minutes once you're pumping, not just having to give yourself a push now and then— are you reducing stress at all? Is there any way to turn what feels like military basic training into a voluntary workout that you actually enjoy?

What is it about exercising at will that makes the difference? First off when we voluntarily exercise, levels of protective repair molecules increase, particularly in the hippocampus, the seat of memory formation. Primary among them is BDNF (brain derived neurotrophic factor). As we learned in Chapter 3, BDNF belongs to a class of compounds called neurotrophins, or growth factors—chemicals in the brain that regulate the growth, proliferation, and survival of certain neurons. In exercising rats, for instance, scientists have consistently observed an increase in cell proliferation in the dentate gyrus, a strip of gray matter in the hippocampus that is one of only two brain regions that support adult neurogenesis. BDNF also spurs the release of internal antioxidants to neutralize those cell-damaging, telomere-eroding reactive oxygen species described in Chapter 2, and it stimulates long-term potentiation (LTP), the strengthening of the communication network between neurons that relates to learning and long-term memory.

Think of LTP this way: You're in your car, driving past a chain of cell phone towers. The towers are neurons, the spaces between them are the junctures, or synapses, and the radio signal connecting your BlackBerry from tower to tower is the neurotransmitter glutamate, zipping your messages along. "Can you hear me now?" you shout, the phone glued to your ear. No response, so you backtrack and drive again from tower A to tower B. "Can you hear me now?" You get a mumbled response. You backtrack again and trace the same path. "Can you hear me now?" "Stop screaming in my ear!" screeches your sister on the other end. That's LTP: With each repeat, the signal transmission gets stronger, and so finally a new fact or skill (or, in this case, sound) sticks.

Indeed, BDNF, writes McEwen in *The End of Stress As We Know It,* "may be the biological go-between that brings about the spectacular results of exercise on the brain."

BDNF, though, isn't the only exercise-induced player. Exercise also sets free other brain growth factors, including insulin-like growth factor (IGF-1), vascular endothelial growth factor (VEGF), and fibroblast growth factor (FGF-2). Studies with rats have shown that IGF-1 and VEGF jump-start the growth of new blood vessels in various parts of the brain. This is called angiogenesis, and it essentially creates additional roads and highways over which to truck nutrients, such as glucose, to those new exercise-launched brain cells. It stimulates the production of insulin receptors, too, which means opening more cell doors to let glucose inside as well as more efficient metabolism of it, averting insulin resistance and type 2 diabetes (see Chapter 4).

All of which leads, of course, to this bottom line: Exercise, by neutralizing the effects of chronic stress, improves cognitive function. Numerous epidemiological and clinical randomized studies, as well as meta-analyses of both types, show that adults (young, old, healthy, and those with signs of early Alzheimer's) who do aerobic exercise think more clearly, remember better, and sustain attention longer than those who don't.

Samples of two of those studies, a giant epidemiological one and a small clinical one:

Using the 18,766 women ages seventy to eighty-one in the Nurses' Health Study, a multi-trial study launched in 1976, a team led by the Harvard School of Public Health's Jennifer Weuve, Sc.D., analyzed physical activity of the subjects as reported twice a year on questionnaires between 1986 and 1995 or 2001. The researchers then administered cognitive tests. Higher levels of physical activity were associated with better cognitive performance in areas ranging from verbal memory to attention. Those who exercised the most had a 20 percent lower risk of cognitive impairment compared to those who exercised the least.

And: A recent MRI study led by Columbia University's Ana C. Pereira, Ph.D., showed that a three-month exercise program (forty minutes of aerobic activity four times a week) led to increased cerebral blood volume in the dentate gyrus of eleven adults ages twenty-one to forty-five. (Recall that the dentate gyrus is that strip of gray matter in the hippocampus that is one of only two brain regions that supports adult neurogenesis.) And the increased blood flow correlated with improvements in verbal learning, including recall, recognition, and memory. Before embarking on the human study, the investigators had run a similar one on mice, with one large difference: They dissected the mice's brains after the trial, revealing significant brain growth in the denate gyrus. It's not a big leap to theorize that in the human subjects the combination of greater blood flow and learning improvements signified brain growth, too.

Even more expansive glimpses into the brains of regular exercisers show whence the growth: Scientists at Sweden's Karolinska Institutet surveyed women and men at midlife regarding their level of physical activity, and—twenty-one years later—when the subjects were in their sixties and seventies, they took brain MRIs of a subset of them. Those who at midlife had broken a sweat exercising at least twice a week had significantly more gray matter—neurons themselves!—than the sedentary folks. And scientists at the University of Illinois found that people ages sixty to seventy-nine who participated in a six-month aerobic-fitness program increased their total brain volume (gray *and* white matter, the latter being the insulated fibers that connect neurons) but that a matched group of adults stretching and toning did not. In both studies, the prefrontal cortex was particularly affected. Recall that the PFC is the seat of executive function—working memory, planning, scheduling, recognition of consequences, and dealing with ambiguity—and is known to show substantial age-related degeneration.

A larger PFC, Fleshner and others note, may confer a greater sense of control over stressors, making the exercise mavens overall less reactive to those nerve-frazzling events that hit them day by day.

An Ounce of Prevention

In rats, uncontrollable tail shocks are a frequently used stressor to induce learned helplessness, an existentialist "no exit" kind of scenario. (For humans, poverty is often cited as a situation of learned helplessness.) But new studies by Fleshner and colleagues show that rats who *voluntarily* run on wheels for six weeks *before* receiving those shocks don't freak out and freeze up twenty-four hours later, the way their sedentary peers do, and they don't get all discombobulated trying to escape from avoidable foot shocks pulsing through the floor of a box.

Why is that? Through exercise, the rats' brains became stress resistant, and a stress-resistant brain directs the body to behave much differently than a stressed-out one does. Fleshner's team got similar results when it compared rats given free wheel access for six weeks to rats left to stew in their cages before both groups were subjected to a daily loud-noise stressor. This time the researchers examined not just the rats' behavior but their corticosterone levels. As early as day four of the eleven-day stressor, the exercised rats had significantly lower corticosterone levels than the sedentary guys.

In both studies, the *duration* of the training, not the intensity, sparked the positive effect: Three and four weeks of running couldn't do for the brain what six weeks could.

Interestingly, the six weeks of training the rats needed for stress protection is roughly equivalent to the five years of training that Ludlow and Roth's subjects needed for telomere protection. Rats' life span is generally two years plus change, compared to humans' eighty years. When I do the math (this is my own personal speculation), it turns out that one week in mouse time is equivalent to forty weeks in human time, which means that six weeks of mouse training is equivalent to 4.6 years of human training—very close to the five years that Ludlow and Roth saw correlated with longer telomeres.

The brains of sedentary rats have no such physiological advantages. When sedentary rats are subjected to uncontrollable stressors, a circuit in their brains involving the amygdala, the bed nucleus of the stria terminalis (BST), and the locus coeruleus (LC) lights up. (The amygdala regulates emotion, including fear; the BST, an area near the hypothalamus, mediates the release of the stress hormone CRH; and the LC is the main source of norepinephrine in the forebrain.) We'll call this the ABC circuit, for easy reference. Nerve fibers connect these regions with a small structure in the brain stem called the dorsal raphe nucleus (DRN). When the ABC circuit switches on, the DRN, which is loaded with serotonin neurons, becomes hypersensitive. The neurotransmitter serotonin causes blood vessels to constrict and works to transmit impulses between nerve cells. With the circuit lit, the serotonin neurons go nuts and release buckets of serotonin into brain regions networked with the DRN, including motor-control areas and limbic structures such as the amygdala. At the same time, boatloads of fight-or-flight's norepinephrine shoot from the locus coeruleus into the DRN. Scientists believe that it is this confluence of events that causes the rat to freeze in its little tracks and become dumb in the face of escapable shocks.

But when voluntary exercise is added to the mix, the serotonin responses are much more constrained when a stressor strikes, particularly an uncontrollable stressor such as tail shocks. "The exercising animals in a stress situation respond, but they don't go overboard and freak out like the sedentary animals," says Fleshner.

Why? Exercise activates the medial prefrontal cortex (mPFC), a part of the prefrontal cortex that dampens the firing of the locus coeruleus into the DRN, thereby keeping serotonin and norepinephrine activity in the DRN at a reasonable level. Remember the larger gray-matter volume in the exercising adults in the Karolinska Institutet MRI study? Exercise, it seems, "immunizes" us (and rats) against stressors: We're less fragile, because our nerves are literally not so exposed. "It's like a shift to the left, so the stress response isn't turned on to the same degree, and it doesn't get turned on to every little freaking thing," says Fleshner.

Exercise physiologist Tinna Traustadóttir, Ph.D., at the University of

Arizona, has taken research like Fleshner's with rats, and carried it over to people—women in particular—and also added the variable of age to the mix.

Traustadóttir's studies may well be the first to compare cortisol, age, and fitness in humans; her findings reflect Fleshner's: The cortisol responses of *older fit* women match those of unfit women *forty-plus* years younger.

As we age, our HPA axis becomes more sensitive to psychological stress. The screeching baby that mildly perturbed us when we were twenty-five sets our teeth on edge at sixty. Nearly three decades of research had shown that aerobic exercise diminishes cardiovascular and catecholamine (epinephrine, norepinephrine) reactivity to stress; Traustadóttir's team wanted to see whether it could diminish HPA-axis reactivity (the glucocorticoid burst)—the stage of the stress response that can really do us in.

They studied three groups of women: nine unfit women ages nineteen to thirty-six (young), thirteen unfit women ages fifty-nine to eighty-one (older), and eleven fit women ages fifty-nine to eighty-one (older). The designations "fit" and "unfit" related to the women's maximal oxygen consumption scores (VO_2), an objective measure of the functioning of cardiovascular, pulmonary, and skeletal muscle systems calculated using a mask and a computer. If a subject's VO_2 max was average or lower for her age group, based on American Heart Association criteria, she fell into the "unfit" category; if her VO_2 max was above average, she fell into the "fit" group.

The young women were tested in the early follicular phase of their menstrual cycles, to minimize the confounding effects of estrogen on cortisol, and the older women were postmenopausal and not on hormone replacement. Everyone was healthy, no one had smoked in the past year, and BMI could not be over thirty.

The women sweated through a stress test combining three types of challenges: mental, which included a color-word task, math in their heads, and anagrams; physical, in which they plunged a hand in ice water for up to three minutes; and psychosocial, in the form of an interview covering a stressful experience. At every turn, the experimenters harassed the subjects to go faster and try harder. Blood was drawn seven times to test cortisol and ACTH levels, and heart rate was recorded at five-second intervals throughout the trial. (See Chapter 1 for a stress-hormone refresher.)

Needless to say, during the stress test, everyone's heart rate, blood pressure, and ACTH and cortisol levels rose. The subjects wouldn't have been alive if they hadn't! The older unfit women had a significantly higher cortisol response than all the others, and their cortisol levels stayed raised longer, too—no surprise there. But that the cortisol levels of the older fit women *did not differ* from those of the young women was a showstopper. "The exercise completely blunted the age effect, which was astonishing," says Traustadóttir.

In the paper, the researchers write: "Our result shows that among unfit women, aging is associated with greater HPA-axis reactivity to psychological stress and that higher aerobic fitness among older women can attenuate these age-related changes as indicated by a blunted cortisol response to psychological stress."

It was as if the brains of the fit older women had dropped forty years in the stress department. Like those of Fleshner's mice, they had become habituated to stress, needing more of it to set them off in the first place.

Traustadóttir speculates that, when stressed, the fit women didn't have to rely on the HPA-axis cortisol response as much as the unfit women did, because aerobic exercise had made their sympathetic nervous system—specifically, the fight-or-flight hormone epinephrine, which boosts the heart rate—more "accustomed to cranking up and then coming back down." That the cortisol levels stayed raised longer in the older unfit women than in the younger unfit and the older fit groups also showed that the HPA-axis feedback mechanism loses elasticity as we age, leaving older cells more likely to soak in cortisol.

Unless we exercise, that is.

"With aging we're not able to respond as well to any kind of perturbation—we're not able to 'get back,'" says Traustadóttir. "The sensitivity isn't there and so everything stays elevated for a longer time." She compares the process to a rubber band being stretched out. Exercise puts elasticity back in the rubber, or slows down its stretching in the first place.

Out with the Old, in with the New

How wonderful that exercise can make our brains resistant to stress and undo damage that chronic stress has wrought. But can it alleviate the burden stress puts on our bodies as well? More new science says that it can—and then some. In our immune and skeletal muscle systems, it can essentially make cells young again.

Cellular Youngbloods

Monika Fleshner was thrilled: The study she'd led in rats on the effects of exercise on stress and immune function translated word for note to people—or, more precisely, antigen to antibody.

When Fleshner's team injected a piece of a novel benign invader, or "antigen" (the sea-mollusk protein KLH), into rats after stressing them, the exercising rats' acquired immune systems made new antibodies to gobble the invader up, but sedentary rats' immune systems did not. They then carried the experiment to humans. They recruited forty-six men in four categories: young (ages twenty-five to thirty) and older (ages sixty to seventy-nine) men who were physically active, and young and older men who were sedentary. They injected them all with KLH. They then took blood samples to measure levels of antibodies to the KLH every seven days for about a month. The higher the KLH levels in the blood, the stronger the immune response. As expected, the older men had lower KLH antibody levels overall than the younger men; immune response to new antigens declines with age. But a happy surprise came when the scientists compared the active older men to their sedentary counterparts.

"We were able to show that the physically active older folks had antibody levels that were just as good as the young people's," says Fleshner. "Exercising had allowed them to maintain a young immune response."

The research opened the door to a possible mechanism behind all those studies showing a reduction in number and severity of infectious diseases among regular exercisers, regardless of age: Exercise may prevent chronic or repeated stress from suppressing the body's immune system.

Jeffrey A. Woods, Ph.D., and colleagues at the University of Illinois followed up Fleshner's cross-sectional study with a longitudinal one that lasted ten months—and backed up the previous results with even more solid evidence. They took sedentary older men and women and randomly assigned them to one of two groups: Thirty were in an aerobic-exercise group; twenty-five were in a flexibility and balance group. Everyone was injected with KLH at eight months, and blood samples were taken two, three, and six weeks later.

Fleshner's results were confirmed: The people in the aerobic-exercise group had a stronger antibody response than the bend-and-stretchers. "Jeff was able to show—not quite as big an effect as we saw because our people had been exercising for years—that an intervention was able to bring an older person's responses closer to a younger person's level," says Fleshner.

Muscular Therapy

Simon Melov, Ph.D., sports big round black glasses and an intentional five o'clock shadow that reflects a moon sliver of close-cropped hair atop his head. The pairing makes him appear scruffy and trim at once. Tiny toy Daleks—extraterrestrial mutant cyborgs of *Doctor Who* fame—sit on a shelf near his desk (they're quiet now, but they do move and talk), and framed covers of 1990s magazines, *Life*'s "Can We Stop Aging?" and *Time*'s "Forever Young," both of which cite him, color the walls.

Melov runs a lab at the Buck Institute for Age Research, in Novato, California, that focuses on how damaging ROS from within mitochondria, the powerhouses of the cell, influence aging and age-related disease.

Melov and McMaster's Mark Tarnopolsky are lead authors on a remarkable study about how weight training reverses muscular aging. The title of the study—surprisingly bold in the scientific lexicon—says it all: "Resistance Exercise Reverses Aging in Human Skeletal Muscle."

And that was after just six months of training, twice a week, on nonconsecutive days.

We've known since the 1970s that resistance training, even among those sixty-five and older, increases strength and improves functioning, such as balance and climbing stairs. Most people see rapid changes in strength in the first two months of training, along with an increase in muscle mass; by about six months, things start to plateau. Particularly apparent in older folks is that with exercise oxidative stress in the body drops and antioxidant activity increases. But *reverse* aging?

Here's what the scientists did: In Canada, Tarnopolsky took muscle biopsies from the thighs of relatively sedentary younger adults (ages twenty to thirty) and relatively active older adults (sixty-five and older). The contrasting activity levels evened out the playing field (active at age sixty-five is similar to relatively sedentary at age twenty), ensuring from the start that any effects could be attributed to aging alone. Janet Noonan, whose story starts this chapter, was among those in the older group. The quick biopsy didn't hurt, but it could be unnerving. "All I could think of was I could be in *The X-Files*," laughs Joan French, another older participant. "They took a needle the size of a small knitting needle and sucked out whatever was in there!"

Then the older adults—fourteen in total—underwent weight training in McMaster's gym for six months, two times a week, on nonconsecutive days, under the supervision of Tarnopolsky's students. They began with a five-minute aerobic warm-up and some stretching, and stretched again following the workout. After the six-month training period, Tarnopolsky took another muscle biopsy from each older participant. He shipped genetic extracts from the biopsied muscle from both groups to

Melov, in sunny California, to be analyzed and compared at the genetic level.

Before the training period, the scientists found, the older adults were 59 percent weaker than the younger adults. But after the six months of pumping iron, they were only 38 percent weaker than the younger adults. That was impressive enough in itself. Yet even more sci-fi in its implications was that the gene-expression profiles for the older subjects reverted back to a younger profile.

Even Melov was surprised. "I thought we'd see an idiosyncratic 'aged-exercise' genetic profile for the older adults," he says. "We were not expecting there to be a recapitulation of the young profile in the old exercisers," he says. "Although everyone understands that exercise is good for you, it's a different thing to show empirically that it actually seems to be altering pathways back to youthful levels. It's amazing—and a very strong catalyst to get people to exercise."

What exactly had happened inside the muscles of the older adults to turn back the clock in just six months?

As we age, our skeletal muscles start to lose mass, a condition known as sarcopenia, Greek for—ghoulishly—"flesh reduction." This atrophy (also a dreadful word) generally begins at about age forty-five and continues at a rate of about 1 percent per year until by age eighty our muscles have lost approximately 50 percent of their fibers (the amount of loss accelerates with each decade). The muscle is replaced by fat, though not noticeably so, as we seem to sag rather than plump up. I began noticing the deterioration in myself at about age forty-three. I had no scientific knowledge of the process at the time and characterized it, with alarm, to friends as: "The muscle is falling off the bone!" It reminded me—not happily—of pork ribs slow-cooked in a smoker.

～～～～

What was driving my *bubbe* arms and flapping thighs?

Mitochondria in my muscle cells, by and large.

Remember the mitochondria sitting in the cytoplasm of our cells from

Chapter 2—the energy powerhouses? The main job of mitochondria is to convert glucose into ATP, the fuel that powers our cells, thereby enabling them to communicate with one another and perform important biochemical processes such as contracting muscles and metabolizing sugar.

But as we age, the mitochondria become impaired: Oxidative damage and other biochemical insults lead to the accumulation of deletions and mutations in their DNA (mtDNA) similar to those suffered by their nuclear-DNA brethren. "Chunks are clipped out of some of the mitochondrial genes," says Tarnopolsky, a competitive athlete and self-described "endurance exercise junkie," who looks much younger than his forty-seven years. Instructions from the genes for important duties—enzyme activity, protein synthesis—get bollixed up. Entire cells even die. Think of a car engine starting to sputter: You floor the ignition to make it up that hill, but what happens? Lots of *rrrevvving*, little power. In mitochondria that lack of oomph translates into less enzyme activity and protein making, and higher oxidative stress. Indeed, mitochondrial dysfunction is the major reason that skeletal muscle atrophies. "Even in our fairly active older people, mitochondrial function is down 20 to 30 percent, and there are lots of mtDNA deletions in the muscle, too," says Tarnopolsky.

When Simon Melov compared the genetic profiles of the younger and older subjects after the initial biopsies (this was before the exercise program), he found about six hundred genes that were expressed differently in the older participants than in the younger participants. Of those, about a third (179) were associated with mitochondrial function; the genes in the older folks just did not "turn on" to the same degree as those in the younger folks. But after the older subjects' six-month training, the picture changed dramatically. "The gene expression profiles for those 179 genes went from the abnormal pattern of aging and reverted back to the gene expression pattern of a young individual," says Tarnopolsky. Adds Melov: "With exercise, those genes were back to normal, back to youthful levels."

Simply put, the profiles of approximately 30 percent of the "old" genes revived and became "young" again. How could this possibly happen?

Tarnopolsky has a theory. Pumping iron, he surmises, may literally pump new life into our muscles.

As described in Chapter 1, mature skeletal muscle cells, unlike white blood cells (leukocytes), are postmitotic; they don't divide. On the outside of skeletal muscle fibers, though, huddled beneath a kind of sheath called the basal lamina, are satellite cells, which do divide and multiply. A satellite cell, similar to a "progenitor" cell, is a "partially committed" stem cell—in this case, a stem cell on the path to becoming a muscle cell but not there yet. In contrast, an embryonic stem cell is a blank slate; it can become any type of cell. As mentioned earlier, as we age, the mtDNA of mature muscle cells accumulates mutations and deletions, leading to reduced mitochondrial function, which means less fuel for the cells. But Tarnopolsky's group found that the mtDNA of those cloistered satellite cells does *not* accumulate mutations and deletions, regardless of whether the cell is from a twentysomething or a septuagenarian. Satellite cells lie quiescent, protected from stressors, beneath their skein of a blanket until they're woken by either muscles contracting or injury to the muscle fiber. Resistance exercise accelerates their activation, and also sparks the release of growth hormone.

Jolted into action, the satellite cells begin to divide and multiply, and to travel up into the mature muscle fiber. There, some of them fuse with the mature muscle cells, pushing their "good" mtDNA into the muscle fiber. Others swim back to the safe haven beneath the basal lamina and pass out again, replenishing the satellite cell pool.

"So there was a dilutional effect," says Tarnopolsky. But there was more: Some of the old "bad" mtDNA, riddled with deletions, actually disappeared. "Out with the old, in with the new," laughs Tarnopolsky.

The far-reaching effect? Worn out genes got new juice from six months of crunches and curls—at least those genes related to mitochondrial function. Hence, mitochondrial function improved and oxidative stress lessened. The process, dubbed mitochondrial DNA shifting, literally breathes new life into old muscle.

Interestingly, the mtDNA shifting does not occur in folks in their twenties. "In young people, their strength goes up, their muscle mass goes up, but their mitochondrial content stays the same," says Tarnopolsky. That's because they don't have the age-related mtDNA deletions to start with. Nor does their oxidative stress seem to improve—but then again, it's not elevated yet.

But what constitutes "young" may be younger than you think. Tarnopolsky notes that his team has seen mtDNA deletions, and thus signs of mitochondrial dysfunction, in folks as young as their thirties. "So would they benefit from activating their satellite cells?" he asks. "Yeah, of course. Can we measure a 3 percent improvement of mitochondrial function? No, we can't from a scientific and statistical perspective. So essentially there's going to be a spectrum along which people are going to derive benefits. But scientifically we just don't have the techniques to be able to detect when that point is where you cross over. Because it's not black or white; it's going to be shades of gray as you start getting older."

Melov and Tarnopolsky's rejuvenation study used people sixty-five and older. Think of the benefits you could reap, says Melov, if you started weight training in your forties. Indeed, a small earlier study led by Sweden's Fawzi Kadi, Ph.D., found that women ages thirty-two to forty-four who participated in a resistance-exercise program targeting neck and shoulder muscles had a 46 percent increase in their number of satellite cells after just ten weeks.

So these days, when I lift those ten-pound free weights in biceps curls or set the lat pull-down to sixty pounds and yank, I can't help but visualize my satellite cells inching out from under their covers and marching upstream, restoring my muscles to a younger state.

The Telomere Connection

Kadi and his colleague Elodie Ponsot, Ph.D., both now at Sweden's Örebro University, wondered what was happening to the telomeres inside those satellite and mature muscle cells. Because mature muscle cells are postmitotic, their telomeres don't shorten as a result of replication (as discussed in Chapter 2). But their precursors, satellite muscle cells, do divide; indeed, they can divide too much. Kadi had read a 2003 paper reporting that severely overtrained athletes—those with exercise-associated chronic fatigue (called fatigued athlete myopathic syndrome, or FAMS)—had abnormally short muscle-cell telomeres. The scientists wanted to know what the effect of *healthful* levels of resistance exercise on telomere length might be.

They pulled out their biopsy needles and got to work. They compared the muscle telomere length of seven *healthy* male power lifters (read: no FAMS) in their twenties and thirties who'd trained for five to eleven years against that of seven healthy active men, also in their twenties and thirties, with no history of strength training.

Telomere length of skeletal muscle cells has two variables compared with that of leukocytes, which have just one. The first variable is the telomere length of the mature muscle cells, which doesn't change after birth; the second is the telomere length of the muscle satellite cells and the satellite cells that are newly incorporated into the mature muscle. Kadi and Ponsot made sure to get measurements for both.

Their results? The telomeres of the power lifters as a group tended to be *longer* than those of the non-lifters. At the group level, "regular power lifting is not associated with an abnormal shortening of skeletal muscle DNA telomere length," the scientists write. You can almost hear their sigh of relief. "On the contrary, skeletal muscle telomeres of power lifters tended to be longer than those in a population of active subjects with no history of strength training."

The new findings are exciting; I've tripled my resistance workouts as a result. But it's important to be realistic, too: New research has shown that as we bulk up our muscles, we can reverse the aging process—but only to a point. "Our study showed that some of the dysfunction with aging is reversible," says Tarnopolsky. But there's only so much a training program can do. Remember that while a third of the mitochondrial aging effects were reversed in the study, two-thirds of them weren't. "Which means that we can improve on the process somewhat, but there's still an inevitable aging component," he says.

It's an important reminder in these days of hype and overblown "solutions": Setting yourself up for impossible goals will only add to your stress, diminishing that crucial sense of control that the longer-telomered among Epel and Blackburn's caregivers had. "What's most important is to exercise on a regular basis," says Kadi over the phone from Sweden. "You have to like what you do—that's the main issue. Pick an exercise form that fits you that has some resistance and endurance, and make sure you increase the intensity and do it on a regular basis."

To Reduce Stress and Slow the Cellular Clock Using Exercise

Endurance and resistance exercise both stimulate muscle protein synthesis, but different kinds: Resistance exercise builds cross-sectional muscle fiber (a structural adaptation), and endurance exercise increases mitochondrial density, boosting oxidative capacity (a metabolic adaptation). Here's how to take advantage of both.

CDC Guidelines for Exercise

Follow the 2008 CDC guidelines for aerobic activity*—the level matched by those with the longest telomeres in Andrew Ludlow and Stephen Roth's new study. As the guidelines say, ten minutes at a time is "fine." Don't forget to warm up and cool down for at least five minutes before and after your session, and to stretch for at least five minutes before and after, to maintain flexibility. Remember: Do not under- or overdo it.

---

* For more information, visit www.health.gov/paguidelines/ and www.acsm.org/physicalactivity.

For Important Health Benefits

Adults need at least:

- two hours and thirty minutes (150 minutes) of moderate-intensity aerobic activity (e.g., brisk walking) every week OR
- one hour and fifteen minutes (75 minutes) of vigorous-intensity aerobic activity (e.g., jogging or running) OR
- an equivalent mix of moderate- and vigorous-intensity aerobic activity

For Even Greater Health Benefits

- five hours (300 minutes) each week of moderate-intensity aerobic activity OR
- two hours and thirty minutes (150 minutes) each week of vigorous-intensity aerobic activity OR
- an equivalent mix of moderate- and vigorous-intensity aerobic activity

The CDC guidelines classify moderate intensity as "working hard enough to raise your heart rate and break a sweat. One way to tell is that you'll be able to talk, but not sing the words to your favorite song." With vigorous-intensity activity, they say, "you're breathing hard and fast, and your heart rate has gone up quite a bit. If you're working at this level, you won't be able to say more than a few words without pausing for a breath."

For the more numbers-oriented among us, tracking our heart rate is another way to know that we're working at the moderate- or vigorous-intensity level. The American College of Sports Medicine (ACSM) just revised its testing prescriptions in February 2009, and recommends calculating maximal heart rate using a formula developed by Ronald L. Gellish, M.S., and colleagues at Oakland University's School of Health Sciences, and then taking a percentage of it, as described on the next page. To paraphrase Mark Tarnopolsky: Forget the old "220 minus your age" formula; it's in with the new.

First, calculate your maximal heart rate using this equation: 206.9 – (0.67 × age) = maximal heart rate. Then take 64 to 74 percent of the maximal (maximal × 0.64 or 0.74) to get your heart-rate range. If you do very little exercise now, start by trying to maintain the lower heart rate (maximal × 0.64) for at least 150 minutes a week. If you already exercise regularly, or have exercised at the lower heart rate (64 percent) for eight to twelve weeks, start increasing your heart rate to the higher end of the range (74 percent), and maintain that rate for at least 150 minutes a week. Following those guidelines will yield health and cardiovascular benefits, says the ACSM—and as I see it, perhaps telomere benefits, too, based on Ludlow and Roth's work. Any activity above that is a bonus, the ACSM adds. As you get accustomed to exercise and can easily sustain the 74 percent of maximal heart rate, recalculate your heart-rate range, first to 84 percent and then to 94 percent of the maximal. "These elevated heart rates, however, are not typically reached by the person who exercises for health benefits," says Walter R. Thompson, Ph.D., senior editor of ACSM's *Guidelines for Exercise Testing and Prescription*, 8th edition. "The safe range for people who are accustomed to exercise, who have not experienced any discomfort during exercise, and who have as their goal good health as opposed to training for an event, should be between 80 and 90 percent of maximal heart rate. It is safer to maintain this level and increase the number of minutes from 150 to 300 each week."

Twice a week, on nonconsecutive days, follow the resistance-exercise protocol Mark Tarnopolsky used in his study on reversing muscle aging.

Do not do too much too fast. To figure out where to start, visit the Testing Page of ExRx.net* or get a one-time assessment at a local exercise facility or from a personal trainer, suggests Kristyn Fales, fitness director at Healthworks Fitness Centers for Women in Chestnut Hill, Massachusetts. If you exercise regularly, evaluate your progress about every two

---

* www.exrx.net/testing

weeks and increase the weight you're lifting and/or the number of repetitions. The ExRx.net site, notes Fales, offers a wealth of information, from a Beginner's Page to full-scale aerobic and resistance workouts.

- Begin with a five-minute aerobic warm-up and some simple stretching.

- Each session, do three sets of ten repetitions each on the following weight machines: leg press, chest press, leg extension, hamstring curls, shoulder press, lat pull-down, seated row, calf raise, abdominal crunch, and back extension. Do one set of ten repetitions each of biceps curls and triceps extensions, either on machines or with free weights.

- Either stretch the body part you've used after each group of three sets for a minute or so, or stretch all body parts for about ten minutes after you complete the cycle. (I prefer stretching after each machine.) Often the machines themselves feature a stretch for the specific muscles you've used.

Figure out a way to be physically active that feels natural to you—or shift your perspective on what you do now—so you'll keep at it and reap the maximum benefits.

Remember, the point is to reduce stress, not increase it by putting unachievable demands on yourself. Personally, I've chosen to fork over a bit more money to join a club that feels like a spa, not like basic training. It's my escape, my "me" time, if only for forty-five minutes at a stretch, with flat-screen TVs bigger than my kitchen table and two movies showing every day (the only way I get to see *any*). What works for you? Three brisk ten-minute walks a day? Taking a class with friends? Biking to work? Remember, *you* are in charge.

CHAPTER 6

Stress and the Mind

If the doors of perception were cleansed everything would appear to man as it is: Infinite.

—William Blake, "A Memorable Fancy,"
in *The Marriage of Heaven and Hell*, 1790

As Elissa Epel and Elizabeth Blackburn so keenly show in their studies on stress (Chapter 2), our biological aging is related to our *perception* of stress, not any objective measure of actual circumstances. Which means that if we can't change the way things are (say, being laid off at age fifty), we *can* change our *response* to those things (a layoff isn't a tragedy: now I can make the leap from editor to college lecturer!). Just as a sense of helplessness—that no-way-out knot in our guts and tornado in our brains—may be the greatest stressor, having a sense of control may be the greatest antidote, both psychologically and physiologically. Its effects reverberate all the way down to the DNA nestled in our cells.

How do we go about getting that sense of control? Or, put another way: How do we alter our view of events when that view seems at once so unconscious and automatic? New research shows that meditation and particular strategies to counter negativity can not only change our minds but actually alter our brains—and by so doing slow the aging process. Take a look.

One Breath at a Time:
Stress, Aging, and Meditation

In the mid-1980s, Maura Santangelo seemed to have it all: She was an ophthalmologist with a thriving practice in upstate New York, happily married to a physician who shared her love of travel, and the mother of two children. She'd also found an outlet for her philanthropic self: In 1991, at age forty-four, she began volunteering with the Seva Foundation, a global service organization based on overseas partnerships. First she performed cataract surgery in Nepal, and then she helped launch the group's Sight Programs, which have helped nearly three million blind people to see. She became so inspired by the work that she took a leave from her clinical practice to earn a degree in public health.

When it came time to return to her job, though, Maura was filled with dread. "I knew all along that my business partnership was flawed on multiple levels," she says. "But once I removed myself, I saw the flaws even more clearly and asked: 'What am I doing here?'"

She sought solace in meditation, specifically Tibetan Buddhist practices. She'd been using the mind-calming techniques, to a greater and lesser extent, since 1965, one year after she arrived in the States from her native Italy and was thrown into a New Jersey high school knowing no English.

"It was while I was meditating that I really admitted that my partnership was not the greatest," she says. "Meditating enabled me to say, 'Whatever my partners do, it's their problem, not my problem. I just have to be able to own up to my part.' It helped me get the distance from daily events so I could deal with them more appropriately—not get angry and fight, but say, 'I'll change what I can and if things get worse, I'm moving on.'"

That's just what she did. In 1998, after seventeen years with the group, she quit. The response was brutal. "My colleagues—people who were not even my partners—reacted to me in a very negative way," recalls Maura. "Who did I think I was? How dare I do this? It's not what I expected." Again she relied on meditation to get her through, turning for support to the nearby Namgyal Monastery, in Ithaca, New York, the North American seat of His Holiness the Dalai Lama.

But it wasn't until 2007, when she participated in a meditation-retreat-cum-study eighty-three hundred feet high in the Colorado Rocky Mountains, that her relationship with stress changed not just in degree but in kind.

Called the Shamatha Project, the three-month retreat in Colorado's Shambhala Mountain Center was a collaboration between a team of scientists, including Blackburn and Epel, neuroscientist Clifford D. Saron, Ph.D., and Buddhist scholar B. Alan Wallace, Ph.D. Its aim was to investigate the long-term effects of Shamatha, a "calm abiding" practice drawn from Buddhist traditions, on a host of biological and psychological indicators.

"After the retreat, I could *see* my projections," says Maura. She became acutely aware that she—and no one else—was responsible for her feelings, regardless of how others treated her. The insight extended to parental blame. "I got really bored with that storyline and focused on my own agency," she says. "And I realized how the normal chatter in our heads actually maintains an identity for us, defining our image of who we think we are." The Shamatha Project allowed the chatter to be not silenced but hushed, clearing her perceptions.

These days, Maura has greater patience and trusts her intuition more. "Before, when I didn't meditate as much, I'd easily lose perspective, get caught up in the emotional second," she says. "It was like being buffeted by the wind—trying to control things and being thrown this way and that. Now I watch from a distance and choose what to try to change and what to walk away from."

Minding Your Mindfulness

Knowing how mindful you are today can help you chart the best stress-reduction path for tomorrow. Answer the twelve questions below to learn your starting point on the road to mindfulness.

People have a variety of ways of relating to their thoughts and feelings. For each of the items below, circle the rating that applies to you. (Notice that the ratings for items 2, 6, and 7 are flipped.)

1. It is easy for me to concentrate on what I am doing.

1	2	3	4
Rarely/Not at all	Sometimes	Often	Almost always

2. I am preoccupied by the future.

4	3	2	1
Rarely/Not at all	Sometimes	Often	Almost always

3. I can tolerate emotional pain.

1	2	3	4
Rarely/Not at all	Sometimes	Often	Almost always

4. I can accept things I cannot change.

1	2	3	4
Rarely/Not at all	Sometimes	Often	Almost always

5. I can usually describe how I feel at the moment in considerable detail.

1	2	3	4
Rarely/Not at all	Sometimes	Often	Almost always

6. I am easily distracted.

4	3	2	1
Rarely/Not at all	Sometimes	Often	Almost always

7. I am preoccupied by the past.

4	3	2	1
Rarely/Not at all	Sometimes	Often	Almost always

8. It's easy for me to keep track of my thoughts and feelings.

1	2	3	4
Rarely/Not at all	Sometimes	Often	Almost always

9. I try to notice my thoughts without judging them.

1	2	3	4
Rarely/Not at all	Sometimes	Often	Almost always

10. I am able to accept the thoughts and feelings I have.

1	2	3	4
Rarely/Not at all	Sometimes	Often	Almost always

11. I am able to focus on the present moment.

1	2	3	4
Rarely/Not at all	Sometimes	Often	Almost always

12. I am able to pay close attention to one thing for a long period of time.

1	2	3	4
Rarely/Not at all	Sometimes	Often	Almost always

Calculating your score:

Add together the values you have circled for all twelve items. Scores range from 12 to 48. Higher values reflect greater mindfulness of thoughts and feelings.

Interpreting your score the *Stress Less* way*:

Scores of 29 or lower reflect below-average levels of mindfulness of thoughts and feelings.
A score of 34 reflects average levels.
Scores of 39 or higher reflect above-average levels.

---

* The *Stress Less* interpretation was developed by the author, not the scientists.

~~~

Psychologist James Carmody, Ph.D., a researcher in mindfulness meditation at the University of Massachusetts Medical School, likens changes
in perception such as Maura's to a fish's awakening to the existence of
water in its bowl. "See the water you're swimming through?" Carmody
asks the fish. "What water?" the fish initially responds. But then, after
intentionally directing its attention to its environment, a lightbulb goes
off: "Ah, now I see."

Along the same lines, how conscious are you that you sit in an ocean
of air?

And more to the point of this book: Is there any scientific evidence
that such awareness can actually affect how you age?

Neuroscientist Clifford Saron, at the University of California, Davis's Center for Mind and Brain, wanted to know the answer to that
question, among many others relating to the neurological and behavioral effects of meditation practice. He led the team of scientists studying
the participants in the Shamatha Project that Maura took part in—an
endeavor, he says, he began planning in 2002 with UC Davis colleagues
and B. Alan Wallace, director of the Santa Barbara Institute for Consciousness Studies. His Holiness the Dalai Lama endorsed the project
seven years later, when the study became open to the public.

Saron's team was charged with designing the longitudinal, randomized, and controlled three-month study, which included a host of physiological and behavioral experiments examining attention and emotion
regulation. They were also to collect and analyze various biological
markers of health, including telomerase, the enzyme that keeps our telomeres up to snuff. Biological markers such as stress hormones have been
measured in meditation trials before, but this was the first time that telomerase was considered.

The scientists tracked telomerase activity against psychological
measures derived from participants' scores on a mindfulness test, from
a personality test assessing neuroticism, and from elements of the Ryff

Scales of Psychological Well-Being, developed by University of Michigan psychologist Carol D. Ryff, Ph.D. The instrument assesses what Ryff calls "the six different dimensions of well-being": environmental mastery, self-acceptance, purpose in life, personal growth, positive relations, and autonomy. These categories, says Ryff, are anything but arbitrary. "They came from my reviewing lots of prior theories of optimal human functioning," she says, "and then developing a measurement tool for the top dimensions that repeatedly came up." Saron's team zeroed in on two of those dimensions: purpose in life and environmental mastery, the latter of which they translated as "perceived control."

The Shamatha retreat was revolutionary not only because it dove into the nascent science of telomere biology but also because it was science driven. "A research team has never set up a three-month retreat before," says Saron, a warm, wry bear of a man who favors khakis and plaid shirts, and totes his laptop in a wheeled suitcase. "The way this has always been done is that the retreat is set up by a meditation center and the researchers show up like filmmakers do and film an event. They have nothing to do with who's in that retreat or with the structure of it. We did something completely unique, which was work with Alan to create essentially an admissions committee, the advertising material, and the retreat logistics. He was in charge of what was taught and the schedule of practice. We were in charge of the testing."

As Alan Wallace speaks, he radiates calm, releasing his clasped hands periodically to shape the air into spirals and tunnels that give a kind of physical volume to his thoughts. Trained for fourteen years as a Buddhist monk, he's the author of many books investigating what science and spirituality share, including the recent *Mind in the Balance: Meditation in Science, Buddhism, and Christianity*. For the Shamatha Project, Wallace led a group meditation every morning and evening aimed at "focusing the development of attention," and supplemented that instruction with the cultivation of the Four Immeasurables: loving-kindness, compassion, empathetic joy, and equanimity. (These practices are described in detail in Wallace's *The Attention Revolution*.) The carefully screened participants then went off to meditate on their own for an average of five hours a day.

"The meditation techniques we used emphasize the cultivating of focused attention," explains Saron. "For instance, how long can you keep your mind on an object without distraction, and how much mental effort is required to do so? What is the quality of that attention? Is it vivid? Is it fuzzy? And are you experiencing a sense of internal relaxation or of striving? Buddhist tradition says that training attention has implications for emotion regulation. Emotion regulation, in turn, should affect how you react to events in your life, and on downstream physiological consequences that we can measure with stress biomarkers."

What exactly is emotion regulation? In a nutshell: If we can view the components of our environment, both external and internal (thoughts, feelings, sensations) as objects, separate from ourselves with no a priori meaning, we can regain control over how we react to them.

There are hundreds of types of meditation practice, some begun thousands of years ago by Eastern cultures, others developed within the past ten years and considered reductionist by those who are classically trained. They range from the classical Buddhist traditions of Mahayana and Theravada to Zen, from compassion meditation to yoga to Integrated Body-Mind Training (IBMT). Those scientifically studied have been shown to elicit what cardiologist Herbert Benson, M.D., nearly forty years ago, dubbed the relaxation response. An antidote to the stress response, the relaxation response slows HPA-axis and sympathetic nervous system activity while increasing parasympathetic activity. It results in lowered oxygen consumption, respiratory rate, and blood pressure, and an increased sense of well-being. Many types of meditation elicit much more than that when practiced long term, including a spiritual connection to what practitioners call "the universal and transcendent Existence."

Still, broadly speaking, most types of meditation accentuate one of two styles: focused attention and open monitoring.

In focused attention, you direct your attention to an object, such as the breath, or a mantra, and you sustain it. Shamatha and Transcendental Meditation (TM) fall into that bucket. In open monitoring, you scan what's happening within your awareness, both inside and outside of you, from moment to moment, without judgment. Mindfulness-Based Stress Reduction (MBSR), a mainstream-oriented practice developed in the late seventies by Jon Kabat-Zinn at the University of Massachusetts Medical School, fits there. Often, open monitoring will start with focused attention to calm the mind and reduce distractions, and then move on to its awareness-monitoring aspect.

For the Shamatha Project, Saron and his colleagues, including UC Davis postdoc Tonya Jacobs, Ph.D., broke the participants, ages twenty-one to sixty-nine, into two groups: an experimental group, whose thirty members would go on the first three-month retreat; and a control "wait-list" group, whose thirty members would remain at their homes living their lives but be flown to the Shambhala Mountain Center and back before, in the middle, and after the end of the retreat to be tested alongside those in the experimental group. Then the people in the control group, having completed their function as controls for both the first retreat group and themselves, would go on their own three-month retreat. Because of technical limitations, telomerase could be tested only post-retreat, from sixteen subjects in the experimental group and twenty-five in the control group—not optimal from a rigorous-trial perspective, say the scientists, but still valid.

Jacobs reported results for the project for the first time at the July 2009 ISPNE conference, in San Francisco. Her presentation blew me away. At retreat's end, the telomerase levels of the experimental group were significantly *higher* than those of the controls. For me, a graph Jacobs flashed on the screen said it all: The telomerase level for the experimental group was 30 percent higher than that of the control group. Driving the rise in telomerase, Jacobs explained, were psychological changes: an increase in perceived control and a decrease in neuroticism. Later, in a paper she submitted for publication, Jacobs reported that the beneficial changes in perceived control and neuroticism in the experimental group were, in turn, explained by increases in both mindfulness and a sense of purpose in life. The latter also corresponded directly with the increase in telomerase activity.

Does this mean that the cells of meditators, influenced by changes in perception, may age more slowly than those of non-meditators? Or looked at another way: Might taking up meditation, with its ability to quash stress and increase well-being, slow the rate at which we age?

Jacobs is a soft-spoken, serious woman in her thirties who's open to argument and remains guarded in her interpretation of the results. "The main group effect is statistically significant, but it is not a strong effect," she says over the clang of forks and cacophony of voices at San Francisco's oldest restaurant, the Tadich Grill, where she, Saron, and I are having dinner. We're lined up at the eatery's gigunda mahogany bar like data points on a graph, my tape recorder in the middle. Despite her caution, I remain thoroughly impressed. So does Saron. "The critical point is that we are demonstrating a relationship between changes in specific psychological traits and telomerase levels that has never been demonstrated before," he says, diving into his pile of scallops and brussels sprouts.

The Shamatha Project provides the first *biological* evidence that training our minds may slow the aging of our cells. Meditation, it tells us, could indeed be life-changing—as in able to actually change the matter of our lives.

Saron's team incorporates into their paper a model developed by Epel, Blackburn, and colleagues that suggests just how the practice may do that. Taking Kabat-Zinn's mindfulness meditation as their starting point, Epel and Blackburn trace how meditation may enable us to turn our view of a threat, which sends our stress response into overdrive, into that of a challenge, a situation whose outcome we not only can control but relish. Indeed, challenge stress (the good kind of stress), as we discussed in the introduction, can actually spur our brains to grow new connections and even new neurons. And a threat, as noted in Chapter 1, does the opposite: It throws our cortisol, insulin, and oxidative stress into high gear, knocks down our production of building-block hormones such as dehydroepiandrosterone (DHEA), insulin-like growth factor, androgens, and growth factor, and decreases the ability of our parasympathetic nervous system to turn off the rapid heart rate and respiration that kick in to cope with emergencies.

That's the type of hormonal imbalance, Epel writes, that can impair telomere length. A challenge, on the other hand, flips that ratio, boosting the building-block hormones and reducing the others. Move beyond challenge to the relaxation that comes with mindfulness and you'll push that ratio even more in your favor.

Epel's team sums up its proposed model this way: Meditation "may have salutary effects on telomere length by reducing cognitive stress and stress arousal and increasing positive states of mind and hormonal factors that may promote telomere maintenance."

Just reading that as I slowly exhale makes me feel younger.

～～～

Scientific study of a subject as gravity-defying as meditation has its challenges. The practice itself is as amorphous as breath, and the guises it comes in are legion. From a logistical standpoint, arranging a credible test for the control group is outrageously difficult. The gold standard is to pair the actual intervention with an analogous but not active program; for example, using sham acupuncture needles on the control group to test against the real acupuncture needles being used on the experimental group. But what can you put in a "fake" meditation program that will keep people coming (let alone convinced) for even eight weeks—the length of MBSR training? As we saw earlier, Saron and Jacobs, like so many other meditation researchers, had to rely on a "wait-list" control group—folks who stood by rather than engaged in a comparable but nonactive program themselves.

Indeed, a rigorous 472-page meta-analysis on the state of meditation research that came out in June 2007—well before Jacobs and Saron's paper—concluded that comparing one practice with another was like setting apples up against oranges (against bananas against pineapples), and that, by and large, the methods of examining the fruit were sorely lacking. The report, prepared for the U.S. Department of Health and Human Services (USDHHS), scrutinized a whopping 813 studies through 2005 in five broad meditation categories, and looked at health outcomes ranging from cardiovascular disease to substance abuse to stress.

Its conclusion? "Scientific research on meditation practices does not appear to have a common theoretical perspective and is characterized by poor methodological quality," write the authors, led by Maria B. Ospina, M.Sc., of the University of Alberta Evidence-Based Practice Center. "Firm conclusions on the effects of meditation practices in health care cannot be drawn based on the available evidence."

And yet tens of thousands of people who've participated in those studies or in myriad meditation-based stress-reduction programs—as well as the scientists and clinicians evaluating their results—attest to the benefits of meditation, regardless of the technique. They point to its success in treating a host of ailments, including chronic pain, insomnia, hot flashes, depression, infertility, and autoimmune diseases such as psoriasis. Many talk about a dose-dependent effect—that is, the longer and more intensely you practice, the greater the benefits.

Using functional magnetic resonance imaging (fMRI), which measures functioning in the brain based on changes in blood flow, scientists such as the University of Michigan's Richard Davidson, Ph.D., have peered into the brains of novice practitioners and Tibetan Buddhist monks, showing that the monks have more gray matter in regions associated with emotion regulation and memory retention (the prefrontal cortex and hippocampus, respectively). Hence the claim for meditation's contribution to brain plasticity—our ability to change our own brains.

Other brain-imaging studies show that the amygdala—the seat of emotional reactivity—is more excitable in non-meditators than in controls (that's Davidson's study, too) and that after an MBSR intervention, gray-matter density in the amygdala actually decreases, along with levels of perceived stress (that one was led by Harvard's Britta Hözel, Ph.D., and Sara Lazar, Ph.D.). Another study points to stronger activity in the ventral anterior cingulate cortex (vACC)—a brain region that controls the parasympathetic arm of the autonomic nervous system (the part that slows us down)—after a mere five days of IBMT (that was run by the University of Oregon's Yi Yuan Tang). Still others point to increased activation in brain areas associated with monitoring (the dorsolateral prefrontal cortex) and engaging attention (the visual cortex), and to greater control of limited attentional resources, enabling meditators to see signals others miss.

Research also shows myriad physiological changes downstream from the neurological ones. Among them are boosted immune function and greater heart-rate variability (as discussed in Chapter 1), and decreases in systolic and diastolic blood pressure, heart rate, oxygen consumption, carbon dioxide elimination, and cortisol levels in response to a stressor.

That meditation reduces stress is a constant in nearly all of the reports. Indeed, two of the most mainstream practices use the stress-reduction concept in their names: Kabat-Zinn's Mindfulness-Based Stress Reduction, and the relaxation response introduced by Harvard's Herbert Benson. UMass's Carmody has shown that people who completed the eight-week MBSR program reduced their levels of perceived stress by more than 20 percent, and those who started out the most stressed reduced their levels by an impressive 30 percent.

What's going on in the brain to permit that? Meditation, say imaging experts such as Davidson, acts on the same neural circuitry as the stress response. "It's a set of interconnected brain regions that play a role in how we regulate emotion," says Davidson. "It includes the anterior cingulate, the prefrontal cortex, the insula—an area critical for communication with visceral organs and bodily functions—the amygdala, and the hippocampus,"

The study of meditation is still in its infancy, despite the fact that it's come a long way since TM burst onto the scene, in the early 1970s, when flocks of consciousness-seeking college students (me included) trucked over to our local maharishi center with forty bucks, a flower, and a white handkerchief to receive our "personalized" mantra. Those were the days when the TM acolytes were claiming the practice could change not just your blood pressure but the state of the economy. But scientific evidence for the benefits of meditation is growing every year as rigorous scientists such as Carmody, Saron, and Davidson continue to plumb the reasons behind its physiological effects.

"The applications continue to expand with promising results, and more and more studies about possible mechanisms of action are being explored," says Kabat-Zinn, citing telomeres as a cutting-edge example. He issues a caveat, too, about throwing disparate practices into one basket, as the USDHHS study did: "If you look at apples, oranges, bananas, and pineapples all together," he says, "you are going to get a fruit salad that doesn't tell you anything meaningful about apples themselves."

Through a Glass, Not Darkly:
Stress, Aging, and Optimism/Pessimism

By all accounts, Eileen Attridge should be chronically stressed. She's the primary caregiver of two challenging daughters. Rosie, who was fifteen when I met her, was diagnosed with severe autism at age two. The now smiling girl bopping to popular tunes in Eileen's San Francisco apartment didn't talk for years or engage with anyone around her. Eileen's other daughter, Teresa, just one year older, is a "typically developing teenager," says Eileen, "with typical teenage issues, which are just hellsome."

Rosie wasn't always so sanguine. During her elementary school years, she went through more than a dozen aides working to socialize her. After each one left, Attridge would watch in horror as her daughter regressed—biting and throwing pots and plates. A devout Catholic, Attridge found solace from her struggles at church, but when Rosie was seven, the pastor asked the family to leave, claiming Rosie was "too disruptive" to attend Sunday Mass. Eileen lost not only her church but the depth of her faith. In addition, the battles—legal and otherwise—with the public school district to secure an appropriate education for Rosie at times became "nightmarish," leading Eileen to yank her daughter out of the classroom for weeks at a stretch.

Still, Eileen, with her glistening black hair and talent for whipping up batches of cookies in her galley kitchen, maintained a "solution-oriented, glass-half-full attitude," she says. In 2008, she—along with some sixty other mothers caring for chronically ill children—participated in Epel and Blackburn's groundbreaking research, described in Chapter 2, which showed that chronic stress may literally gnaw at our DNA, speeding up the rate at which our cells age by ten years or more. Eileen had joined the study hoping to contribute to the understanding of autism's effects on family and friends. It turned out she contributed even more.

Eileen became the symbol of the good news the scientists uncovered. As you'll recall, what matters in cell aging is the level of *perceived* stress, they reported, not an objective measure of circumstances. To wit: Despite Eileen's many years caring for Rosie, her DNA "age," as measured by the length of her telomeres, matched that of the study's controls, not that of the harried caregivers. Attitude, not circumstance, made the difference.

"I was the exception," says Eileen with a laugh. "When it comes to Rosie, it's never 'Why me?' It's always 'Why not me?'" she says. "No one can take care of Rosie better than I can. I can deal."

How Full—or Empty—Is Your Glass?

The way we see the world has a huge effect on how much events stress us—psychologically and physiologically. The following test provides a window onto where you fall on the optimism-pessimism continuum.

Please answer the following questions about yourself by indicating the extent of your agreement using the scale following each question. Be as honest as you can throughout, and try not to let your responses to one question influence your response to other questions. There are no right or wrong answers. (Please note that responses to items 2, 4, and 5 are reversed.)

1. In uncertain times, I usually expect the best.

    0 = Strongly disagree   1 = Disagree   2 = Neutral
    3 = Agree   4 = Strongly agree

2. If something can go wrong for me, it will.

    4 = Strongly disagree   3 = Disagree   2 = Neutral
    1 = Agree   0 = Strongly agree

3. I'm always optimistic about my future.

    0 = Strongly disagree   1 = Disagree   2 = Neutral
    3 = Agree   4 = Strongly agree

4. I hardly ever expect things to go my way.

    4 = Strongly disagree   3 = Disagree   2 = Neutral
    1 = Agree   0 = Strongly agree

5. I rarely count on good things happening to me.

    4 = Strongly disagree   3 = Disagree   2 = Neutral
    1 = Agree   0 = Strongly agree

6. Overall, I expect more good things to happen to me than bad.

    0 = Strongly disagree   1 = Disagree   2 = Neutral
    3 = Agree   4 = Strongly agree

Calculating and interpreting your score:

Add up your responses to items 1 through 6. Scores will range from 0 to 24. *Higher scores indicate greater optimism.* The average score for the 2,204 men and women given the test to judge its validity was 15.

The "values" for optimism and pessimism are not absolute but relative, notes test author Michael F. Scheier, Ph.D., head of Carnegie Mellon University's Department of Psychology. "We think of optimism and pessimism as being continuous in nature—one is either lower or higher than someone else," he says.

Where do you fall relative to that average of 15? More optimistic or less?

~~~~~~

That optimism correlates with reduced stress levels and physical benefits is not news. Numerous scientific studies from around the globe have linked optimism and its relatives ("feeling," or "affective" states such as well-being, emotional vitality, and happiness) with decreased rates of everything from heart disease to diabetes to mortality. But that optimism or pessimism may influence the very aging of our cells is an eye-opener. The findings confirm that slowing aging lies, at least in part, in the mindset with which we approach the world.

In August 2009, two studies emerged that essentially summed up the history of optimism research.

Heather N. Rasmussen, Ph.D., and colleagues at Carnegie Mellon University raked the scientific literature for both observational and experimental papers on the topic published through April 2009. They then re-crunched all the data to discern general patterns. They ended up analyzing data from eighty-three studies that met strict criteria. All came from peer-reviewed English-language journals. Most were longitudinal and prospective—that is, forward looking and therefore not colored by memory—and used the Life Orientation Test (LOT) or Life Orientation Test-Revised (LOT-R), the quiz at the start of this section, to measure optimism and pessimism. The paper, called "Optimism and Physical Health: A Meta-analytic Review," includes all the heavies in the field in its pages.*

Rasmussen minces no words in her conclusion: "The results from the overall analysis help to document the positive role that optimism plays in physical well-being," she writes. Moreover, her separate analy-

---

* In addition to authors Michael F. Scheier, Ph.D., and Joel B. Greenhouse, Ph.D., both from Carnegie Mellon, there are, among others, Andrew Steptoe, Ph.D., and Yoichi Chida, Ph.D., at the University College London; Laura D. Kubzansky, Ph.D., at the Harvard School of Public Health; Suzanne C. Segerstrom, Ph.D., at the University of Kentucky; Sheldon Cohen, Ph.D., at Carnegie Mellon University, and Erik J. Giltay, Ph.D., M.D., at Leiden University Medical Center, in the Netherlands. Rasmussen herself, a graduate student when she spearheaded the study, is now at the University of Kansas.

ses of studies with specific outcomes—survival, mortality, heart health, immune function, cancer, pregnancy—also showed significant links between optimism and good health. Optimism, she concluded, borrowing a phrase from the business world, "provides value added."

Hilary A. Tindle, M.D., M.P.H., an internist at the University of Pittsburgh School of Medicine, heartily agrees. She was lead author of a huge epidemiological study that looked at the influence of optimism on heart disease and mortality over eight years. It analyzed data from ninety-seven thousand of the postmenopausal women enrolled in the Women's Health Initiative, an NIH-funded study that has been following women ages fifty to seventy-nine since 1994.

Tindle compared female optimists to female pessimists, also using the LOT-R, and found that the optimists were 14 percent less likely to die from any cause and 30 percent less likely to die from coronary heart disease than the pessimists. This was after adjusting for various demographic, health-risk, and psychosocial factors, including age, race, education, income, hypertension, smoking, diabetes, high cholesterol, depression, alcohol use, hormone replacement therapy, physical activity, and BMI.

The adjustments are important. "What they say is, the results are not just from education, not just from income, not just from smoking, diabetes, exercise, or depression," says Tindle. "They're from something else."

Yet an observational study such as Tindle's can go only so far. It took startling research by UCSF's Aoife O'Donovan, Ph.D., to tie optimism and pessimism not just to physical health but to biological aging.

O'Donovan was a first-year graduate student in her native Ireland when Epel and Blackburn's findings linking leukocyte telomere attrition and chronic stress came out. She'd run a study there showing that optimism and pessimism were both linked with mental-health outcomes—specifically, anxiety and depression (optimism with less, pessimism with more)—but that pessimism alone was associated with physical ailments, as measured largely by absence from work due to sickness. The Blackburn and Epel paper inspired her to look deeper, to see where the biological effects of stress fit into the picture. But it wasn't until several years later, when she was a visiting grad student in Epel's UCSF lab, that she had the chance to design a study to do just that.

For her subjects she used thirty-six healthy women ages fifty-one to seventy-nine, who were in the stressful situation of caring for a spouse with dementia. Twenty-three were caregivers; thirteen were controls. She analyzed their blood, taken at the start of the study, to assess telomere length and levels of the pro-inflammatory cytokine IL-6, as well as their answers on several tests, including the Perceived Stress Scale, the LOT-R, and inventories of emotional stability, physical activity, and sleep difficulties.

Why did O'Donovan measure IL-6, a marker of inflammation? To O'Donovan, inflammatory markers reflect how "old" a person's immune systems is, a critical variable in assessing how stress might age us. Levels of IL-6 rise, remember, to battle infection or disease—a good thing in the short term but a bad thing in the long term, as continued overproduction of IL-6, or chronic inflammation, can make the immune system vulnerable to invaders and more susceptible to diseases of aging such as cardiovascular disease, type 2 diabetes, and certain cancers. Recall, too, that both acute and chronic psychological stress have been associated with increased IL-6, and that repeated inflammation has been linked with shorter leukocyte telomeres, likely because it indicates higher rates of immune-cell turnover and greater oxidative stress. The bottom line, according to O'Donovan, is that inflammation may be a driver that is aging us overall.

"For me, it's all about inflammation," says O'Donovan, via Skype, from Dublin. "We know that immune-system markers predict health outcomes and mortality. And—this is very controversial—the immunologic theory of aging suggests that immune-system aging is core to general-systems aging."

O'Donovan's results drew a clear line between such aging and a person's outlook. Specifically, her team found that pessimism was strongly associated with both shorter telomeres and higher IL-6 concentrations, even after controlling for age and the length of time each woman had been a caregiver. And the results stood firm even after the effects of perceived stress were taken into account. This means that in and of itself—separate from all other factors—the more pessimistic a caregiver was, the "older" her immune system.

Indeed, those with the highest pessimism scores had telomeres that were roughly eleven to twenty-three years shorter than those with the lowest pessimism scores. Add stress to the mix and you've got an aging double whammy.

What might be going on? It could be that a pessimistic outlook makes you more vulnerable to stress, leading you to perceive an event as threatening that an optimist may brush off. And when you feel threatened, as we saw in Chapter 1, your pro-inflammatory response turns on high in preparation for a possible injury.

Psychologists classify optimism and pessimism as personality traits—as opposed to emotions or affective states, such as happiness and depression. That means they generally remain stable across time, unless there's an intervention. An argument rages among researchers as to whether optimism and pessimism are opposite poles on a continuum, or two different constructs altogether, activating different parts of the brain. O'Donovan subscribes to the latter view, pointing out a recent study by Tali Sharot, Ph.D., and colleagues at New York University, that used fMRIs to show that specific parts of the brain—the amygdala and the rostral anterior cingulate cortex (rACC)—light up when subjects imagine *positive* future events. Indeed, the rACC's brilliance, Sharot found, depends on how high the subjects scored as optimists.

Why does the traits' definition matter? "From an intervention point of view, if optimism and pessimism are entirely different systems, it may not be important to encourage people to think positive things, but it may be important to help them to counter their overly negative expectations," says O'Donovan. It's a new but subtle way of assessing the so-called positive-psychology movement.

O'Donovan's take eschews adopting a Pollyanna attitude—or, as psychologist Seymour Epstein dubbed it in 1989, naive optimism; that is, denying what is real. "That's where people just think that everything's going to be fine," says UCLA psychologist Shelley E. Taylor, Ph.D., who specializes in how social relationships affect stress levels (more on how social support affects stress in Chapter 7). "They're people who are in denial, who aren't processing, versus most optimists, who actually think things are going to go well because they're pretty good at this—they have control."

It also eschews the slip down the slope to the place where people blame themselves for illnesses such as cancer, or for the inability to combat those illnesses. Cultural commentator Barbara Ehrenreich got that right in her witty, stinging (though decidedly one-sided) *Bright-Sided: How the Relentless Promotion of Positive Thinking Has Undermined America.* Seeking help online and elsewhere when she got her own breast-cancer diagnosis, Ehrenreich was overrun by positivity proselytizers, chiding her for her anger and urging her to "embrace" her cancer as a "gift." She was having none of it: "Breast cancer, I can now report, did not make me prettier or stronger, more feminine or spiritual," she writes. "What it gave me, if you want to call this a 'gift,' was a very personal, agonizing encounter with an ideological force in American culture that I had not been aware of before—one that encourages us to deny reality, submit cheerfully to misfortune, and blame only ourselves for our fate."

What O'Donovan's take does advocate is assessing the new science on optimism/pessimism and positive affect with clear eyes, to take to heart the studies that are rigorously designed and analyzed by serious scientists, and to apply the results appropriately: The way you approach the world may alter the way the world affects you.

The University of Michigan's Carol Ryff sums up the complexities this way: "Aristotle wrote about *eudaimonia* as the ultimate objective in life," she says. "What he meant by that was not 'happiness.' In fact, he likens happiness to sort of cows grazing in the field and feeling content, and the higher level of well-being that humans are capable of involves striving in the face of adversity, working hard to make the most of your talent and potential. So *eudaimonia* in Aristotle's formulation is really about what he calls the 'realization of your true potential.' That requires hard work, and you don't always feel good when you're in the middle of what may be major life pursuits, whether it's raising your kids or doing a good job at work or whatever. John Stuart Mill probably said one of the wisest things ever about happiness when he said happiness will not be achieved if you make it an end in itself; it's a by-product of other, more noble pursuits."

As Mill put it in his autobiography: "Those only are happy (I thought) who have their minds fixed on some object other than their own happiness; on the happiness of others, on the improvement of mankind, even on some art or pursuit, followed not as a means, but as itself an ideal end. Aiming thus at something else, they find happiness by the way."

To Reduce Stress and Slow
the Cellular Clock Using Your Mind

My Meditation, Myself

1. Recollect Awareness

Jason Siff, author of the recently released *Unlearning Meditation: What to Do When the Instructions Get in the Way*, has developed a new approach to meditation that takes the practice out of the hands of experts and puts it squarely in our own. In doing so, the practice, called Recollective Awareness (translated from the Pali word *anupassana*), speaks directly to the central tenet of this book: When we feel that *we* are in control of a circumstance, our stress levels drop—regardless of whether that circumstance is our meditation method, our diet, or our exercise or sleep regimen.

Siff, a Buddhist monk in Sri Lanka in the late 1980s and cofounder of the not-for-profit Skillful Meditation Project, in Los Angeles, has written the following meditation instructions *specifically* for readers of this book: smart, active, *stressed* people sandwiched between caring for children and caring for elderly parents, between the demands of work and a commitment to physical and psychological well-being, between balancing budgets and giving their kids everything they themselves never had.*

From Jason Siff to you:

Recollective Awareness Meditation is an open and "allowing" approach to meditation. It initially develops gentleness, tolerance, patience, and acceptance, and it can also lead to relaxation. In contrast to other forms of meditation, it allows thoughts and feelings, and adapts to each individual's experience as he or she practices. It also includes a period of "recollecting" the meditation experience, which is a way of bringing awareness to what happens during practice. This kind of recollection helps you develop greater familiarity with your meditative experiences, thus leading to a fuller understanding of how the mind works in both meditation and daily life.

Instructions for Recollective Awareness Meditation

Sit in a comfortable posture with your eyes closed. Bring your attention to the touch of your hands on your lap or your knees, but do not try to hold your attention there. Instead allow your thoughts, feelings, sensations, and breathing (and whatever else may be going on) to continue uninterrupted.

You are not trying to stop your thoughts or feelings; rather, you are learning to *show preference* for the touch of the hands while allowing those thoughts and feelings to come, stay, and leave on their own. You are, essentially, showing preference for being with the experience of your body sitting still, even though your mind may be drawn into that still-

* If you want to contact a teacher or learn more about his method, visit www.skill fulmeditation.org.

ness for only a few seconds at a time. Remember, if your thoughts and feelings continue to occupy much of your attention, that is just what you are experiencing and it does not need to be changed.

Following these instructions, you may experience lengthy periods when your mind is very active, making it difficult for you to stay with the touch of the hands for even a few seconds. You may wonder if sitting with all this mental chatter is really meditating; I assure you it is. If you force your mind to be still, that will just create agitation, tension, aggression, and self-dislike. In this path of gaining greater peace and tranquility, you are using peaceful means from the very beginning.

Since you are giving up much of your control over your experience, you may find that your attention shifts from one thing to the next. Let it. If your attention is drawn to sounds, let it be with sounds. If you become aware of the breath, you can let your attention stay with your breathing. When your attention moves to something else, allow it to leave the breath.

PRACTICAL CONSIDERATIONS FOR MEDITATING

There is no one right meditation posture for everyone all the time. Start off by sitting in a comfortable position, whether on a chair or a cushion. You can even lie down if you need to, but try to adopt a lying-down posture that is not used for sleep, such as lying flat on your back. If you need to change position during the meditation period, try to do it slowly and quietly, and remain in the new posture for some time before moving again.

People new to meditation should try to sit for fifteen to twenty minutes. Those who have meditated before can start with thirty minutes. You can use a pleasant-sounding timer or have a clock in view, which you can check periodically during the meditation period.

You don't need to have a perfectly quiet and peaceful environment, but in general try not to sit in a noisy or crowded place. Choose a time of day when you are less likely to be disturbed. Remember to turn off the ringer on your phone.

WHEN THE MEDITATION PERIOD IS OVER

After each meditation sitting, take a few moments to silently recollect what went on during your practice. Start by recalling what is easy to remember and then try to recall parts of the sitting that are more difficult to bring back to mind. A good deal of each meditation sitting may be difficult to retrieve afterward, so be satisfied with a simple recollection of what you truly remember.

To aid in this process of recollection, you might want to keep a meditation journal. If you decide to write down your meditation experiences, give yourself an extra five to ten minutes after the sitting to do so. Try to write a narrative of what you experienced in the meditation sitting. You can also list your experiences. In both cases, try to capture your thoughts, feelings, images, and sensations—you may find that similes and longer descriptions are more accurate than single words. Try to be as honest as you can about what you experienced, as that is more important than getting all the details right.

For each journal entry, include the day and time of the meditation sitting. Try to keep the journal for at least five meditation sittings so you get a sense of your journey. If while meditating you find that you are often thinking about what you are going to write in your journal, stop keeping a journal for a few meditation sittings and then pick it up again.

2. Breath of life

Even practiced meditators such as those in the Shamatha Project need help slowing down. Notes Cliff Saron, "When Alan was teaching people at the retreat, they would say things like, 'I can't focus at all. I can't find my breath.' And the answer would be, 'Can you find one breath?' It's not 'Can you sit for forty-five minutes or twenty minutes or five minutes.' This is a developmental process of learning."

We'd all do well to heed that gentle advice.

The role of the breath is central in most meditation practices. The reason is as much physiological as psychological. "Whenever you inhale, you turn on the sympathetic nervous system slightly, minutely speeding up your heart," writes Robert Sapolsky in *Why Zebras Don't Get Ulcers.* "And when you exhale, the parasympathetic half turns on, activating your vagus nerve to slow things down. This is why many forms of meditation are built around extended exhalations."

Recall the giant vagus nerve from Chapter 1: It snakes from the brain stem to the colon, with multitudinous fibers attached to various organs, including the heart and lungs, and slows the heart and respiratory rates, among other functions, once a stressor has passed.

Here are the instructions that Sat Bir Singh Khalsa, Ph.D., assistant professor of medicine at Harvard Medical School, gives to participants in his research studies, which concentrate on the psychophysiological mechanisms underlying the practice of meditation and yoga techniques. Try following them for at least ten minutes.

> As you inhale, the belly extends out as though it were being filled with air (it is not). Then, as the inhale continues and the belly extends fully, the chest expands. At the end of the inhale, pause very briefly, and then as you start to exhale, let the chest collapse first. As the exhale continues, the belly pulls in slightly as though it were being emptied of air. Then pause very briefly at the end of the exhale before beginning the next inhale. The breath rate should be four breaths per minute or slower (fifteen seconds or longer for each breath), but even six breaths per minute is therapeutic. It is important that this breathing is done through the nose. The eyes are closed during this exercise, and your mental attention is focused on the flow of the breath.

Counter Negativity

UCSF psychologist Judith T. Moskowitz, Ph.D., M.P.H., studies ways to "plant seeds of resilience" in people under extreme stress because they've recently been diagnosed with a chronic illness, in particular HIV. She knows, through years of research, that positive and negative emotions "co-occur" under conditions of stress but that people need help countering the negative and allowing the positive to rise through the muck. After scouring the scientific literature, she identified eight cognitive behavioral skills that are especially effective at helping people achieve this. "No one's saying these skills cure a disease," she says. "Rather, they give people additional resources for coping with stress, which may keep them healthier."

Moskowitz's theories jump off from the "broaden and build" function of positive emotion developed by Barbara L. Fredrickson, Ph.D., a professor at the University of North Carolina at Chapel Hill and author of the popular book *Positivity*. Negative affect gives us tunnel vision, Fredrickson says, while positive affect opens our vistas—both cognitive and behavioral—enabling us to look past a current stressor to creative ways to cope.

"Positive constructs, such as optimism and positive emotions, buffer negativity by building your resources—resilience, social connectedness—over time," says Fredrickson. "You broaden your outlook."

That's not to say there isn't a place for "necessary negativity," she adds. You're turned down for a job, so of course you're sad—angry at yourself, even. You figure out what went wrong (my ideas really are too renegade for a corporate boss) and move on. What works against us is "gratuitous negativity"— going global from a place of dishonesty fueled by hurt feelings (I suck as a writer because my editor kicked back my story). Blast gratuitous negativity apart "by examining the *facts*," writes Fredrickson. "Dispute it the way a good lawyer would."

Here, then, are the skills Moskowitz recommends developing. "Find at least one of these that works for you, and do it every day," she advises.

- **Notice something good that happened to you today, and tell someone about it or write it down.** The "event" can be as small as drinking an excellent cup of coffee or climbing out of bed when you planned to. "When you're under serious stress, it's particularly hard to see good things," says Moskowitz. "We focus on what's bad. In many ways that's adaptive: If something's going wrong, you need to address it." But evolutionary adaptations can work against us if the bad never lets up. Sharing a good event by telling it to someone or writing it down brings it out into the world and helps put the negative in perspective.

- **Keep a "gratitude" record.** Every day, to counter shortfalls, write down one thing you're grateful for. Again, it doesn't have to be earth shattering, or even big. Me? I'm grateful today that my daughter gave me one of her Pocky chocolate-covered Japanese dessert sticks. Truly. It's not just the chocolate I'm grateful for; it's her generosity to me (a rare thing).

- **Concentrate on being mindful for at least ten minutes a day.** Forget the past, forget the future: Take in, without judgment, your thoughts, feelings, and physical sensations *right now*. Go for a ten-minute walk and zero in on the crunch of gravel beneath your feet and the wind on your face. OK, it may sound corny. But if you're molecularly deciphering gravel, you're not hearing your 401(k) tank. Or sit in a comfortable chair and use the Recollective Awareness or breathing instructions described earlier. Moskowitz reports that a 2003 fMRI study by University of Michigan's Richard Davidson found that twenty-five subjects who did mindfulness meditation showed significant increases in left-sided anterior brain activation—an area that correlates with positive affect—as compared to sixteen subjects who did not meditate. And a team led by Fredrickson found that seven weeks of loving-kindness meditation increased subjects' daily positivity compared to a control group. This positivity was in turn linked to increased life satisfaction, decreased depression, and improved health even three months after the study began.

- **Reinterpret a negative experience.** This does not mean donning rose-colored glasses, stresses Moskowitz. It just means finding that "small, good thing"—to borrow a phrase from Raymond

Carver's marvelous short story—in the midst of the turmoil. The reinterpretation must be "do-able," says Moskowitz. You miss the bus to work and are sure you're going to be reprimanded for being late. But then another bus comes along, and you sit next to a woman who tells a terrific joke, and you laugh and laugh. Sure, it's not so great to see your boss's scowl when you arrive at the office at nine fifteen. But you can still remember that joke. In a meta-analysis of studies about coping with HIV, Moskowitz found that reappraisal was one of the skills most effective at reducing negativity.

- **Redirect your attention to your strengths.** Yes, I got furious with my eleven-year-old daughter when she rolled her eyes at me for the seventh time in an hour and then answered me in The Voice (you know, the one that says: "You are the stupidest human being on the planet"). I got very quiet and then stormed out of the neighborhood gift shop where we were shopping for her friend's birthday present. I even got in my car and moved it to another spot in the lot, so she could see me driving away. "What a horrible mother I am!" I wailed internally, going global on cue. But then I remembered: I sit with her every night while she does her homework, and I actually understand and can teach her sixth-grade math. I drive her hither and yon, and will drop anything when she needs me. I cook her the foods she wants (a very limited repertoire) and make sure she's rich in books she loves. My breathing slows, my chest relaxes. I can go back in the store now.

- **Make a list of *attainable* goals for the week, and work toward achieving *one* every day.** Think how good you'll feel when you can cross that item off that list! I struggle with this one all the time. Sure, I tell myself upon awakening, I can write five thousand words of this book today. Er, wait. Experience has shown me that one thousand is a reach; how about, say, five hundred? And then a bit of coaching: The words don't have to be good (I can always rewrite); they don't even have to be good *enough*. They just have to be. Best-selling author Anne Lamott perhaps puts it best, in her hilarious 1994 guide on writing, *Bird by Bird*, whose title sprang from her father's advice to her brother, age ten, as he struggled with a book report on birds: "Just take it bird by bird." Bird by bird. Word by word.

- **Do something nice for someone else.** Elizabeth W. Dunn, Ph.D., of the University of British Columbia, has done several studies showing that giving can make people happier. In one, she had forty-six UBC students rate their happiness and then gave them envelopes containing either five dollars or twenty dollars and instructed them either to spend the money on themselves or toward a bill, or to give the money to charity or as a gift. At the end of the day, the students again rated their happiness. Those who gave the money away, she found, were happier than those who kept it for themselves. In another study, Dunn's team gathered data on income, spending, and happiness from 632 men and women across the United States. It turned out that happiness correlated with the amount of money people spent on others rather than how much money they made. Dunn concluded that "intentional activities—practices in which people actively and effortfully choose to engage—may represent a more promising route to lasting happiness." There's that element of control again, which affects everything, it seems, from our stress levels to how fast we age.

CHAPTER 7

Stress and Social Support

There is something in staying close to men and women and
  looking on them, and in the contact and odour of them,
  that pleases the soul well,
All things please the soul, but these please the soul well.

—Walt Whitman, *Leaves of Grass*, 1921

In 2001, shortly after she'd moved her mother into a nursing home, Emily Lewis received devastating news: Jay, her best friend of eight years, her "number one cheerleader," had died tragically in a fire while on a hunting expedition. He was fifty years old.

"Jay was my go-to, my safety net," says Emily. "As long as he was around, I could call and say, 'I don't know what to do about A, B, or C.' And he would help me with it." She took a month off from her job as an intensive-care nurse at the Ohio State University Medical Center to recover. "Who's going to tell me now that everything's all right?" she wondered.

There had been lots of reasons to call Jay. Emily was the primary caregiver for her mother, who was diagnosed with Alzheimer's disease in 1993, at age seventy-one. They lived together on the family farm—420 acres of rolling fields in tiny Rushville, Ohio—along with Emily's two surviving aunts and an uncle. Emily managed the property, which included three houses and a barn full of horses.

After the last aunt died, in 1997, Emily stitched together a "patchwork quilt" of part-time help to care for her mother while she was at work. On weekends and holidays, Emily took charge round-the-clock herself. She'd turn on her mother's beloved classical music and settle her in a glide rocker—even in the barn, to have her near as Emily cleaned the stalls. She used aromatherapy with her mother after reading that it helped calm folks with "exacerbated emotions." She sat beside her at doctor's appointments, watching her slog through "mini-mental health tests" that required her to count backward and write sentences. "My favorite sentence she wrote was 'Let's get out of here,'" laughs Emily, with characteristic humor.

When her mother's mobility hit rock bottom, Emily moved her to the nursing facility to keep her safe. "It was like musical chairs," says Emily, recalling the once-bustling household. "Then the music stopped. And now there's nobody here."

At night Emily would wake up with a start, terrified: Her mother's care cost some six thousand dollars a month, and the trust her father had left them was dwindling. "I can bluff my way through a lot, but the reality was, How was I going to pay for next month?" she says. Her blood pressure soared—"160s, 170s over like 110," she says—and for the first time in her life she had to take blood-pressure medication.

She began seeing a therapist on the advice of her mother's geriatric specialist and turned to her three dogs for comfort. After Jay died, Emily even took the dogs to therapy. "I'd call and say, 'I'm not feeling loved today. They love me; they're coming with me.'" My therapist would go, 'All righty!' She became my safe person."

Emily's German shepherd, Knight, developed almost a sixth sense about her. "If my lip starts to quiver, and I get a little sad, Knight spoons with me in bed at night," says Emily.

She coped, too, by *giving* support. "I'm like my mother," she says. "If I help people, that's a good thing for Emily."

While still caring for her mother at home, Emily volunteered as an assistant dog trainer once a month at a nearby dog-training club. And she joined a program that taught prison inmates to care for abandoned dogs, preparing the dogs for adoption. "We call it Second Chance

Companions," says Emily. "It's not only for the four-legged but for the two-legged." And later, after her mother died, in 2008, she also became a medical guardian for the local branch of the Honor Flight Network, which flies World War II veterans to Washington, D.C., to visit their memorials. Emily pays her own way; the veterans go for free. Soon after, she was able to cut her blood-pressure dose by half.

Throughout those long years of caregiving and loss, Emily also found solace in her church and the tight-knit community of Rushville, a village of just 262 residents whose families have lived there for generations. "I distanced myself from the Eeyores of the world," she says, laughing.

"Rushville is kind of like Mayberry, is how we put it," she says. "It's a blessing, beyond words."

Getting by with a Little Help . . .

When the going gets tough, do you have people you can turn to? Answer these questions to learn the strength of your social-support safety net.

1. In general, how many people do you feel close to—that is, friends and family members with whom you feel at ease, can talk to about private matters, and can call on for help?

   0   1   2   3   4   5 or more

2. How often do you feel you have a definite place in your family and among your friends?

   1 (never)   2 (rarely)   3 (sometimes)   4 (frequently)
   5 (always)   0 (don't know or n/a)

3. When you're with your family and friends, how often do you feel you *don't belong*?

   1 (always)   2 (frequently)   3 (sometimes)   4 (rarely)
   5 (never)   0 (don't know or n/a)

4. How often do you wish you knew more people you could talk to about personal matters—that is, people who made you feel cared for?

    1 (always)   2 (frequently)   3 (sometimes)   4 (rarely)
    5 (never)   0 (don't know or n/a)

5. Do you feel that, on the whole, you did more for others in the last twelve months than others did for you, or did others do more for you?

    1 (I did more)   2 (about equal)   3 (others did more)
    0 (don't know or n/a)

6. How satisfied are you with the relationships you have with your relatives and friends?

    1 (not at all satisfied) 2 (not very satisfied) 3 (somewhat satisfied)
    4 (very satisfied)   5 (completely satisfied)

7. a. How often does your spouse/partner make you feel loved and cared for?

    1 (never)   2 (rarely)   3 (sometimes)   4 (frequently)
    5 (always)   0 (don't know or n/a)

  b. Your children? (If you don't have children, circle "0.")

    1 (never)   2 (rarely)   3 (sometimes)   4 (frequently)
    5 (always)   0 (don't know or n/a)

  c. Your extended family?

    1 (never)   2 (rarely)   3 (sometimes)   4 (frequently)
    5 (always)   0 (don't know or n/a)

  d. Your friends?

    1 (never)   2 (rarely)   3 (sometimes)   4 (frequently)
    5 (always)   0 (don't know or n/a)

8. a. How often is your spouse/partner willing to listen when you need to talk about your worries?

    1 (never)   2 (rarely)   3 (sometimes)   4 (frequently)
    5 (always)   0 (don't know or n/a)

b. Your children?

    1 (never)   2 (rarely)   3 (sometimes)   4 (frequently)
    5 (always)   0 (don't know or n/a)

c. Your extended family?

    1 (never)   2 (rarely)   3 (sometimes)   4 (frequently)
    5 (always)   0 (don't know or n/a)

d. Your friends?

    1 (never)   2 (rarely)   3 (sometimes)   4 (frequently)
    5 (always)   0 (don't know or n/a)

9. a. How often is your spouse/partner critical of what you do?

    1 (always)   2 (frequently)   3 (sometimes)   4 (rarely)
    5 (never)   0 (don't know or n/a)

b. Your children?

    1 (always)   2 (frequently)   3 (sometimes)   4 (rarely)
    5 (never)   0 (don't know or n/a)

c. Your extended family?

    1 (always)   2 (frequently)   3 (sometimes)   4 (rarely)
    5 (never)   0 (don't know or n/a)

d. Your friends?

    1 (always)   2 (frequently)   3 (sometimes)   4 (rarely)
    5 (never)   0 (don't know or n/a)

10. All things taken together, how satisfied are you with your

a. marriage/partnership?

    1 (not at all satisfied) 2 (not very satisfied) 3 (somewhat satisfied)
    4 (very satisfied)   5 (completely satisfied)

b. relationship with your children?

    1 (not at all satisfied) 2 (not very satisfied) 3 (somewhat satisfied)
    4 (very satisfied)   5 (completely satisfied)

c. relationship with your extended family?

    1 (not at all satisfied) 2 (not very satisfied) 3 (somewhat satisfied)
    4 (very satisfied)   5 (completely satisfied)

d. relationship with your friends?

    1 (not at all satisfied) 2 (not very satisfied) 3 (somewhat satisfied)
    4 (very satisfied)   5 (completely satisfied)

Calculating your score:

Add up the scores for your answers to all the questions. Scores will range from 5 to 108. Higher scores indicate greater social support.

Interpreting your score the *Stress Less* way*:

5–29: No to little social support
30–56: Low social support
57–82: Moderate social support
83–108: High social support

In 1972, my sophomore year in college, Bette Midler—a.k.a. the Divine Miss M—released a song that, along with the Rolling Stones' "Jumpin' Jack Flash" and Don McLean's "American Pie," became emblematic of our commune-driven era: "You got to have friends," the Divine One sang in that throaty twang, as we shouted the words ourselves and danced around our dorm rooms. "The feeling's oh so strong/You got to have friends/To make that day last long."

Like Emily Lewis, we knew in our tie-dyed hearts that Bette was right. And soon, science began to catch up.

In 1979, social epidemiologists Lisa F. Berkman, Ph.D., and S. Leonard Syme, Ph.D., both then at the Yale School of Medicine, published a seminal paper showing that social relationships do indeed contribute to longevity. Using data from a huge survey (6,928 residents of Califor-

---

* The *Stress Less* interpretation was developed by the author, not the scientists.

nia's Alameda County) and a follow-up survey given nine years later, Berkman and Syme found that the participants with the fewest social contacts were two to three times more likely to die than those with the most. Such isolation, noted James S. House, Ph.D., and colleagues nine years later, as we slid into the Me Generation, was as much a risk factor for mortality as smoking, obesity, and high blood pressure.

Since then, a database's worth of research from around the globe—on subjects from mice to undergraduates to elderly housemates—has buttressed the claim: Social support is good for your health and increases longevity (in Bette's words: can "make that day last long"). And the positive results are independent of health behaviors—meaning that it truly is not what you do but whom (and how many) you know that matters when it comes to improving everything from heart rate and blood pressure to immune function. An illustration from a paper by UCLA's Teresa E. Seeman (see figure 5) socks home the relationship in black and white.

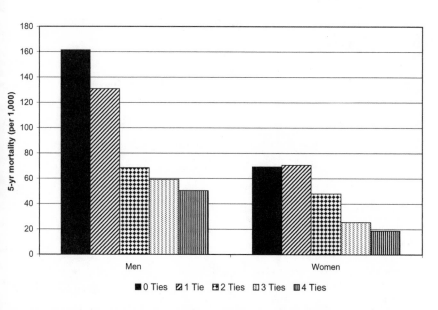

Figure 5. Connect 4: Sex-specific 5-year Mortality (per 1,000) by Level of Social Integrastion: New Haven EPESE cohort (adapted from Seeman et al., 1993).

For every one thousand women, nearly seventy with just one or two social ties had died after five years while only about nineteen with four social ties had. A later study of Seeman's that tracked Wisconsin high school graduates for some forty years linked positive social experiences with lower allostatic load for both women and men across the board.

"The degree to which having emotional support, the perception that this exists and the reality of its being there, basically means that your brain is bathed in lesser amounts of stress hormones," says Seeman over the phone from California. "That as you interpret your world, the brain's responses hinge less on perceptions of threat, fear, anxiety, and you experience fewer of the biological downstream consequences that come with that, including the cognitive problems that show later in life."

The reverse is true as well. For example, a 2009 study by Rebecca C. Thurston, Ph.D., at the University of Pittsburgh, and Laura Kubzansky, at the Harvard School of Public Health, found that during a nineteen-year follow-up period, "high loneliness" was associated with increased risk of coronary heart disease among women after controlling for variables ranging from age and income to physical activity, alcohol use, and cholesterol levels.

How does social support get under our skin to permit our stress levels to drop and everything from our immune to our cardiovascular systems to slow their aging processes? It happens through a kind of domino effect, with our brains being the first tile to fall and the DNA in our cells likely soaking up the reverberations. While there have been no studies to date that directly investigate how social support affects telomere length, it is easy to speculate how the lack of it may erode our cells and how an abundance of it may do the opposite.

Socially isolated folks, report scientists such as Ohio State's Janice Kiecolt-Glaser, have both stronger stress responses than their well-connected counterparts and longer-lasting ones—that is, increased levels of cortisol flood their bloodstreams for longer periods of time. One physical repercussion of this is an impaired immune system: Recall those hydrocortisol creams described in Chapter 1—how we use them to combat skin rashes and other inflammatory processes? Well, they do that by inhibiting the trafficking of pro-inflammatory cytokines (messenger proteins) to wound sites, where they would call forth white blood cells to fight any invaders. Likewise, when your body produces its *own* excess cortisol, cytokine trafficking slows to a crawl: The cytokines stay in the bloodstream, hanging out like teenagers at a mall, rather than heading over to the wound that needs them and calling forth immune-cell troops. Hence the higher level of pro-inflammatory cytokines (IL-6 and C-reactive protein) in the *blood* of socially isolated and other chronically stressed folks—a risk factor for everything from cardiovascular disease to arthritis—but slower healing at the site of a wound.

On the flip side, other researchers have shown that folks who cope by seeking social support have lower cortisol levels throughout the day than those who don't. Katie O'Donnell, Ph.D., and Andrew Steptoe, both at University College London, are among those investigating this angle. It's not that people who look for social support are healthier from the get-go, says Steptoe. They're not less likely to be smokers, depressed, younger, and so on. "No, it's a direct association between the coping response and cortisol," he says. "Now, this measure is not the same as having social support," he cautions. "It has to do with responding to stress by *mobilizing* support. But it's likely that people who say they cope in this way also enjoy adequate levels of support—or else they wouldn't find this a useful strategy for dealing with stress."

Under the Social-Support Influence: Your Brain

UCLA's Naomi Eisenberger, Ph.D., wanted to track such results to their source. So she designed a three-pronged study that investigated how people's social-support status affected both their cortisol levels *and* the brain activity that drove that biochemical response.

First, she and her colleagues took thirty men and women ages eighteen to thirty-six and assessed their cortisol levels before and after a grueling task: delivering a speech to blank-faced evaluators and then counting backward from 2,083 by 13 at accelerating speeds in front of the same chilly judges. If subjects made a mistake, they had to start over.

The researchers then handed participants Palm Pilots and over a ten-day period, contacted them at random intervals to ask about the level and quality of support of their most recent partner.

A week later, each participant crawled into an fMRI scanner and played a virtual ball-tossing game, supposedly with two others (depicted as cartoon animations on the screen) but in truth with a preset computer program. (Think Wii but with the subject pressing keys rather than swinging a remote.) As described earlier, an fMRI tracks blood flow to various parts of the brain. In the first scan, the fake players threw the participant the ball about half the time. But in the second scan, they excluded him or her early on, keeping the game to themselves (junior high all over again). The participant then filled out a questionnaire noting his or her level of social distress.

Eisenberger crunched and cross-correlated all the data and found that the participants with more social support in their everyday lives had significantly lower levels of cortisol during the speech and math stressors, even though no supports were physically present during the ordeal. Moreover, the levels were dose dependent: "The more social support, the less of a cortisol response they showed," says Eisenberger.

Eisenberger pushed further, seeking the neurological pathways driving the reduced cortisol levels.

Remarkably, the same brain circuitry that lights up when we feel physical pain lights up when we experience emotional pain such as social rejection or unfair treatment. The area is the dorsal anterior cingulate cortex (dACC), deep in the limbic region of the brain. Studies with rhesus monkeys have shown that the dACC also lights up in infants when they're separated from their moms, as does a region called Brodmann area 8 (BA8), an area in the frontal cortex involved in managing uncertainty. And when researchers directly stimulate the dACC in rats, cortisol levels rise. From the brain's perspective, it seems, the pain of separation is as real as the sting of a needle.

Likewise, the same brain circuitry that kicks in when we feel physical pleasure kicks in when we feel emotional pleasure—that is, the reward-system circuitry, including the ventral striatum, which houses the nucleus accumbens, described in Chapter 4. The very same "pleasure center" that glows with a hit of starchy, fatty foods and—more intensely—with cocaine or other drugs of abuse also glows from warm and fuzzy feelings, regardless of whether they arise from a friend's lending us an ear or our donating to a cause we believe in.

Recently, Hidehiko Takahashi, M.D., at Japan's National Institute of Radiological Sciences, showed both sides of this neural-circuitry coin. In an fMRI study of nineteen young men and women, he noted that going green with envy at another's success activated that same pain circuitry, the dACC, whereas experiencing schadenfreude (glee that the envied person has failed) activated the corresponding reward-system circuitry, the ventral striatum/nucleus accumbens.

Eisenberger recorded similar results. Greater social distress at being excluded from the ball-tossing game correlated with greater activity in subjects' dACCs. Increased activity in the dACC and the BA8 correlated with both lower levels of social support and increased cortisol reactivity to the speech/math stress task. Those who reported interacting with supportive individuals on a daily basis showed less dACC and BA8 activity during the social-rejection episode, and this reduced activity was associated with lower cortisol levels during a social stress task.

"What we found is that people who had more social support in their everyday lives showed less sensitivity to the rejection experience," says Eisenberger. "So they showed less activity in the pain-related neural circuitry that we typically find activated in these studies of social rejection. They just weren't activating the pain circuitry to the same extent as people who were less supported."

Social support, in other words, actually changes your brain, which in turn leads to less cortisol release.

"We thought starting off that people with more social support were going to show more activity in the prefrontal regulatory region, so that they would be the ones *coping* better with the stressor," says Eisenberger. "But what we saw was that the people with more social support were in a very basic way just responding less. They were *interpreting* the stressor differently."

Recall from Epel and Blackburn's studies in Chapter 2 that interpretation is key in the stress–biological aging story. The caregiving moms who perceived themselves as being under the least stress had the longest telomeres, by the equivalent of ten years or more. And the telomeres actually *lengthened* in the caregiving spouses who saw their stress levels drop over the course of the year.

If I were to trace a speculative path of how social support affects biological aging, I'd do it this way:

Social Support ➡ Reduced perception of stress ➡ Less active brain pain circuit, more active brain reward circuit ➡ Lowered cortisol ➡ Slowed, or reversed, biological aging

Amazing. Social support physiologically dampens our brain's and body's reactivity to psychological stressors.

So the question becomes: How can we pump up our social connections (in the real world, that is, not in the cyber-ether of Facebook and LinkedIn, Plaxo, and Classmates.com)? Michelle C. Carlson, Ph.D., and Teresa Seeman may have found one answer.

Give to Receive:
The Neurobiology of Volunteering

Social support, of course, goes two ways: We can give it, and we can receive it. New research suggests that its stress-reducing benefits accrue regardless of which end we're on.

Michelle Carlson, an associate professor at the Johns Hopkins

Bloomberg School of Public Health, knew from the scientific literature that giving of ourselves contributes to improved health and longer life, but she wanted to drill deeper: *How* does it do that? Can it actually *change* our brains, reversing some of the broken connections that come with aging?

To find out, she turned to a program called Experience Corps, which was co-founded in 1995 by Linda P. Fried, Ph.D., then also at Johns Hopkins. Experience Corps places volunteers ages fifty-five and older into underserved public elementary schools across the United States to work as tutors and mentors to youngsters through third grade. Volunteers work fifteen hours a week for at least one school year. The giving and getting goes both ways: The kids get one-on-one help with reading, library activities, and conflict resolution from men and women who care, and the adults increase their social engagement, thereby exercising both their bodies (supervising recess, shelving library books) and brains (working memory, problem-solving skills, and brain flexibility). It's the antithesis of those sedentary, solitary computer games that promise you'll "Improve your IQ!" or "Develop a photographic memory!"

"The goal of the program is to provide the older adults with social, cognitive, psychological, and physical engagement to hopefully enhance their aging," says Teresa Seeman, who collaborated with Carlson on a pilot study investigating how integrated programs such as EC affect cognition. "To what degree did they make new friends and have increased social interaction with people both in school and outside? Does being involved in something like this enhance their sense of mastery and efficacy because they feel they're doing something important? At the same time the aim is to benefit the children by improving their academic achievement."

Carlson recruited eight female EC volunteers from the Baltimore community and matched them with a control group, women who would become EC volunteers the following year. All participants were African American and had low income, a low education level, and a "marginally normal" score on a cognitive test. Mental state was only so-so, indicating risk for cognitive impairment. In particular, Carlson wanted to learn if over the six-month trial the EC volunteers would show increased activity in the prefrontal cortex, which oversees executive functions, including working memory, planning, scheduling, recognition of consequences, and dealing with ambiguity. It's a region known to show substantial age-related degeneration.

"We wanted to see if those at greatest risk for dementia as exhibited through memory impairments could, through this intervention, have enduring changes in brain plasticity," says Carlson. Earlier studies had shown that, as a group, those who scored lower on executive-function measures showed the most benefit short-term because they had so much room for improvement. Think of folks in their twenties lifting weights versus those in their sixties. Muscle bulking in the sixtysomethings will be more apparent quicker because they're starting with essentially nil.

At the start of the study, Carlson did fMRIs of all the participants, and noted similar brain patterns for both the volunteers and the controls. She then scanned them all again, after the EC volunteers had been working with students in the Baltimore schools for six months.

She was "pretty shocked" at the results. The EC volunteers—but not the controls—showed increases in brain activity precisely in the areas targeted by the intervention: the left prefrontal cortex (executive-function territory) and the anterior cingulate cortex, an area implicated in efficient filtering or inhibiting of conflicting information—say, focusing on a single voice amid a cacophony of exuberant conversations, and remembering what page you're on in *Chicken Little*. In other words, volunteering in Experience Corps *reversed* cognitive decline by waking up neurons that had been napping.

The scientists acknowledge that the sample size was small and specific to women. But it provided "proof of concept" and lay the groundwork for a larger, even more rigorous trial. "The Experience Corps volunteers reduce this chronic stress burden—the allostatic load," says the Rockefeller University's Bruce McEwen, whom, you'll recall, coined the term. "People who are not depressed, who have a meaning and purpose in life, clearly have a different physiology."

Priming Our Nervous Systems
to Engage with Others

Experience Corps helped the volunteers increase their social engagement, but what if we're so hyped up we can't engage to start with?

Stephen W. Porges, Ph.D., head of the of the Brain-Body Center at the University of Illinois at Chicago, has developed a theory that helps reduce stress by opening the door to social interaction. Porges doesn't use the expression "reducing stress" in his work but rather "what it is that makes us feel safe with another." He refers to our "social engagement system" to describe the interlocking neurological and muscular elements that enable us to connect with people in a "reciprocal" way: that is, to toss the ball of conversation——talking *and* listening—back and forth as we not only share information but alter the other's physiological state. He considers dancing (eye-to-eye contact, dipping your partner low), playing (tag, you're it!), and singing or playing musical instruments the crème de la crème of social engagement.

When we're "stressed" (as I put it) or "dysregulated" (as he puts it), our social engagement system is off kilter—or even, in the worst case scenario, kaput. Porges has recommendations for how to re-engage it, so to speak, based on a rethinking (or, better put, a "reawakening") of our understanding of how the autonomic nervous system functions. He calls that renewed thinking the Polyvagal Theory. Here, briefly, is what it says:

Remember the vagus nerve—the major nerve of the parasympathetic nervous system—from Chapter 1? It's that giant snaking thing with seemingly endless fibers that exits the brain stem and has tentacles that innervate everything from the heart and respiratory tract to the liver and gastrointestinal tract. Unlike older theories of the autonomic nervous system, which see the play between the sympathetic and parasympathetic nervous systems as an attempt at "balance" (the SNS cranks things up, and the PNS—controlled by the vagus nerve—slows them down, restoring balance), Polyvagal Theory looks to the PNS—

specifically, the vagus nerve—as the regulator, and speaks to a "hierarchy" within it.

To start, Porges sketches out a more complex picture of the very anatomy of the vagus nerve itself.

The vagus nerve, says Porges, is not a single solid rod. Rather, it's more like a bifurcated pipe, with two hollow pathways comprising its core. Dangling into the pipe are myriad nerve fibers, each originating in a different part of the brain stem. For instance, the fibers that go through the pipe to the colon come from one part of the brain, and the fibers that go to the heart come from another. Before any messages can travel through those fibers, though, the brain must tell them which pathway to follow.

One of those pathways is *myelinated*, that is, it is cushioned with myelin, a fatty substance that enables messages to move faster and stay more accurate. This is the newer pathway—only mammals, high up on the evolutionary food chain, have it. When we feel safe, brain circuits involved in controlling facial muscles (necessary for our expressions), motor activity of the middle ear (necessary for listening), and pitch and tone of our vocalizations send messages through this myelinated pathway. The messages move quickly and arrive at their destinations intact.

The other pathway is *unmyelinated*——it's ancient, reptilian. When we *don't* feel safe, brain circuits related to functions such as those listed earlier (our expressions, our vocalizations) bypass the myelinated pathway and, by default, turn to this one. It's a defensive maneuver, says Porges. This pathway can "shut us down like a reptile," to make us safe. Our facial muscles go slack, our ears stop hearing human voices, our own voice clanks to a monotone. We may even pass out. This pathway takes over particularly fast in people who've been traumatized in the past—and who have experienced the "learned helplessness" described in Chapter 5.

Obviously, the myelinated pathway is crucial to the social engagement system. Thus, before we can even begin to take advantage of the social support that might be out there, we have to make sure our social engagement system is in working order—or, as Porges puts it technically, we have to "recruit the neural circuits that promote social behavior." Our autonomic nervous system kicks in to *automatically* determine whether a social situation is safe or not. But there are ways to prime the social engagement system to increase our sense of control. Using the muscles in our face and middle ear, Porges recently told *Nexus* magazine, "will actively change our physiological state by increasing vagal influences on the heart and actively blunt the sympathetic adrenal system. Then we can be more in contact with reality, more alert and engaged."

See the end of this chapter for other ways to develop your social engagement system.

Oxytocin: The Yin-Yang Hormone of Social Relationships

Health psychologist Shelley Taylor's corner office at UCLA sings with light and air. She designed it that way: Green linen shades cap the long windows, a leafy tree sports a papier-mâché "bird of happiness" at its base, a solid blond wood desk spreads between us. The place is nurturing yet cool, like Taylor herself.

That stolid way of being has served her well. In 2000, with then-postdoc Laura Klein, Ph.D., Taylor turned the fight-or-flight theory inside out by introducing a new stress-response concept that applied specifically to women. She called it, lyrically, tend and befriend.

Until 1995, Taylor explains, women constituted only about 17 percent of subjects in stress experiments. So why, she wondered, did researchers assume that women's stress responses matched those of the men being tested in the lab? Yes, fight-or-flight kicks in for women, too—initially. It's an instinctive physiological response. But after that, women's behavior differs markedly from that of their spear-wielding-drown-my-sorrows counterparts: Women rush to protect their children and themselves and to establish a safe haven (that's tending). Then they reach out to others for help and support (befriending).

Sounds familiar, yes?

"Men and women both experience fight-or-flight," says Taylor, her blond hair curving neatly under her chin. "But women are more likely to turn sooner to social means for controlling their stress. They call somebody up. And it's very soothing. It doesn't always work, but it certainly works better than drinking!"

Tend and befriend made a media splash and led to Taylor's 2002 book on the subject, *The Tending Instinct*. Since developing the theory, she's spent countless hours in the lab trying to understand the biological basis of that affiliative response. Based on studies with animals and her own research, she's found that it's driven partly by how the hormone oxytocin—which, despite what you may have heard, is *not* the "cuddly" hormone—affects the release of dopamine and endogenous opioids in the brain (as described in Chapter 4). "Oxytocin is not," she says seriously, "a straightforward hormone."

Although much research (mostly in animals, some in humans) has shown that blood levels of oxytocin rise with social bonding—affection between partners, sex, giving birth, breast-feeding, early maternal bonding, and even reuniting with a dog after work—the hormone plays the converse role, too: When adult females, young and old, are socially isolated or distressed, it spikes, signaling that it's time to rally support.

Oxytocin, says Taylor, acts like a "social thermostat," in tandem with other indicators: When we experience relationship stress—say, we're lonely or our mate just doesn't "get it"—blood levels of oxytocin rise, signaling us to seek out people who can help. Once we connect *positively*, our stress hormones subside and our psyches calm down. If the connection is negative, though, our stress response intensifies.

"What we have seen is that when people's social relationships are suffering in some way or they're socially isolated, they get an increase in oxytocin, which we believe acts as a stimulus to affiliating with others," says Taylor. "And so it's basically a neurochemical signal that says: 'You do not have enough people around you or you have the wrong types of people around you; you need to find relationships that will protect you.'"

Taylor's latest foray into the oxytocin thicket proves the point. She and her colleagues looked at eighty-five young adults, women and men, in committed couple relationships. The subjects filled out surveys on everything from perceived stress levels and optimism to depression and anxiety, and also reported on the nature of their relationships, whether supportive or unsupportive. Then the scientists took blood to measure oxytocin and vasopressin levels in the women and men. Vasopressin, animal studies show, is essentially the male counterpart to oxytocin; its molecular structure differs by just one amino acid, and it helps regulate *male* bonding behavior, including controlling and guarding territory, mates, and offspring (very he-man).

As the scientists expected, the oxytocin levels were higher for the women distressed about their relationships, but they were not higher for the distressed men. Rather, the study showed for the first time in humans that vasopressin's trajectory followed a similar pattern: Vasopressin levels were higher for the distressed men but not for the distressed women. Estrogen and testosterone do play a role: Estrogen facilitates oxytocin's action, and testosterone does the same for vasopressin. But even taking those hormones out of the mix didn't alter the findings. Taylor concluded that "plasma oxytocin in women and plasma vasopressin in men may be biomarkers of distressed pair-bond relationships."

There's an evolutionary reason for Taylor's conclusion. The crucial relationship for a monogamous species like ours is—what else?—bonding with a significant other. It's essential for survival. Multitudinous reproductive technologies notwithstanding these days, we've historically needed a mate to reproduce, as well as to help gather food and remain safe. That our brains send out a biological alarm to ensure that we continue doing so makes perfect evolutionary sense.

~~~

Structurally, oxytocin is a neuropeptide, like NPY in Chapter 4; it's made up of a small chain of amino acids. It's produced in the hypothalamus—that tooth-shaped gland deep in the brain that also sparks the stress response—and travels to the pituitary, which sends it into the body through the bloodstream and to various parts of the brain (refer back to Chapter 1 for more on the hypothalamus and pituitary). That it acts both within the brain and in the greater world of the body is important to remember, as that twofold distribution may be what accounts for its yin-yang personality.

Research by neurobiologist C. Sue Carter, Ph.D., at the University of Illinois at Chicago, has enlightened us terrifically about oxytocin's dual nature. Carter studies prairie voles, rodents indigenous to the central plains of the United States and southern Canada. Why prairie voles? Because, unlike 95 percent of mammals, they remain monogamous for life after mating, raising pups together with the confidence of Donna and Alex Stone on *The Donna Reed Show*. Physiologically, they are built that way: Their oxytocin receptors overlap with their dopamine receptors in their nucleus accumbens—the pleasure center of the brain. Simply put, to prairie voles, being Mr. (or Ms.) Mom *feels good*. It turns out that we humans *also* have oxytocin receptors within dopamine-rich brain areas. Hence *our* animal magnetism—one partner at a time. (There are, of course, exceptions.)

Where does oxytocin's apparent ability to reduce stress fit into the mix? People in experiments in which oxytocin is administered exogenously—through, say, a nasal spray that reaches the brain—become calmer, less fearful, more trusting, and more empathetic. Their sympathetic-nervous-system activity decreases, and their cortisol secretion drops. Imaging studies show that under such influence, activity in the amygdala—the area in the brain that helps process social information and recognize threats—decreases as well. Ever wonder how the "love drug," Ecstasy, works? In part, it sparks oxytocin release in the brain.

All of which highlights the question: How do we reconcile this boosted cuddle quotient with clear evidence that oxytocin *rises* when we're stressing out about our relationships? In a nutshell, high oxytocin levels in the *blood* are different from high oxytocin levels in the *brain*. Taylor theorizes that it is not oxytocin itself that alleviates relationship stress but rather oxytocin's ability to kick off the brain's reward circuitry, the dopamine and endogenous opioid systems mentioned earlier. When we find a satisfying relationship, oxytocin levels rise in both the blood *and* the brain, and the reward circuitry snaps into action. But if we fail to find such a relationship or our partner disappoints, the oxytocin may bypass the brain and its reward systems and go straight into the blood, jacking up levels there, indicating the need to "befriend" someone else.

It could be, Taylor writes in her new paper, that the reduced stress responses attributed to oxytocin in the past are due instead to the oxytocin boost that comes with cozying up to someone who cares, as well as the hormone's "modulation" of reward pathways, such as the dopamine and opioid systems.

As we age, whom we reach out to for support changes, too. "Early in life, girls play with other girls," says Taylor, whose work with the Mac-Arthur Study of Successful Aging, a seven-year trial investigating influences on physical and cognitive functioning, concentrates on adults ages seventy to seventy-nine. "And then, there's an important period of life where everybody is oriented toward the other sex and toward finding partners, getting hitched up in one way or another, having children. As they age, men report that they turn to their wives for social support. But women report that as they age, they turn to everybody *but* their husbands—their children, friends, other relatives. Yes, their husbands are a main source of support, but they're also a main source of frustration. The big story in older women's lives is their women friends."

Bette Midler, now a robust sixty-four, may be singing about that soon, too.

STRESS LESS

To Reduce Stress and Slow the Cellular Clock Using Social Support

Volunteer

Find a cause you believe in. As Michelle Carlson's pilot study showed, volunteering can reverse cognitive decline by revitalizing slumbering neurons. Your local library and houses of worship are great places to learn about volunteer opportunities. So is the Internet: Type in "local volunteer work" and the name of your city, and thousands of hits will likely come up (my search for Boston yielded fifty-nine hundred). Following the Experience Corps model,* find a place where you can be physically and mentally active and engage with other volunteers.

Meditate to increase your sense of compassion

A recent study led by Jennifer Crocker, Ph.D., at the University of Michigan, found that students who rated high on "compassionate goals"— that is, those who aimed to support others not for selfish reasons but to improve others' well-being—had increased social support themselves. Their very intentions, the researchers noted, helped create a supportive environment that went both ways. Studies have shown that meditation is one way. But how to increase our sense of compassion? There is even a type of meditation called compassion meditation, which concentrates on challenging our traditional assumptions about relationships with others, highlighting the illusory nature of our judgments. Emory University psychiatrist Charles L. Raison, M.D., who has done extensive research on the subject, explains how a feeling as powerful as, say, hate for another, can be illusory. "The conventional reality of the feeling is true, the way the wave on a river is true," he says. "You see a ripple go by. The wave

* To learn more about Experience Corps and possibly become a volunteer, visit www
.experiencecorps.org.

has a certain phenomenological existence, but you watch the river for a second, and the wave is swallowed up and gone. True like that, whereas the river would be truer." (For a refresher on meditation, see Chapter 6.)

Seek out a "safe person"

This is what Emily Lewis did. The person could be a therapist, a member of the clergy, or a spiritual counselor, a friend. Optimally, this is someone you can meet with, but talking by phone can help, too. Communicating online will not do the trick.

Develop your social engagement system

UIC's Stephen Porges has developed some specific ways to do this:

- Respect what your body is doing, even when it goes into withdrawal mode. Remind yourself that it's trying to protect you, albeit according to an ancient code. Be gentle with yourself.

- Retreat to a quiet room for a bit. "Perhaps the most profound social engagement disrupters are background sounds, especially low-frequency background sounds," says Porges, enjoining me to hear Chicago's L rumbling down the tracks through the phone. "When the system is downregulated, your heart rate is faster, you're getting into that sympathetic mode, and you become more acutely sensitive to low-frequency sounds because you've lost neural regulation of middle-ear muscles. You don't hear what people are saying; you hear the rumble. Everyone has that experience when they're really wiped out. They react not to the verbal content, but they become hypersensitive. It's an adaptive function all mammals have."

- Simply sit with someone you know and trust. If no one is around, look at pictures of people you know and trust.

- Listen to vocal music, preferably female vocalists, because they "express a range of acoustic frequencies that 'triggers' the social engagement system," says Porges. Remember, the muscles of the middle ear connect to the brain circuits that enable social engagement.

- Find someone to talk with and listen to you. Begin to toss that verbal ball. When you're comfortable, make eye contact. (If you're uncomfortable and make eye contact, you may appear to be staring, which will disrupt the social flow.) "The social engagement system is a dyad, just like dance," says Porges. "Features of it are the prosody of the human voice, the sequencing of listening and talking, moving and stopping, the intonation, the rhythm, and facial expressivity." (Botox, he says, only half-joking, may be seriously impeding recipients' social engagement systems with its freezing of the upper face muscles, particularly around the eyes.) "When you're talking and as the feedback from the reciprocal dialogue occurs, you're starting to expand the range of frequencies that you use. As you listen, the middle-ear muscles engage, and in turn you modulate your tone and vocal rhythms. It's a feedback mechanism. Look at the acoustic properties of conversations that begin with one person's being stressed out. You know when they're ready to say good-bye because their words become more melodic, the tone of their voice has changed."

- Sing or play a musical instrument. "When people sing, they must listen to their articulations in order to adjust them," says Porges. "That's a wonderful exercise." Porges suggests singing lessons to parents of autistic children, not just to get the children singing, but to help them engage on a musical level with another. Singing also uses the breath in a conscious way. "Singing is cheap pranayama yoga," he laughs.

- Exercise your facial muscles. Again, the muscles of your face connect via nerves to the brain circuits that enable social engagement.

Spend time with friends face-to-face

Facebook and other social networking sites are great, but communications online and via texting tend to run to the six-word-memoir genre ("On tenterhooks waiting for test results") rather than the verbal and physical give-and-take that can soothe our nervous systems and reverse the aging of our brains.

CHAPTER 8

Stress and Sleep

. . . O sleep! O gentle sleep!
Nature's soft nurse, how have I frighted thee,
That thou no more wilt weigh my eyelids down,
And steep my senses in forgetfulness?

—William Shakespeare, *Henry IV*, part 2, act 3, scene 1, 1600

Laura Maskell knows from stress and missed sleep. She's been an emergency room doctor in Oregon for more than twenty-two years, working twelve-hour shifts, often alternating days and nights. She's also the single mother of a twelve-year-old daughter—a demographic filled with its own special brand of Sturm und Drang, as those of us likewise blessed know.

Until her thirties, Laura could balance the strains of missed z's with exercise—lots of exercise. She'd taken up fencing when she entered the U.S. Naval Academy in Annapolis, Maryland, as part of the first class of women. Though she didn't stay at the academy past freshman year, she continued with the sport back in Oregon, as a member of the U.S. Fencing team, throughout college and medical school. It wasn't just the physical workout that helped; it was the mental calisthenics, too. "Fencing is like chess," says Laura. "You're setting people up to make a mistake or you're devising openings for yourself." Wielding that sword hours a day, Laura offset the damage that sleep deprivation wreaks on our brains, including memory problems (disastrous in medical school) and difficulty making decisions (ditto).

But during her internship, exercise alone wasn't enough. "When I was an intern, we'd do twenty-four hours on and twenty-four hours off, and I'd go places with friends and just sleep," she says. "We'd go to Sauvie Island and my friends would take pictures of me sleeping. We'd go to the beach, and I'd be sleeping there."

Laura needed a release, and a boyfriend introduced her to one: cocaine. She didn't use it during work or while training for fencing competitions, but it sure came in handy afterward. When she finished her internship and started her first job, in the ER at a hospital in Seaside, Oregon, her schedule got even more lopsided. She would work one forty-eight-hour shift a week so she could take off for World Cup games in Europe. Returning stateside, she'd jump into another two straight days on the job. "I had really screwed up sleep back then," she says.

Needless to say, her judgment wasn't what it had been back when she was a young teetotaler eschewing her parents' addiction path. The hospital found out about the drug use and she was out. That was her low point. "I started taking typing lessons on the computer," she says. "I thought I'd have to be a secretary." With the help of a twelve-step program, she climbed back into the world, eventually landing a job at a Portland emergency room, where she stayed until the hospital shut down, ten years later.

Losing that long-term job threw Laura for a loop: She had no severance and a six-year-old daughter to support. Her sleep suffered as much as her pocketbook. The job she finally found was an hour and a half away, in Lebanon, Oregon, and custody arrangements for her daughter required that she not move. So she worked nights—three in a row, napping during the day and returning home early on the fourth day, grateful for her full-time nanny. She loved the job but the fragmented sleep got to her: Her exercise practice slipped from five to three times a week, and she put on fifty pounds. "You know how I put myself to sleep?" she asks. "I eat a big meal—tofu burritos and tomato-basil quiche. It's exactly what you're not supposed to do. But when I can catch that wave of being soporific after eating, I sleep really well."

Working three nights in a row is her limit. Push her into four, and her patience snaps or she might forget to finish writing instructions in a patient's chart if she's interrupted midstream. "My tolerance goes way down on the fourth day. I've gotten complaints from patients that I was not being nice—never anything about my competence, but my body language gets real loud," she says. "I have lots of compassion, but if you're not really sick, in my mind I'm going, 'If you're drug seeking, I'm not your girl.'"

Getting Through the Night

Sleep deprivation, say sleep experts, is one of the strongest stressors, fraying both our brains and our bodies. How does your time in the Land of Nod measure up?

For each question below, please circle the number corresponding to your response.

1. Please rate the current (i.e., last two weeks) severity of your insomnia problem(s).

	None	Mild	Moderate	Severe	Very severe
a) Difficulty falling asleep:	0	1	2	3	4
b) Difficulty staying asleep:	0	1	2	3	4
c) Problem waking up too early:	0	1	2	3	4

2. How satisfied/dissatisfied are you with your current sleep pattern?

Very satisfied	Satisfied	Neutral	Dissatisfied	Very dissatisfied
0	1	2	3	4

3. To what extent do you consider your sleep problem to interfere with your daily functioning (e.g., daytime fatigue, ability to function at work/ daily chores, concentration, memory, mood, etc.).

Not at all Interfering	A little	Somewhat	Much	Very Much Interfering
0	1	2	3	4

4. How noticeable to others do you think your sleeping problem is in terms of impairing the quality of your life?

Not at all Noticeable	A little	Somewhat	Much	Very Much Noticeable
0	1	2	3	4

5. How worried/distressed are you about your current sleep problem?

Not at all Worried	A Little	Somewhat	Much	Very Much Worried
0	1	2	3	4

Calculating and interpreting your score:

Add your scores for all seven items (1a+1b+1c+2+3+4+5) = _____
Total scores range from 0 to 28.

0–7: No clinically significant insomnia
8–14: Subthreshold insomnia
15–21: Clinical insomnia (moderate severity)
22–28: Clinical insomnia (severe)

~~~~~~

We know that lack of sleep works against us; we feel it in our bones (and hearts and stomachs and brains). Sans sleep, manageable stressors—for Laura, say, a patient with a fake bellyache seeking Vicodin—can send us on a tirade, if not verbal, then gestural. Our eyes roll, our jaws clench, we storm about. Our brains, perceiving a threat, announce "all HPA-affected systems go!" and everything ratchets up. Now that we're in revved-up mode, at bedtime our heads hit the pillow, but our bodies and brains are in overdrive. We toss, we turn, we swear, maybe we drink a glass of wine (my own preference). Sleep, when it comes, is fragmented—and not only because we're waking up to pee.

And so stress, once again, kicks off another of its seemingly endless cycles: Poor sleep begets stress begets poor sleep . . . It's a variation on the stress–comfort food theme outlined in Chapter 4.

"Here's how chronic stress and insomnia relate," says sleep-and-stress expert Jessica D. Payne, Ph.D., now at University of Notre Dame. "Let's say you are really unhappy with your job. With time that starts to eat away at you, you are ruminating all the time, you're not sleeping very well. That stress triggers the lack of sleep. Now, sleep deprivation is one of the most potent stressors—that's why it's used as a torture technique. It elevates cortisol through the roof. So now you get into this negative feedback loop: You can't sleep, which elevates stress hormones, which then makes it harder to sleep, which then makes you even more stressed the next day."

Indeed, in its 2008 report on sleep among U.S. adults, based on more than four hundred thousand respondents, the Centers for Disease Control reported that approximately 29 percent of us sleep less than seven hours a night—the minimum required, on average—and fifty million to seventy million of us have chronic sleep disorders. Scarily, 11 percent of respondents had not had a single night of sufficient sleep in the preceding month. More women than men were sleep deprived—no surprise for me, given the snoring hulk of a husband I lie next to every night. The ratio of insomnia in women to men? Approximately 1.4 to 1.0, according to a recent study in the *Journal of Women's Health*.

How is all this night wakefulness aging us before our time? Studies have shown that people who don't get enough sleep have elevated levels of stress hormones as well as the pro-inflammatory cytokine IL-6, an indicator of suppressed immune function. (IL-6, recall from Chapter 2, is an immune-system messenger protein.) And levels of growth hormone, a restorative chemical, drop. That means we're at greater risk for a slew of bodily ailments, from heart disease to type 2 diabetes, from infections to obesity. In the brain, the hippocampus (the seat of memory consolidation and retrieval) becomes sluggish without sleep and in extreme cases may even atrophy, leaving us less able to form new memories and consolidate old ones. Indeed, a new study by Anna L. Marsland, Ph.D., and colleagues at the University of Pittsburgh showed that increased levels of IL-6 in middle-aged adults corresponded with a smaller volume of hippocampal gray matter.

These biochemical changes, as we've seen in previous chapters, often correspond with shorter telomeres and lower levels of the restorative enzyme telomerase. Might that mean that missed sleep, too, contributes to aging all the way down to our cells?

There don't appear to be any studies published yet that directly investigate the sleep-telomere link. But missed sleep, as Payne notes, is a huge stressor; when it's persistent, it calls forth the same erosive characters as chronic stress: long-term high levels of cortisol, the catecholamines, and IL-6, as well as inflammation, hippocampal sensitivity. My speculation? Folks who are chronically sleep deprived and have no way of making up for it (with, say, an afternoon nap) have shorter telomeres, on average, than those who snooze peacefully through the night.

The fact that chronic lack of sleep may lead to older cells is enough to make me put my head down on my keyboard and count sheep. Before I do, though, here's a look at the how of sleep, the way our brains and bodies respond to restless nights. The more we know about the physiological effects of stress on sleep (and vice versa), the greater our incentive to buck the modern trend to squeeze ever more activity into the twenty-four-hour day. With our gadgets of choice (BlackBerrys, iPhones, iPads, etc.) feeding the frenzy, we may be connecting to one another at the expense of staying together ourselves.

Your Brain on Sleep Loss

A university sleep lab is nothing to write home about, despite how homey its researchers try to make it feel. The Center for Sleep and Cognition, in Boston's Beth Israel Deaconess Medical Center, is no exception. Sure, a cool pattern of intersecting rectangles—soothing gray, non-stimulating beige—covers the white bedspread, and a huge photo print of orange orchids spreads upward from the headboard. But it's hard to get away from the institutional blue of the walls and the research cameras watching your every snuggle and toss.

It's in this room that Jessica Payne, working as a postdoc in the lab of sleep-and-memory guru Robert Stickgold, Ph.D., strapped recording electrodes onto volunteers' heads to learn what went on beneath their skulls as they slept—in particular, how stress and sleep influence memory and psychological function.

Payne is fresh faced and athletic, and talks as fast as I do; as the conversation warms up, each of our remarks seems to set a new record for the other's response, launching an accelerating verbal volley. Payne's doctoral thesis explored sleep and stress, including the influence of cortisol on the nature of dreaming. Cortisol, she notes, peaks late in the night, when rapid eye movement (REM) sleep predominates and dreams send us walking through walls and turn our tears into rain. Might dreaming, then—with its sharded, colliding quasi-real images—be a window into the memory-forming process itself?

The question fascinates Payne, but she's yet to move beyond theorizing into evidence. What she *has* shown in the lab is how increased stress hormones and lack of sleep each bollix up our memories. She's now intent on learning not just why that is but whether the mechanisms driving the deficits—high cortisol among them—might be what drive aging, too.

To Sleep, Perchance to Remember

We have two major types of sleep: REM (rapid eye movement) sleep and NREM (nonrapid eye movement) sleep. NREM is divided into three substages, 1 through 3, with each stage progressively deeper. Throughout the night, REM and NREM alternate in ninety-minute cycles. As the night continues, this cycle length remains stable, but the *ratio* of REM to NREM sleep changes. Early in the night, stage 3 of NREM predominates; this is deep sleep, also called slow wave sleep—when you're essentially a log. More than 80 percent of slow wave sleep occurs in the first half of the typical eight-hour night.

Cortisol, controlled by the body's inner clock, deep in the hypo-thalamus, is at its low point during slow wave sleep. Growth hormone, rich in restorative powers, and melatonin, a brain hormone that makes us sleepy, are at their height then. In the second half of the night, lighter sleep (stage 2 of NREM and REM) predominates. Cortisol levels increas-ingly rise, peaking near morning, to mobilize energy (glucose) so we can tear ourselves out of bed. Growth hormone and melatonin, meanwhile, drop precipitously.

This, scientists say, is the "architecture of sleep"—a fitting nomen-clature, it seems to me, for a state of being that lets us build castles in the air.

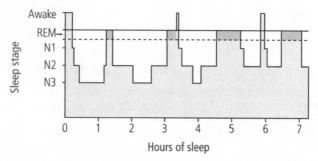

Figure 6. Castles in the Air: The stages of sleep—REM to NREM 1, 2, and 3.

But starting at about age thirty (yes, that young), our sleep architecture begins to change: Slow wave sleep isn't quite as deep, for instance, and so becomes shorter and more fragmented. A paper by the University of Chicago's Eve Van Cauter, Ph.D., a giant in the sleep-and-metabolism field, looked at data from a series of studies on changes during aging in 149 healthy men. She found that slow wave sleep decreased from 18.9 percent of the night's sleep for folks in early adulthood (ages 16 to 25) to a measly 3.4 percent for those at midlife (36 to 50 years). While it remained at that 3.4 percent from midlife on, another change came to bear: With every passing decade starting at midlife, we lose twenty-eight minutes from our sleep schedule.

No wonder we're so tired! And it's not just quality and quantity of sleep that's affected by stress and the aging process. Scanning technology, including fMRI, has revealed that different parts of our brains kick in for different phases of sleep. Which means that particular functions suffer more or less, too.

In NREM sleep, including that deep slow wave sleep, the hypothalamus (a springboard for the stress response), prefrontal cortex (seat of executive function), and regions associated with muscle movement nod off. The hippocampus (memory making and retrieval) stays active, but many pathways connecting it to the neocortex—the part of the giant cerebral cortex involved in higher mental functions—slow down.

During REM sleep, when our eyelids twitch and most dreaming occurs, regions such as the amygdala (regulates emotion, including fear), the anterior cingulate cortex (regulates the sympathetic nervous system), and areas regulating muscles, breathing, heart rate, vision, and hearing kick up their heels (hence those Technicolor dreams). Levels of various brain chemicals shift, too: During REM, the neurotransmitter acetylcholine, which excites brain cells and activates muscles, may be as high as when we're awake. During NREM slow wave sleep, serotonin (which can calm us) and norepinephrine (in the brain, also important for sleeping) are at near-normal levels, while feisty acetylcholine virtually evaporates.

Memories, it turns out, are processed primarily during early NREM slow wave sleep. It's a two-step process: First they must be encoded, and then they must be consolidated.

Briefly, a memory is encoded when a chemical/electrical representation of it is stored in the brain. This applies to both declarative memories (memories of an experience, an event, or a fact) and procedural memories (memories of physical acts, such as riding a bike). "What your wedding day was like—that's a declarative memory, specifically an episodic memory," says Payne. The steps of the hora I danced after the vows? That's procedural memory. For any memory to last over time, from minutes to years, it must be consolidated. And consolidation occurs only when we are zonked out.

Different types of memory are consolidated during different sleep phases. Declarative memories require NREM slow wave sleep to be con-solidated. Procedural memories require both REM and NREM. Disrupt early sleep and you may flunk that test you studied so hard for; disrupt late sleep and you may hit the dance floor with two left feet. Matthew P. Walker, Ph.D., at the University of California, Berkeley, has had hun-dreds of subjects perform a simple test: Type a series of four numbers again and again with their left hand, making a new procedural memory. He tests some subjects in the morning after they have practiced the task, and then again twelve hours later. He has others learn the task late in the day, tests them, and then lets them get a good night's sleep. Performance for the same-dayers remains about the same for both tests; performance for those who get to "sleep on it" improves by 20 to 30 percent.

All of this means that if you're lying in bed stressing away, with your cortisol levels soaring just when they should be low, you're going to cut short your memory-making slow wave sleep and instead slide mostly into NREM stage 2, a much lighter, more raucous state of being.

Many fMRI studies have shown that even *one* night of missed sleep can disrupt the parts of the brain needed to make memories of events and facts. Back when Matthew Walker was affiliated with Harvard, he and colleagues randomly assigned twenty-eight subjects ages eighteen to thirty to either a sleep-deprivation or a control group. The sleep-deprived folks stayed awake for thirty-five hours in the lab setting, while the controls went home to snuggle in their beds. The next day, each participant slipped into an fMRI machine and viewed a series of picture slides. Two days later, after everyone had logged in two nights of sleep, all of the participants returned and were tested to see if they could pick out the original slides from a series now infiltrated with new slides. De-spite the intervening two nights of shut-eye, the sleep-deprived group showed a 19 percent drop in recall compared to their well-rested coun-terparts. The fMRI scans backed up the findings: The hippocampi of the sleep-deprived were much less active than those of the controls.

Walker and colleagues recently reported that even a nap during the day can boost the ability to remember. The scientists had thirty-nine subjects undergo two separate learning sessions, six hours apart. After the first session, they divided the subjects into two groups: an experimental group that took a hundred-minute nap before the second learning session, and a control group that stayed awake before the second session. Over just those six hours, the control group showed a "marked deterioration" in learning ability, while the experimental group actually *improved* their ability to learn.

What might the hippocampus be doing to implant memories while we snooze? One study using positron-emission tomography (PET), a scanning technique that uses short-lived radioactive substances to produce 3-D colored images of body function and metabolism, takes us deep inside the brain. The scientists scanned subjects' brains both as they lay still and learned the route in a virtual maze and then later while they slept. Remarkably, during early slow wave sleep, the *very same* parts of each subject's hippocampus lit up as when the subject was tracking the maze with eyes wide open. The hippocampus was effectively replaying the events from the day *exactly as they had occurred* and chattering away to the neocortex about them, which chattered back using electrical impulses of its own. It was this "conversation" that embedded the maze's route into the subjects' higher-level brain circuits for the long haul, freeing up the hippocampus to process even more new material. Strikingly, the amount of activity in the hippocampus during sleep correlated with the amount of improvement the subjects showed the next day in running the maze they'd learned. "By literally reactivating the experience in a chemical and electrical sense, you're helping to consolidate the memory," says Payne.

Finally, sleep helps us become wise in the long term. It enables the brain to take newly acquired information and integrate it with the old, establishing the associative links that let us abstract and conceptualize, synthesize, and have insight—including those eureka moments following a restful night.

Radiologist Seung-Schik Yoo, Ph.D., is a self-described tech junkie. When I visit his lab, in Boston's Brigham and Women's Hospital, he shows me with pride his latest achievement: a skinny robotic arm that people can move with their thoughts alone via real-time fMRI and a computer. He instructs me to imagine moving my left arm up. The real-time fMRI will pick up the brain areas I've engaged, he explains, translate the signals, and voilà: The robotic arm will rise. Very cool—but a little bit scary. I keep my arms close to my sides.

When he is not crafting a place where brains meet machines, Yoo concentrates on the neuroimaging piece of sleep studies. One that rocked the sleep world shed new light on why people—including Laura Maskell (and me!) —have hair-trigger tempers when we miss too much sleep.

The amygdala processes emotional material. It's particularly sensitive to the bad, scary stuff; part of its evolutionary role is to alert us to danger so we can protect ourselves. You see a snake flick through the brush and your amygdala wigs out. The amygdala is part of the limbic system, the more primitive part of our brain. It has connections running everywhere, including to the prefrontal cortex, the seat of logic and reason. One job of our prefrontal cortex—particularly the middle part, the medial prefrontal cortex—is to bring the amygdala back to its senses, so to speak, so we will respond appropriately to events.

Yoo and his colleagues wanted to learn how lack of sleep affects the *emotional* brain. So they recruited twenty-six participants ages eighteen to thirty, and had fourteen of them stay awake for thirty-five hours in the lab setting while twelve controls went home to sleep in their beds. The next day, each volunteer crawled into an fMRI machine for a scan, where he or she looked at one hundred images ranging from emotionally neutral to grisly—everything from flowers to buildings to children with tumors and mutilated bodies. The subjects classified how each image struck them emotionally by clicking a button.

Everyone's amygdala lit up in response to the disturbing images. But what sent the scientists' minds spinning was that the amygdalas of the sleep-deprived group nearly caught fire: They were *over 60 percent* more reactive than the amygdalas of the control group. Indeed, the scientists, in their paper, called the results "remarkable"—not a word used casually in scientific literature. Moreover, the amount of the amygdala activated in the sleep-deprived folks when they viewed the most disturbing images was three times larger than the amount activated in the controls. Finally, the scientists saw a distinct difference in the brain connections of the two groups: The connection between the amygdala and the medial prefrontal cortex in the controls was significantly stronger than in those who'd stayed awake.

"It just went nuts!" says Yoo about the amygdala of the sleep-deprived participants. "Somehow, the prefrontal cortex, which is considered to be a housekeeper and big brother of our lower brain, loses connection to the more primitive amygdala when we lose sleep. It's a functional disconnect. It means your wires are there, but there's not much current or electricity going through, temporarily."

When You Sleep—but Not Enough

Loss of sleep, for most of us, doesn't mean propping our eyelids open with toothpicks for nights on end but rather cutting our sleep time per night to five or six hours rather than the recommended seven. But numerous research papers, including a new review by the University of Pennsylvania's David F. Dinges, Ph.D., report that even four nights with just three to six hours of sleep not only leaves us nodding off at our desks but also makes us more forgetful, our brains operate more slowly, and our attention frays. Indeed, Dinges notes, after just two weeks of sleeping four hours a night, "deficits in attention, working memory, and cognitive throughput were equivalent to those seen after two nights of total sleep deprivation." Two weeks of sleeping six hours a night—not uncommon for many of us—left people with cognitive deficits equivalent to those found in folks who hadn't slept a wink all night. That's because the damage is cumulative, he writes, with each additional night of truncated sleep adding to the brain-drain burden.

For me this is a huge wake-up call (no pun intended). Sleeping six hours a night can wrack my brain to the same extent as no sleep at all? Might that extra hour per night help me keep my train of thought mid-sentence or get that idiom right (I was left "hung out to dry," not "hung out drying")?

And it's not only mature neurons that take a hit. Miss too much sleep and you may be impeding the birth of *new* brain cells, exactly the fate of a brain that stresses too much (see Chapter 3). Using rats as their subjects, a group led by Peter Meerlo, Ph.D., at the University of Groningen, found that prolonged shortened or missed nights of sleep cumulatively led to "a major decrease" in the survival, maturation, and generation of new cells in the hippocampus—one of two places in the adult brain, you'll recall, where neurogenesis takes place. Yet excessive glucocorticoids, noted Meerlo, may not be the only assassins. Chronically sleep-deprived rats have lower levels of the growth factors IGF-1 (insulin-like growth factor 1) and BDNF (brain-derived neurotrophic factor) than rats with adequate sleep. Remember, too, that BDNF also stimulates long-term potentiation and spurs the release of internal anti-oxidants to neutralize the cell-damaging and telomere-eroding reactive oxygen species described in Chapter 2.

Dinges and others are careful to note that exactly how much sleep each of us needs, and how vulnerable we are to the cognitive deficits of sleep loss, varies from person to person. Research suggests that there's even a genetic component to the calculation. But no matter what your genetic predisposition, consider these words of the University of Chicago's Allan Rechtschaffen, Ph.D., from more than thirty years ago: "If sleep does not serve an absolutely vital function, then it is the biggest mistake the evolutionary process has ever made."

Your Body on Sleep Loss

We've all had the experience: When we sleep less, we eat more, often ravenously. I succumbed with every all-nighter I pulled in college, jamming my mouth full of bulging tuna-fish sandwiches (lots o' mayonnaise) once I'd turned in that paper on Wordsworth or Alan Bullock's giant Hitler book. Intuition told me that my growling stomach was a result of calories burned from extra activity—an important reason to eat. But science gives the lie to that explanation. Those hunger pangs were false signals, the result of the hormones leptin and ghrelin having been thrown out of balance from lack of sleep.

Leptin, as we've seen in Chapter 4, is an appetite-depressing hormone secreted by fat tissue. It signals "energy balance" to the brain, telling us when we're full. Ghrelin does the opposite: It's an appetite-stimulating hormone released by cells in the stomach. It tells the brain, *Better eat now!* In healthy folks, ghrelin levels rise rapidly before meals and fall just as rapidly after they've cleared their plates. Numerous studies have shown that people who are sleep deprived or chronically have too little sleep have significantly decreased levels of leptin and significantly increased levels of ghrelin—regardless of how many calories they take in. Their insulin levels are raised, too, putting them at greater risk for insulin resistance and type 2 diabetes.

Shahrad Taheri, Ph.D., now at the UK's University of Bristol, led a particularly large longitudinal—and therefore convincing—study on the effect of lost sleep on leptin and ghrelin levels. Taheri followed 1,024 men and women from the Wisconsin Sleep Cohort Study, which ran from 1989 until 2000. The subjects filled out questionnaires and kept diaries on their sleep habits. Every four years they gave blood and underwent tests while they slept to assess their sleep states and their breathing and heart rates. The leptin levels of the participants who consistently slept five hours or less a night took a nosedive: They were 15.5 percent lower than the levels of the controls, who logged in a good eight hours of sleep. Conversely, the ghrelin levels of the short-sleepers shot up: They were nearly 15 percent higher than those of their well-rested counterparts. No wonder the short-sleepers were chowing down. In addition, their body mass indexes (BMI) were higher than the BMIs of the controls, and proportionally so: the less sleep, the higher the BMI.

In fact, chronic short sleep leaves us not just hungrier, but thanks to those cortisol spikes, hungrier for—you guessed it—the simple carbs and the fatty sweets. In a study led by the University of Chicago's Van Cauter, subjects whose sleep was restricted to four hours per night for just six nights wound up in a pre-diabetic state, their insulin soaring. And, Van Cauter has shown, it's not just sleep quantity that matters; it's quality, too. If we don't get enough of that NREM slow wave sleep, our ability to metabolize glucose sinks. Studies in young healthy adults show that merely suppressing slow wave sleep with no cuts in sleep time lead to increased risk of type 2 diabetes.

Those experimental results are backed up—and broadened—by much epidemiological research on folks of all ages. The largest may be the previously mentioned Nurses' Health Study, which followed 70,026 women for ten years. It found that those who slept five hours or less a night had a significantly higher risk of being diagnosed with diabetes compared to those who slept a sound eight. Sounds familiar, no?

Indeed, the closer you look, the more the price we pay for chronic sleep loss looks like the price we pay for chronic stress: Obesity is another condition falling on the sleep-stress continuum. Population-based studies involving more than five hundred thousand adults and twenty-eight thousand children have tagged truncated sleep as an important risk factor for obesity, and a recent review of both cross-sectional and longitudinal studies by Case Western Reserve University's Sanjay R. Patel, M.D., concludes that "short sleep duration appears independently associated with weight gain." Although Patel doesn't conclusively pin that added weight on imbalances in ghrelin and leptin, he does point to research that links it to an increase in light NREM sleep and a corresponding decrease in NREM slow wave sleep—regardless of how long the subjects slept. In one, the participants who had the least slow wave sleep had an alarming 40 percent increased risk of obesity compared to those who had the most.

"When you get less than optimal amounts of sleep, say, five or six hours per night rather than seven or eight, your blood pressure rises, your pro-inflammatory cytokines rise, and cortisol levels, which are normally low in the evening, become elevated," says the Rockefeller University's Bruce McEwen, summing up the evidence. "This raises insulin levels—it is moving the body toward the metabolic imbalance that can lead to type 2 diabetes. The elevated cytokines contribute to the hardening of the arteries and other degenerative processes that accumulate very slowly in the brain and the body. We suddenly see our waistline increasing, and when we go to the doctor we learn that our cholesterol levels and our blood pressure are high. These are indications that this allostatic load is progressing. The question, of course, is: Can we change our lifestyle to slow that process down?"

To Reduce Stress and Slow the Cellular Clock Using Sleep

Getting some shut-eye

Lawrence J. Epstein, M.D, is chief medical officer of Sleep HealthCenters, a network of twenty-five sleep diagnosis and treatment facilities affiliated with academic hospitals in Massachusetts, New York, Connecticut, Arizona, and Rhode Island. In his book, *The Harvard Medical School Guide to a Good Night's Sleep*, Epstein outlines a six-step program to help those of us with trouble sleeping descend into the Land of Nod.

"Everyone is prone to having something occur that disrupts their sleep; for example, job loss, moving, or final exams," he tells me from the company's headquarters, in Brighton, Massachusetts. "Disturbing events can lead to hyperarousal—increased heart rate and stress hormones, among other things—which is exactly the opposite of what we need to go to sleep." For most people, when the stimulus resolves, the sleeping problems go away. But for some, the process can be self-perpetuating, a kind of learned response. "Going to bed becomes a *stimulus* for the arousal response," he says. Caffeine compounds the problem, as does alcohol, which may lull us to sleep but can come back to bite us when it wears off. "Chronic insomnia," says Epstein, "takes on a life of its own."

Studies comparing cognitive behavioral therapy and prescription sleep aids show the two run pretty much neck and neck in improving sleep, but cognitive behavioral therapy, research indicates, is longer lasting. (If you choose to go the medication route, be sure to talk to your doctor about a drug that won't reduce slow wave sleep. As Sanjay Patel notes in his review, many prescribed sleep aids, including some common antianxiety drugs and certain antidepressants, may not boost that deep, slow wave sleep and actually may reduce it.)

Unfortunately, though, it can be tough to find cognitive behavioral therapy for sleep. Behavioral sleep medicine is a new specialty, says Epstein, with only about 150 board-certified practitioners across the country to date.

Lee M. Ritterband, Ph.D., a psychologist and computer specialist, aims to change that. Ritterband's team at the University of Virginia has developed a tailored, interactive Internet-based intervention for treating sleep problems called SHUTi (Sleep Healthy Using the Internet). It's based on interventions for insomnia developed over the past twenty years in numerous scientific studies. SHUTi users keep sleep diaries, which the program uses to calculate how much sleep they should get and when they should sleep, based on how well they slept the previous week. They learn how to restrict time in bed to improve sleep quality, and are guided through developing a pre-sleep routine, controlling behaviors that work against sleep, making their bedrooms optimal for sleep, and altering their negative beliefs about sleep ("If I don't fall asleep *right now*, I'll totally screw up that presentation tomorrow!). "It's all fully automated," says Ritterband, who's spent most of the day at home shoveling out from a giant February snowstorm that hit the Washington, D.C., area (which probably helped him sleep that night!). "The goal is to eliminate any human involvement so we can disseminate the program on large scale."

As this book was going to press, Ritterband's team was preparing to launch a huge clinical trial in 2011 to follow up a wildly successful smaller one in which 95 percent of the participants said the program had helped not just their sleep but their "overall quality of life."

You, as a reader of this book, have special access to SHUTi through the personal address www.theasinger.com/shuti. There you can learn about the upcoming availability of the program for consumers, as well as how to participate in a clinical trial.

Going it on your own

If you want to launch your own sleep program *now*, here's an annotated version of the six-step program Epstein discusses in his book.

- **Remember, sleep is important.** For starters, says Epstein, stop thinking of sleep as a catch-as-catch-can experience. Instead, block out sleep time—and don't cut corners. Think of the number of hours you need to sleep to feel refreshed as nonnegotiable as the number of minutes you need in the shower. You don't shut off the water before you've rinsed off the soap, do you? Sleep deserves the same commitment.

- **Consider your lifestyle.** Research has shown that exercise not only helps you fall asleep faster; it also promotes deep, slow wave sleep and keeps you snoozing through the night. (Refer back to Chapter 5 for exercise guidelines.) Be sure, though, to end your workout at least two hours before you turn in, or the stimulatory effect of all that thumping could make it harder to fall asleep. Diet makes a difference, too, in how ready your body and mind will be for bed. Use Walter Willett's Healthy Eating Pyramid, in Chapter

4, as your guide, as well as the other takeaways there. Anything more than a light snack an hour or two before bedtime is a no-no, as digestion takes a lot of work and could keep you awake. A glass of wine is fine—as long as you finish drinking at least three hours before you turn in.

- **Maintain the five habits of good sleep.**

  ◊ **Go to bed and wake up at around the same time every day.** This will ensure that you'll keep your biological clock—keeper of the circadian rhythm introduced in Chapter 1—in good working order. If you want to treat yourself on weekends, grab the extra shut-eye in the morning—and limit it to an hour at most.

  ◊ **Plan—and follow!—a bedtime routine.** Consistency may be the "hobgoblin of small minds," as Ralph Waldo Emerson saw it, but where sleep's concerned, it's the sandman. You want to train your body to anticipate sleep. Turn off the computer and for about an hour do things you find relaxing—reading, listening to music, watching TV, meditating. If you're a before-sleep ruminator, Epstein suggests writing down those nonstop thoughts before you slip between the sheets and keeping a pad nearby in case others arise afterward. If you find yourself in tussles with your kids about *their* bedtime and yours follows soon after, consider developing a shared routine with them (say, TV, reading together in the living room, then lights out).

  ◊ **Use the bedroom for sleep and sex—only.** Again, association is the name of the game. The goal is to be able to look at your bed and feel a yawn coming on (for the sleep part, that is—not the sex part). No reading, no TV, no long discussions or working through fights with your mate once you crawl into bed.

  ◊ **Limit naps.** Naps are not verboten; they just need to be parceled out appropriately—and taken only during the day. Pennsylvania State University's Alexandros N. Vgontzas, M.D., has found that daytime napping (a two-hour nap at midafternoon following a sleepless night) improves alertness and performance, and reverses the out-of-whack cortisol and IL-6 levels described earlier that are brought on by lack of sleep. The body's need for sleep (called the homeostatic drive) increases with every hour you're awake, so don't dampen it by napping too close to bedtime.

◊ **If you're tossing and turning, or even staring at the ceiling, for twenty minutes or more, get out of bed.** At a certain point, *trying* to sleep can work against you. You begin to associate "bed" not with "rest" but with "frustration," a state of being that's anathema to sleep. This habit helps drive the concept of so-called sleep restriction. "If you sleep five hours a night but are in bed for ten, your sleep efficiency is just 50 percent, whereas 'normal' is 85 percent," says Lee Ritterband. SHUTi, he explains, looks at users' sleep diaries and assigns a "sleep window" that corresponds with their actual snooze time. They're in bed less, but soon sleeping more. "People get pretty tired, so their sleep efficiency goes up," he says. As sleep efficiency increases, the program widens the sleep window by twenty minutes per week. So if you can't sleep, go do something soothing outside the bedroom until your eyes start to close: Read, drink herbal tea, listen to calming music.

• **Design your bedroom for sleep.** Be sure your bed is cozy, control noise (maybe turn off that cell phone), and block light— remember, light tells the biological clock that it's time to raise cortisol so you can get out of bed and start the day. Keep the room cool and well ventilated. If your clock mocks you from the shelf, turn it around or throw a pillowcase over it.

• **Put the kibosh on what Epstein calls sleep saboteurs.** Particular offenders: **Caffeine** jacks us up because it blocks the effect of the neurotransmitter adenosine, which promotes sleep. Coffee is wonderful in the morning; I can't start the day without my grande soy latte (extra hot, no foam). But imbibing caffeine less than three hours before bedtime makes it harder both to fall asleep and to maintain slow wave sleep. That's because it takes three to five hours for caffeine to clear your system. **Alcohol**, as mentioned earlier, may soothe you into sleep but fragments sleep once it starts to wear off. It reduces both NREM slow wave sleep and REM sleep, which means you're left floating lightly in stages 1 and 2 of NREM—not a restorative place to be. Epstein suggests having no more than one or two drinks a day, and taking that last sip at least three hours before bedtime. **Smoking**, for an untold number of reasons, is terrible for you. (I quit twenty-seven years ago, and it was the hardest, smartest thing I've ever done.) But smoking even close to bedtime is akin to taking Ambien to wake up: Nicotine is a central nervous system stimulant, so it works directly against your cardiovascular, neurological, and other systems when you're intent is to wind down. Nor do you want to be **hungry** or **full** at bedtime: Both can keep you awake, whether the cause is your digestive system pumping away, heartburn, or a growling stomach. Finish dinner several hours before you retire.

- **If your sleep problems persist, find help.** This is where practitioners in your area, as well as SHUTi, come into the picture. Studies have shown that as little as four to eight weeks of cognitive behavioral therapy improves sleep.

Hot Tip

Notre Dame's Jessica Payne suggests a hot bath about ninety minutes before bedtime if you anticipate sleeping problems, or if you find yourself absolutely unable to sleep. "It sounds hokey, but this really, really works, particularly as we age," she says. The mechanism at work is thermoregulation: Good slow wave sleep regulates body temperature, and our bodies have to be relatively cool for us to get high-quality slow wave sleep. Soaking in a hot bath elevates your body temperature, and when you get out thermoregulation kicks in and your temperature drops rapidly. It's that drop, says Payne, that helps you not only fall asleep but move quickly into slow wave sleep. Payne has introduced the home remedy during presentations and is amazed at the response. "I had so many people writing me and saying, 'Wow, it actually does work!'" she says.

CONCLUSION

I Should Have Danced All Night

All cultures dance. You don't have to teach people to dance. Basically people learn not to dance.

—Choreographer Mark Morris, keynote address,
2008 Society for Neuroscience conference

Choreographer Sara Rudner's Dancing-on-View: The ICA Variations *has the rock-solid architecture of a skyscraper and the brushed spontaneity of a child's kiss. It is four hours of continuous, glorious dancing that seem to pass in an eyeblink—even while embracing, I'd swear, the world's entire variety of movement in its thirty-five announced segments.*

That's how, in July 2008, I opened my *Boston Globe* review of Rudner's window on to, as she put it, "dance as an ongoing activity" (the audience was free to come and go). It was a paean to the day-in, day-out sweat and tears, laughter and camaraderie and singleness of purpose out of which dances and dancers make it into the light of day.

The process, as I know from having danced myself, is at once prosaic and magical. It's as mundane as counting out a movement phrase or blocking out you-go-here-while-she-goes-there spacing. It's also as wondrous as the action of a child's magic slate, in reverse: Replace the plastic cover so a new world—with its own ever-shifting dynamics, tempi, traffic, *and* personalities—comes into focus.

Rudner, a member of Twyla Tharp's famous company for some twenty years, was sixty-five when she made and danced in *The ICA Variations,* whose layers of complexity—temporally, spatially, rhythmically—left me bug-eyed. Peggy Gould, a standout in the eighteen-member cast, was fifty. Gould sent everyone howling with a face clinic, in which she instructed a clump of dancers to "find a rhythmic component" to—yes—their nostrils ("maybe staccato?") or "directional possibilities" for their lips ("swing side to side?" "set up a counterpoint?").

Go ahead. Try it. You're guaranteed to stretch your brain—not to mention your nose. Do it in front of a mirror and you'll be rolling on the floor.

As a dance critic for some twenty-five years, I've long been aware that choreographers and dancers seem to age, mentally and physically, so much more slowly than the rest of us. The observation left me wondering: What is the connection between how dancers spin magic out of intricate physical movement and how they keep their cells humming along vigorously well into their eighties and nineties? What are the mechanisms that keep their brains, muscles, bones, and organs so much more vital and active than the same parts in the rest of us?

Consider that dance pioneer Martha Graham performed in her own *Cortege of Eagles* when she was seventy-six and was choreographing a new dance, *The Eye of the Goddess*, at the time of her death, at age ninety-six. The revolutionary Merce Cunningham premiered his newest creation, *Nearly Ninety*, on—you guessed it—his ninetieth birthday, three months before he died. At age eighty, he danced a duet with Mikhail Baryshnikov at Lincoln Center, grasping a bar because of severe arthritis; at eighty-four, he'd tap-dance in his wheelchair ("That was a way to be active," he told me in a 2003 interview for *Boston* magazine); at eighty-nine he still taught "fabulous" classes, says June Finch, seventy herself, who's been teaching at the Cunningham studio for four decades. Dancer Carmen de Lavallade, whom Alvin Ailey came to New York to partner in the 1954 production of *House of Flowers*, is now seventy. She continues to perform, in a troupe named Paradigm, whose youngest member, founder Gus Solomons, is a robust sixty-nine. And those are just a few of the better-known never-say-quit terpsichoreans around.

Dancing, as I came to realize researching this book, combines many of the elements of longevity revealed in the latest scientific research on stress and aging: intensely focused mental and physical attention; grappling with novelty (to build new neural pathways rather than just etch existing ones deeper); aerobic and resistance exercise *together*; the elimination of abdominal fat; dealing with risk but within a controlled environment; meditative practices (talk about mindfulness!); a sense of spirituality; powerful social relationships; as well as eating healthful diets rich in fruits, veggies, and whole grains.

Indeed, dancers have taken the pursuit of new perspectives that neuroscientists tout as the way to keep the mind and body nimble and made it as essential, as unconsciously necessary, as breathing.

"You're solving new problems all the time," says Rudner over tea the morning after her last *ICA* performance. She's casual in soft capris, a fanny pack around her waist, and reading glasses dangling from a chain around her neck. "You're constantly being challenged and going, 'Oh, I can't do that, but I'm going to try.'" You don't want arms and legs in sync, she tells me, but one set of limbs outrunning the other, so you can jump outside of the box. "What does it feel like to be in that activity where you're really like, 'I don't know where anything is'?" she asks. "You have to learn a new skill—body and mind."

Cunningham—who choreographed more than 150 dances and eight hundred events, starting in the 1940s—strived as the years passed to grow not so much the intent of his dances but their density. "I have a great inclination to go toward complexity," he said in that 2003 interview. "So something that we thought in the beginning was very complex, now seems utterly simple." His definition of complexity? He laughed. "More inches of movement per centimeter."

Cunningham famously ordered his dances through the chance throwing of coins or eight-sided dice he had unearthed in Minneapolis, or by consulting the *I Ching* (the Chinese Book of Changes). "Instead of deciding something for yourself, you use chance operations to bring up a situation you wouldn't know anything about," he said. "You use them to find out something more. In other words, you accept the gamble." In so doing, he changed the way viewers saw not just his dances but the world. One example that turns my mind inside out: He exploited positive and negative space equally—that is, he drew your eye not just to the shapes made by flesh-and-blood bodies but to the spaces of air and light between and surrounding those impenetrable parts.

Scientific research on dance and the brain provides evidence for the cognitive benefits of such practices. At the University of Toronto, Melody S. Berens, Ph.D., and Laura-Ann Petitto, Ed.D., recently ran a randomized controlled brain-imaging trial showing that trained dancers were significantly more accurate in performing an attention task than non-dancers. They were better able to pick the salient bits out of competing information and to remember more acutely. Mind you, the task had nothing to do with dancing—evidence that training in the arts can benefit learning overall. In a follow-up study using cheek swabs of DNA, Berens and Petitto found that trained dancers had particular variants of genes, related to dopamine reward-system pathways, that play a role in, for example, reasoning, pleasure, and motor processing. "Education in the arts," the scientists conclude in their presentation abstract, "may afford cognitive benefits beyond the specific arts at hand."

Indeed, in a new three-year study at seven universities sponsored by the Dana Foundation, researchers led by Michael S. Gazzaniga, Ph.D., of the University of California, Santa Barbara, found that arts training overall facilitates sustained attention and an increased ability to manipulate information in both working and long-term memory.

Using monkeys, early research had shown that brain cells called mirror neurons, which lie in the inferior parietal and premotor cortices of the brain—lit up both when the monkeys picked up an object and when they just watched someone pick up the thing. Recent MRI studies by neuroscientists such as Daniel Glaser, Ph.D., and Beatriz Calvo-Merino, Ph.D., at the University College London; and Emily S. Cross, Ph.D. (an accomplished dancer herself), at the Max Planck Institute of Cognitive Neuroscience, not only carry the phenomenon over to people but also show how dance training can sensitize that outside-inside transfer: The mirror neurons of trained dancers, research has shown, fairly kick up their heels when dancers detect movements they've been trained to perform; for instance, pirouettes for ballet dancers and the promenade for tango dancers.

"Actively learning anything is always good for the whole brain, right?" says Brandeis neuroscientist Eve Marder, Ph.D., whose office is presided over by a life-size cardboard cutout of Xena, the warrior princess. A long-time dance lover, Marder is the one who brought choreographer Mark Morris to the 2008 Society for Neuroscience conference to be the keynote speaker. "And the incredibly complex feat of sensory-motor integration necessary to know thirty or forty dances at any moment in time, as Mark's dancers do, is bound to engage large regions of the brain. It's a prodigious act of memory."

But there are benefits, too, for those of us with a much more limited repertoire. Science has shown, Marder notes, that exercise produces brain-derived neurotrophic factor (BDNF), a growth factor that increases brain plasticity. "So coupling the exercise-induced changes with the intellectual challenge would maximally promote enhanced plasticity and rebirthing, if you will, of brain connections," she says. "You're not just sitting doing crossword puzzles, where you're inactive, or just walking on a treadmill, where you're active. It's putting those two things together. That's why I think dance is so optimal. If you were to, say, take X number of sixty-year-olds and have them dance three times a week for the rest of their life, would you be less likely to see dementia in that population? I would argue: possibly. Who knows? But I would expect from the basis of what we know that it's probably the best thing you could do."

~~~~~

Dean Ornish, M.D., founder of the Preventive Medicine Research Institute in Sausalito, California, has published, to my knowledge, the only clinical scientific study to date that links cellular aging with the type of integrated lifestyle behaviors that dance naturally embraces. Mind you,

I am bringing the two worlds together here; scientists are intensely particular about not generalizing beyond what the evidence shows. But you can't help but see the parallels . . . and speculate.

Ornish is likely best known to the public for his best-selling books, the most recent of which is *The Spectrum: A Scientifically Proven Program to Feel Better, Live Longer, Lose Weight, and Gain Health*, based on the "comprehensive lifestyle intervention" he initially developed in the lab for people with heart disease. The intervention includes an extremely low-fat (only 10 percent of calories from fat), plant-based, whole-foods diet; moderate aerobic exercise (say, brisk walking thirty minutes a day, six days a week); stress management (gentle yoga, meditation, imagery, and progressive-relaxation techniques an hour a day, six days a week); and group support (one hour a week). It's the kind of regimen dancers are familiar with intuitively—except, of course, they ramp up the exercise component.

Ornish recently published a pilot study that investigated whether three months of those intensive lifestyle changes would affect white-blood-cell telomerase activity. (Three months wasn't long enough for changes in telomere length to show.) UCSF's Elizabeth Blackburn, Elissa Epel, and Jennifer Daubenmier collaborated with him. His subjects were thirty men ages forty-nine to eighty, all of whom had been diagnosed by biopsy with low-risk prostate cancer but had chosen not to pursue aggressive treatment. Ornish took blood for several measures, including telomerase levels at the start and again at the end of the three-month intervention.

Remarkably, overall, telomerase activity significantly increased—by nearly 30 percent!—during the course of the intervention, indicating perhaps a slower aging of the participants, all the way down to their cells.* The scientists associated the increase with two factors: decreases in both LDL ("bad") cholesterol and psychological distress, particularly intrusive thoughts. That is, as LDL dropped and as intrusive thoughts

---

* Twenty-four of the thirty subjects had enough cells for telomerase testing.

diminished over the three months, telomerase levels rose. Apparently, it wasn't one lifestyle change that made the difference but the interaction of the four. Other improvements included decreases in BMI and blood pressure. No one's cancer progressed. While total PSA (prostate-specific antigen, a measure for prostate-cancer risk) did not change significantly, the "relevant PSA," as Blackburn put it to me—that is, the percent of free PSA—improved.

There were limitations. The study was small, and because of logistical issues, it did not have a control group, notwithstanding hard work on the part of the researchers to get one. So despite the rigorous execution of the study, Ornish and his team are careful to cite the results as preliminary. "Our findings suggest but do not prove conclusively, the possibility that some or all aspects of the combined lifestyle changes in this study might be responsible for the recorded increase in telomerase activity," they conclude.

The statement is immensely provocative, both for people with various diagnoses and for the many of us who are stressed to the limit and watching birthdays zip by. Indeed, in commenting to me on the study, Elizabeth Blackburn draws a direct line between telomerase levels and the reduction of a typical feature of stress: intrusive thoughts. "The more the telomerase went up, the greater the improvement in intrusive thoughts," she says. This was a situation in which people "actively did something," she says, and telomerase levels rose.

~~~

The science of telomeres has remained largely at the level of molecules and cells, and in some animals, but studying telomeres in people is still terrifically new. Yet it is one of the most rapidly growing fields in aging research. Right now, hundreds of scientists around the world are busy discovering new insights into how telomeres work in our bodies and how they are connected to our lives and longevity. Indeed, I expect to see an explosion of interest in telomere research regarding not just stress and aging but all dimensions of aging.

Today, we all go for our annual checkups to keep careful track of various metabolic and other measures: levels of cholesterol, triglycerides, glucose, and inflammatory markers such as C-reactive protein. These are supposed to give us a snapshot of our overall health. But in the not-too-distant future, clinicians will likely be looking to a new, more accurate and all-encompassing measure of our general health, risk for disease, and even where we stand on the aging spectrum: levels of telomerase and telomere length.

You now have the tools to start influencing that measure even before tests for it arrive at your health provider's office. Recall from the preceding chapters how crucial having a sense of control is in reducing stress— and how central reducing stress is to slowing the aging process, all the way down to the DNA in our cells. Stress may be the new biological clock, but we also hold within us the means to slow and even rewind its springs. We have the ability to change how we perceive the world.

In his New York office, Bruce McEwen ticks off the lifestyle factors addressed in this book: "Exercise, sleep, social support, feeling part of a community, diet," he says. "Much of this is in our own hands."

Unwind/Rewind

When it comes to controlling how stress ages us, what matters is not just our stress resistance but our stress *resilience*—how well we can bounce back from stress. Our lifestyle choices play a significant role in determining that. Take the test below for a measure of your own resilience. Then, after using the suggestions in this book that "speak" to you for three weeks, take it again. Watch your score rise.

Please indicate the extent to which you agree with each of the statements below by using the following scale:

1 = Strongly disagree   2 = Disagree   3 = Neutral
4 = Agree   5 = Strongly agree

1. I tend to bounce back quickly after hard times.

    1   2   3   4   5

2. I have a hard time making it through stressful events. (R)

    1   2   3   4   5

3. It does not take me long to recover from a stressful event.

    1   2   3   4   5

4. It is hard for me to snap back when something bad happens. (R)

    1   2   3   4   5

5. I usually come through difficult times with little trouble.

    1   2   3   4   5

6. I tend to take a long time to get over setbacks in my life. (R)

    1   2   3   4   5

Calculating your score:

1. Take your responses to questions 2, 4, and 6 and *reverse* each one. That is, if you circled 1, give the response the value of 5; if you circled 2, give the response the value of 4; and so on: 3 = 3, 4 = 2, 5 = 1. Add up the *reversed* values. (Reverse scoring is what makes many tests scientifically valid, as opposed to the guesswork of many popular tests.)

2. Add up your responses to the remaining questions: 1, 3, and 5.

3. Add the sums from points 1 and 2 to get your total score.

Scores will range from 5 to 30. The higher your score, the greater your resilience.

Interpreting your score the *Stress Less* way*:

26–30: Very resilient
20–25: Resilient
15–19: Moderately resilient
9–14: Fairly resilient
5–8: Not resilient

* The *Stress Less* interpretation was developed by the author, not the scientists.

SELECTED BIBLIOGRAPHY

The field of stress, aging, and telomeres is very new but growing at a rapid pace. What follows is a selected bibliography of the books and scientific studies I used in researching and writing *Stress Less*. I've listed the books separately, as I used many of them for various chapters.

To keep up to date on developments in this hot area, visit my Web site at www.theasinger.com and search the National Institute of Health's online publication library www.ncbi.nlm.nih.gov/pubmed/. At the latter, you can track individual scientists or areas of interest using key words.

BOOKS

Begley, Sharon. *Train Your Mind, Change Your Brain: How a New Science Reveals Our Extraordinary Potential to Transform Ourselves*. New York: Ballantine Books, 2007.

Blakeslee, Sandra, and Matthew Blakeslee. *The Body Has a Mind of Its Own: How Body Maps in Your Brain Help You Do (Almost) Everything Better*. New York: Random House, 2007.

Brady, Catherine. *Elizabeth Blackburn and the Story of Telomeres: Deciphering the Ends of DNA*. Cambridge, MA: MIT Press, 2007.

Brown, Carolyn. *Chance and Circumstance: Twenty Years with Cage and Cunningham*. New York: Alfred A. Knopf, 2007.

Carstensen, Laura L. *A Long Bright Future: An Action Plan for a Lifetime of Happiness, Health, and Financial Security*. New York: Broadway Books, 2009.

Ehrenreich, Barbara. *Bright-Sided: How the Relentless Promotion of Positive Thinking Has Undermined America*. New York: Metropolitan Books/Henry Holt and Co., 2009.

Epstein, Lawrence, with Steven Mardon. *The Harvard Medical School Guide to a Good Night's Sleep*. New York: McGraw Hill, 2007.

Finch, Caleb E. *The Biology of Human Longevity: Inflammation, Nutrition, and Aging in the Evolution of Lifespans*. Burlington, MA: Academic Press, 2007

Fink, George, ed. *Encyclopedia of Stress*, Second Edition. Four-volume set. Oxford, UK. Academic Press/Elsevier. 2007.

Fredrickson, Barbara L. *Positivity: Groundbreaking Research Reveals How to Embrace the Hidden Strength of Positive Emotions, Overcome Negativity, and Thrive.* New York: Crown Publishers, 2009.

Gage F. and Christen Y., eds. *Retrotransposition, Diversity and the Brain,* "Telomeres and telomerase in human health and disease," by Jue Lin, Elissa S. Epel, and Elizabeth H. Blackburn. Springer-Verlag Berlin Heidelberg, 2008: 1–12.

Guarente, Leonard P. *Ageless Quest: One Scientist's Search for Genes That Prolong Youth.* Cold Spring Harbor, NY: Cold Spring Harbor Laboratory Press, 2003.

Guarante, Leonard P., Linda Partridge, and Douglas C. Wallace., eds. *Molecular Biology of Aging.* Cold Spring Harbor, NY: Cold Spring Harbor Laboratory Press, 2008.

Joseph, James A, Daniel A. Dadeau, and Anne Underwood. *The Color Code: A Revolutionary Eating Plan for Optimum Health.* New York: Hyperion. 2002.

Kabat-Zinn, Jon. *Full Catastrophe Living: Using the Wisdom of Your Body and Mind to Face Stress, Pain, and Illness.* New York: Delta Trade Paperbacks, 1990.

Katzen, Mollie, and Walter C. Willett. *Eat, Drink and Weigh Less: A Flexible and Delicious Way to Shrink Your Waist Without Going Hungry.* New York: Hyperion, 2006: 22.

Kessler, David A. *The End of Overeating: Taking Control of the Insatiable American Appetite.* New York: Rodale, 2009.

Levitin, Daniel J. *This Is Your Brain on Music: The Science of a Human Obsession.* New York: Plume, 2007.

McEwen, Bruce S., with Elizabeth Norton Lasley. *The End of Stress As We Know It.* Washington, DC: Joseph Henry Press, 2002.

Mill, John S. *The Autobiography of John Stuart Mill.* New York: Columbia University Press, 1994.

Ornish, D. The Spectrum: *A Scientifically Proven Program to Feel Better, Live Longer, Lose Weight, and Gain Health.* New York: Ballantine Books; 2008.

Ratey, John J., with Eric Hagerman. *Spark: The Revolutionary New Science of Exercise and the Brain.* New York: Little, Brown and Co., 2008.

Ricklefs, Robert E., and Caleb E. Finch. *Aging: A Natural History.* New York: Scientific American Library, 1995.

Sacks, Oliver. *Musicophilia: Tales of Music and the Brain.* New York: Random House, 2007.

Sapolsky, Robert M. *Why Zebras Don't Get Ulcers: The Acclaimed Guide to Stress, Stress-Related Diseases, and Coping,* third ed. New York: Owl Books/Henry Holt and Co., 2004.

Seligman, Martin E. P. *Learned Optimism: How to Change Your Mind and Your Life.* New York: Vintage, 2006.

Willett, Walter C., with Patrick J. Skerrett. *Eat, Drink, and Be Healthy: The Harvard Medical School Guide to Healthy Eating.* New York: Free Press, 2005.

STUDIES BY CHAPTER

Introduction: Stress—The New Biological Clock: How You Can Turn It Back

Almeida, David M. "Resilience and vulnerability to daily stressors assessed via diary methods." *Current Directions in Psychological Science,* 2005, vol. 11, no. 2: 64–68.

Almeida, David M., and Melanie C. Horn. "Is daily life more stressful during middle adult-hood?" In *How healthy are we?: a national study of well-being at midlife*. Brim, Orville Gilbert, et al., eds. Chicago: University of Chicago Press, 2004: 425–51.

Becker, J. B., L. M. Monteggia, T. S. Perrot-Sinal, R. D. Romeo, J. R. Taylor, R. Yehuda, and T. L. Bale. "Stress and disease: is being female a predisposing factor?" *The Journal of Neuroscience*. October 31, 2007, vol. 27, no. 44: 11851–5.

Benedetti, M. G., A. L. Foster, M. C. Vantipalli, M. P. White, J. N. Sampayo, M. S. Gill, A. Olsen, and G. J. Lithgow. "Compounds that confer thermal stress resistance and extended lifespan." *Experimental Gerontology*. October 2008, vol. 43, no. 10: 882–91.

Charles, S. T., D. M. Almeida. "Genetic and environmental effects on daily life stressors: more evidence for greater variation in later life." *Psychology and Aging*. June 2007, vol. 22, no. 2: 331–40.

Epel, E. S. "Telomeres in a life-span perspective: A new 'psychobiomarker'?" *Current Directions in Psychological Science*. 2009 Association for Psychological Science. Vol. 18, no. 1: 6–10.

Khaw, K. T., N. Wareham, S. Bingham, A. Welch, R. Luben, N. Day. "Combined impact of health behaviours and mortality in men and women: the EPIC-Norfolk prospective population study." *PLoS Medicine*. January 8, 2008, vol. 5, no. 1: e12. Erratum in: *PLoS Medicine*. March 18, 2008, vol. 5, no. 3: e70.

Lachman, M. E. "Development in midlife." *Annual Review of Psychology*. 2004, vol. 55: 305–31.

Longo, V. D., and B. K. Kennedy. "Sirtuins in aging and age-related disease." *Cell*. July 28, 2006, vol. 126, no. 2: 257–68.

Mackin, J. "Women, stress, and midlife." *Human Ecology*. Cornell University, College of Human Ecology, Fall 1995, vol. 23, issue 4.

Mather, M., and L. L. Carstensen. "Aging and motivated cognition: the positivity effect in attention and memory." *Trends in Cognitive Sciences*. October 9, 2005, vol. 10: 496–502. Review.

Neupert, S. D., D. M. Almeida, and S. T. Charles. "Age differences in reactivity to daily stressors: the role of personal control." *The Journals of Gerontology, Series B: Psychological Sciences*. July 2007, vol. 62, no. 4: P216–25.

Olsen, A., M. C. Vantipalli, and G. J. Lithgow. "Lifespan extension of *Caenorhabditis elegans* following repeated mild hormetic heat treatments." *Biogerontology*. August 2007, vol. 7, no. 4: 221–30.

Serido, J., D. M. Almeida, and E. Wethington. "Chronic stressors and daily hassles: unique and interactive relationships with psychological distress." *Journal of Health and Social Behavior*. March 4, 2004, vol. 5, no. 1: 17–33.

Shellenbarger, Sue. "The female midlife crisis; More women than men now report upheaval by age 50; the ATV tipping point." *Wall Street Journal* (Eastern edition). New York: April 7, 2005. P D.1.

Sinclair, D. A., and L. Guarente. "Unlocking the secrets of longevity genes." *Scientific American*. March 2006, vol. 294, no. 3: 48–51, 54–7.

Singer, T. "The Midlife Confidence Surge." *MORE*. February 2008.

Smith, E. D., M. Tsuchiya, L. A. Fox, N. Dang, D. Hu, E. O. Kerr, E. D. Johnston, B. N. Tchao, D. N. Pak, K. L. Welton, D. E. Promislow, J. H. Thomas, M. Kaeberlein, and B. K. Kennedy. "Quantitative evidence for conserved longevity pathways between divergent eukaryotic species." *Genome Research*. April 2008, vol. 18, no. 4: 564–70.

Stroud, L. R., P. Salovey, E. S. Epel. "Sex differences in stress responses: social rejection versus achievement stress." *Biological Psychiatry*. August 15, 2002, vol. 52, no. 4: 318–27.

Chapter 1: The Old Science of Stress

Abe, K, J. U. Tilan, and Z. Zukowska. "NPY and NPY receptors in vascular remodeling." *Current Topics in Medicinal Chemistry*. 2007, vol. 7, no. 17: 1704–9.

American Heart Association Statistics Committee and Stroke Statistics Subcommittee. "Heart disease and stroke statistics—2010 update: a report from the American Heart Association." *Circulation*. February 23, 2010, vol. 121, no. 7: e46–e215.

Bertok, L., and Hans Selye. *Annals of the New York Academy of Sciences*, vol. 851, issue 1. "Stress of Life," June 1998: xv–xv.

Burleson, M. H., K. M. Poehlmann, L. C. Hawkley, J. M. Ernst, G. G. Berntson, W. B. Malarkey, J. K. Kiecolt-Glaser, R. Glaser, and J. T. Cacioppo. "Neuroendocrine and cardiovascular reactivity to stress in mid-aged and older women: long-term temporal consistency of individual differences." *Psychophysiology*. May 2003, vol. 40 no. 3: 358–69.

Bybee, K. A., and A. Prasad. "Stress-related cardiomyopathy syndromes." *Circulation*. July 22, 2008, vol. 118, no. 4: 397–409.

Campisi, J., T. H. Leem, and M. Fleshner. "Acute stress decreases inflammation at the site of infection. A role for nitric oxide." *Physiology and Behavior*. November 2002, vol. 77, nos. 2–3: 291–9.

Campisi J, T. H. Leem, B. N. Greenwood, M. K. Hansen, A. Moraska, K. Higgins, T. P. Smith, and M. Fleshner. "Habitual physical activity facilitates stress-induced HSP72 induction in brain, peripheral, and immune tissues." *American Journal of Physiology— Regulatory, Integrative, and Comparative Physiology*. February 2003, vol. 284, no. 2: R520–30.

Centers for Disease Control and Prevention. 2007 National Diabetes Fact Sheet, 1–7 (http://www.cdc.gov/diabetes/pubs/estimataes07htm).

Centers for Disease Control and Prevention. Faststats – Diabetes, 1–3 (http://www.cdc .gov/nchs/fastats/diabetes.htm).

Chida, Y., and A. Steptoe. "Greater cardiovascular responses to laboratory mental stress are associated with poor subsequent cardiovascular risk status: a meta-analysis of prospective evidence." *Hypertension*. April 2010, vol. 55, no. 4: 1026–32.

Chida, Y., and A. Steptoe. "The association of anger and hostility with future coronary heart disease: a meta-analytic review of prospective evidence." *Journal of the American College of Cardiology*. March 17, 2009, vol. 53, no. 11: 936–46.

Christian, L. M., J. E. Graham, D. A. Padgett, R. Glaser, and J. K. Kiecolt-Glaser. "Stress and wound healing." *Neuroimmunomodulation*. 2006, vol. 13, nos. 5–6: 337–46.

Collins, S. M. "Stress and the Gastrointestinal tract. IV. Modulation of intestinal inflammation by stress: basic mechanisms and clinical relevance." *American Journal of Physiology: Gastrointestinal and Liver Physiology*. 2001, vol. 280: G315–G318.

Collins, S. M., and P. Bercik. "The relationship between intestinal microbiota and the central nervous system in normal gastrointestinal function and disease." *Gastroenterology*. 2009, vol. 136: 2003–2014.

Collins, S. M. "Translating symptoms into mechanisms: functional GI disorders." *Advances in Physiology Education*. 2007, vol. 31: 329–31.

Crimmins, E. M., and C. E. Finch. "Infection, inflammation, height, and longevity." *Proceedings of the National Academy of Sciences.* January 10, 2006, vol. 103, no. 2: 498–503.

Dhabhar, F. S. "Enhancing versus suppressive effects of stress on immune function: implications for immunoprotection and immunopathology." *Neuroimmunomodulation.* 2009, vol. 16, no. 5: 300–17.

Dhabhar, F. S., and K. Viswanathan. "Short-term stress experienced at time of immunization induces a long-lasting increase in immunologic memory." *American Journal of Physiology: Regulatory, Integrative, and Comparative Physiology.* September 2005, vol. 289, no. 3: R738–44.

Dimsdale, J. E. "Psychological stress and cardiovascular disease." *Journal of the American College of Cardiology.* April 1 2008, vol. 51, no. 13: 1237–46.

Eppel, Elissa S., Heather M. Burke, and Owen M. Wolkowitz. "The *Psychoneuroendocrinology* of aging: Anabolic and catabolic hormones." *Handbook of Health Psychology and Aging.* C. M. Aldwin, C. L. Park, and A. Spiro, eds. The Guilford Press, 2007: 119–141.

Erusalimsky, J. D., and D. J. Kurz. "Cellular senescence in vivo: its relevance in ageing and cardiovascular disease." *Experimental Gerontology.* August-September 2005, vol. 40, nos. 8–9: 634–42.

Gimeno, D., M. G. Marmot, and A. Singh-Manoux. "Inflammatory markers and cognitive function in middle-aged adults: the Whitehall II study." *Psychoneuroendocrinology.* November 2008, vol. 33, no. 10: 1322–34.

Glaser, R., R. C. MacCallum, B. F. Laskowski, W. B. Malarkey, J. F. Sheridan, and J. K. Kiecolt-Glaser. "Evidence for a shift in the Th-1 to Th-2 cytokine response associated with chronic stress and aging." *Journals of Gerontology: Biological Sciences and Medical Sciences.* August 2001, vol. 56, no. 8: M477–82. Erratum in: *Journals of Gerontology: Biological Sciences and Medical Sciences.* November 2001, vol. 56, no. 11: M673.

Glaser, R., and J. K. Kiecolt-Glaser. "Stress-induced immune dysfunction: implications for health." *Nature Reviews Immunology.* March 2005, vol. 5, no. 3: 243–51.

Gouin, J. P., L. Hantsoo, and J. K. Kiecolt-Glaser. "Immune dysregulation and chronic stress among older adults: a review." *Neuroimmunomodulation.* 2008, vol. 15, nos. 4–6: 251–9.

Gould, E. "How widespread is adult neurogenesis in mammals?" *Nature Reviews Neuroscience.* June 2007, vol. 8, no. 6: 481–8.

Graham, J. E., L. M. Christian, and J. K. Kiecolt-Glaser. "Stress, age, and immune function: toward a lifespan approach." *Journal of Behavioral Medicine.* August 2006, vol. 29, no. 4: 389–400.

Harvard School of Public Health. "The Nutrition Source. Simple steps to preventing diabetes." 2009: 1–8 (http://www.hsph.harvard.edu/nutritionsource/more/diabetes-fullstory.index.html).

Johnson, J. D., J. Campisi, C. M. Sharkey, S. L. Kennedy, M. Nickerson, and M. Fleshner. "Adrenergic receptors mediate stress-induced elevations in extracellular Hsp72." *Journal of Applied Physiology.* November 2005, vol. 99, no. 5: 1789–95.

Johnson, J. D., and M. Fleshner. "Releasing signals, secretory pathways, and immune function of endogenous extracellular heat shock protein 72." *Journal of Leukocyte Biology.* March 2006, vol. 79, no. 3: 425–34.

Juster, R. P., B. S. McEwen, and S. J. Lupien. "Allostatic load biomarkers of chronic stress and impact on health and cognition." *Neuroscience and Behavioral Reviews.* October 12, 2009.

Kemeny, M. E. "Psychobiological responses to social threat: evolution of a psychological model in psychoneuroimmunology." *Brain, Behavior, and Immunity.* January 2009, vol. 23, no. 1: 1–9.

Kiecolt-Glaser, J. K., T. J. Loving, J. R. Stowell, W. B. Malarkey, S. Lemeshow, S. L. Dickinson, and R. Glaser. "Hostile marital interactions, proinflammatory cytokine production, and wound healing." *Archives of General Psychiatry.* December 2005, 62(12): 1377–84.

Kiecolt-Glaser, J. K., J. P. Gouin, and L. Hantsoo. "Close relationships, inflammation, and health." *Neuroscience and Biobehavioral Reviews.* September 12, 2009.

Kiecolt-Glaser, J. K., K. J. Preacher, R. C. MacCallum, C. Atkinson, W. B. Malarkey, and R. Glaser. "Chronic stress and age-related increases in the proinflammatory cytokine IL-6." *Proceedings of the National Academy of Sciences.* July 22, 2003, vol. 100, no. 15: 9090–5.

Kiecolt-Glaser, J. K., M. A. Belury, K. Porter, D. Q. Beversdorf, S. Lemeshow, and R. Glaser. "Depressive symptoms, omega-6:omega-3 fatty acids, and inflammation in older adults." *Psychosomatic Medicine.* April 2007, vol. 69, no. 3: 217–24.

Kiecolt-Glaser, J. K., and R. Yehuda. "Toward optimal health: Janice K. Kiecolt-Glaser, Ph.D. and Rachel Yehuda, Ph.D. discuss chronic stress in women." Interview by Jodi R. Godfrey. *Journal of Womens Health (Larchmt).* May 2005, vol. 14, no. 4: 294–8.

Kroenke, C. H., L. D. Kubzansky, N. Adler, and I. Kawachi. "Prospective change in health-related quality of life and subsequent mortality among middle-aged and older women." *American Journal of Public Health.* November 2008, vol. 98, no. 11: 2085–91.

Kubzansky, L. D., I. Kawachi, S. T. Weiss, and D. Sparrow. "Anxiety and coronary heart disease: a synthesis of epidemiological, psychological, and experimental evidence." *Annals of Behavioral Medicine.* Spring 1998, vol. 20, no. 2: 47–58.

Kubzansky, L. D., and I. Kawachi. "Going to the heart of the matter: do negative emotions cause coronary heart disease?" *Journal of Psychosomatic Research.* April-May 2000, vol. 48, no. 4–5: 323–37.

Kubzansky, L. D., I. Kawachi, A. Spiro 3rd, S. T. Weiss, P. S. Vokonas, and D. Sparrow. "Is worrying bad for your heart? A prospective study of worry and coronary heart disease in the Normative Aging Study." *Circulation.* February 18, 1997, vol. 95, no. 4: 818–24.

Kubzansky, L. D., S. R. Cole, I. Kawachi, P. Vokonas, and D. Sparrow. "Shared and unique contributions of anger, anxiety, and depression to coronary heart disease: a prospective study in the normative aging study." *Annals of Behavioral Medicine.* February 2006, vol. 31, no. 1: 21–9.

Kubzansky, L. D., I. Kawachi, and D. Sparrow. "Socioeconomic status, hostility, and risk factor clustering in the Normative Aging Study: any help from the concept of allostatic load?" *Annals of Behavioral Medicine.* Fall 1999, vol. 21, no. 4: 330–8.

Kuo, L. E., K. Abe, and Z. Zukowska. "Stress, NPY and vascular remodeling: Implications for stress-related diseases." *Peptides.* February 2007, vol. 28, no. 2: 435–40. Erratum in: *Peptides.* April 2007, vol. 28, no. 4: 949. Abe, Ken [added].

Lightman, S. L., C. C. Wiles, H. C. Atkinson, D. E. Henley, G. M. Russell, J. A. Leendertz, M. A. McKenna, F. Spiga, S. A. Wood, and B. L. Conway-Campbell. "The significance of glucocorticoid pulsatility." *European Journal of Pharmacology*. April 7, 2008, vol. 583, nos. 2–3: 255–62.

Mackay, F. "Stress and immunity: From starving cavemen to stressed-out scientists." The Dana Foundation. *Cerebrum*. October 17, 2007: 1–4.

Maier, S. F., L. R. Watkins, and M. Fleshner. "Psychoneuroimmunology. The interface between behavior, brain, and immunity." *American Psychologist*. December 1994, vol. 49, no. 12: 1004–17.

Maninger, N., O. M. Wolkowitz, V. I. Reus, E. S. Epel, and S. H. Mellon. "Neurobiological and neuropsychiatric effects of dehydroepiandrosterone (DHEA) and DHEA sulfate (DHEAS)." *Frontiers in Neuroendocrinology*. January 2009, vol. 30, no. 1: 65–91.

Maselko, J., and L. D. Kubzansky. "Gender differences in religious practices, spiritual experiences and health: results from the U.S. General Social Survey." *Social Science and Medicine*. June 2006, vol. 62, no. 11: 2848–60.

Maselko, J., L. D. Kubzansky, I. Kawachi, T. Seeman, and L. Berkman. "Religious service attendance and allostatic load among high-functioning elderly." *Psychosomatic Medicine*. June 2007, vol. 69, no. 5: 464–72.

McEwen, B. S. "Hormones as regulators of brain development: life-long effects related to health and disease." *Acta Pædiatrica Supplement*. July 1997, vol. 422: 41–4.

McEwen, B. S. "Stress, adaptation, and disease. Allostasis and allostatic load." *Annals of the New York Academy of Sciences*. May 1, 1998, vol. 840: 33–44.

McEwen, B. S., and E. Stellar. "Stress and the individual. Mechanisms leading to disease." *Archives of Internal Medicine*. September 27, 1993, vol. 153, no. 18: 2093–101.

McEwen, B. S., and T. A. Milner. "Hippocampal formation: shedding light on the influence of sex and stress on the brain." *Brain Research Reviews*. October 2007, vol. 55, no. 2: 343–55.

McEwen, B. S., and J. C. Wingfield. "What is in a name? Integrating homeostasis, allostasis and stress." Hormones and Behavior. February 2010, vol. 57, no. 2: 105–11.

McEwen, B. S. "The brain is the central organ of stress and adaptation." *Neuroimage*. September 2009, vol. 47, no. 3: 911–3.

Mendelson T., R. C. Thurston, and L. D. Kubzansky. "Affective and cardiovascular effects of experimentally-induced social status." *Journal of Health Psychology*. July 2008, vol. 27, no. 4: 482–9.

Mirescu, C., and E. Gould. "Stress and adult neurogenesis." *Hippocampus*. 2006, vol. 16, no. 3: 233–8.

Mirescu, C., J. D. Peters, and E. Gould. "Early life experience alters response of adult neurogenesis to stress." *Nature Neuroscience*. August 2004, vol. 7, no. 8: 841–6.

Otte, C., S. Hart, T. C. Neylan, C. R. Marmar, K. Yaffe, D. C. Mohr. "A meta-analysis of cortisol response to challenge in human aging: importance of gender." *Psychoneuroendocrinology*. January 2005, vol. 30, no. 1: 80–91.

Robles, T. F., R. Glaser, and J. K. Kiecolt-Glaser. "Out of balance: A new look at chronic stress, depression, and immunity." *Current Directions in Psychological Science*. 2005, vol. 14:2: 111–115.

Rosenberger, P. H., J. R. Ickovics, E. Epel, E. Nadler, P. Jokl, J. P. Fulkerson, J. M. Tillie, and F. S. Dhabhar. "Surgical stress-induced immune cell redistribution profiles predict short-term and long-term postsurgical recovery. A prospective study." *Journal of Bone and Joint Surgery*. December 2009, vol. 91, no. 12: 2783–94.

Rozanski, A., J. A. Blumenthal, K. W. Davidson, P. G. Saab, and L. Kubzansky. "The epidemiology, pathophysiology, and management of psychosocial risk factors in cardiac practice: the emerging field of behavioral cardiology." *Journal of the American College of Cardiology.* March 1, 2005, vol. 45, no. 5: 637–51.

Schubert, C., M. Lambertz, R. A. Nelesen, W. Bardwell, J. B. Choi, and J. E. Dimsdale. "Effects of stress on heart rate complexity—a comparison between short-term and chronic stress." *Biological Psychology.* March 2009, vol. 80, no. 3: 325–32.

Seeman, T. E., B. S. McEwen, J. W. Rowe, and B. H. Singer. "Allostatic load as a marker of cumulative biological risk: MacArthur studies of successful aging." *Proceedings of the National Academy of Sciences.* April 10, 2001, vol. 98, no. 8: 4770–5.

Segerstrom, S. C., and G.. E. Miller. "Psychological stress and the human immune system: a meta-analytic study of 30 years of inquiry." *Psychology Bulletin.* July 2004, vol. 130, no. 4: 601–30.

Selye, H. "A syndrome produced by diverse nocuous agents." *Nature.* July 4, 1936, vol. 138: 32.

Sharkey, S. W., J. R. Lesser, A. G. Zenovich, M. S. Maron, J. Lindberg, T. F. Longe, and B. J. Maron. "Acute and reversible cardiomyopathy provoked by stress in women from the United States. Circulation." February 1, 2005, vol. 111, no. 4: 472–9.

Shively, C. A., D. L. Musselman, and S. L. Willard." Stress, depression, and coronary artery disease: modeling comorbidity in female primates." *Neuroscience and Biobehavioral Reviews.* February 2009, vol. 33, no. 2: 133–44.

Stam, R., K. Ekkelenkamp, A. C. Frankhuijzen, A. W. Bruijnzeel, L. M. Akkermans, and V. M. Wiegant. "Long-lasting changes in central nervous system responsivity to colonic distention after stress in rats." *Gastroenterology.* October 2002; vol. 123, no. 4: 1216–25.

Steptoe, A. "Psychophysiological stress reactivity and hypertension." *Hypertension.* 2008, vol. 52: 220–21.

Steptoe, A., M. Hamer, and Y. Chida. "The effects of acute psychological stress on circulating inflammatory factors in humans: a review and meta-analysis." *Brain, Behavior, and Immunity.* October 2007, vol. 21, no. 7: 901–12.

Stewart, J. C., D. L. Janicki, M. F. Muldoon, K. Sutton-Tyrrell, and T. W. Kamarck. "Negative emotions and 3-year progression of subclinical atherosclerosis." *Archives of General Psychiatry.* February 2007, vol. 64, no. 2: 225–33.

Szabo, S. "Hans Selye and the development of the stress concept: special reference to gastroduodenal ulcerogenesis." *Annals of the New York Academy of Sciences.* June 30, 1998, vol. 851: 19–27.

Thurston, R. C., and L. D. Kubzansky. "Women, loneliness, and incident coronary heart disease." *Psychosomatic Medicine.* October 2009, vol. 71, no. 8: 836–42.

Viswanathan, K., and F. S. Dhabhar. "Stress-induced enhancement of leukocyte trafficking into sites of surgery or immune activation." *Proceedings of the National Academy of Sciences.* April 19, 2005, vol. 102, no. 16: 5808–13.

Weng, N. P. "Aging of the immune system: how much can the adaptive immune system adapt?" *Immunity.* May 2006, vol. 24, no. 5: 495–9.

Wheway, J., H. Herzog, and F. Mackay. "NPY and receptors in immune and inflammatory diseases." *Current Topics in Medicinal Chemistry.* 2007, vol. 7, no. 17: 1743–52.

Wheway, J., C. R. Mackay, R. A. Newton, A. Sainsbury, D. Boey, H. Herzog, and F. Mackay. "A fundamental bimodal role for neuropeptide Y1 receptor in the immune system." *The Journal of Experimental Medicine.* December 5, 2005, vol. 202, no. 11: 1527–38.

Wittstein, I. S. "Acute stress cardiomyopathy." *Current Heart Failure Reports.* June 2008, vol. 5, no. 2: 61–8.

Wolkowitz. O. M., E. S. Epel, and S. Mellon. "When blue turns to grey: do stress and depression accelerate cell aging?" *World Journal of Biological Psychiatry.* 2008, vol. 9, no. 1: 2–5.

Wolf, S. A., A. Melnik, T. P. Waltinger, A. Akpirnali, R. Sapolsky, and G. Kempermann. "The prenatal immunological environment modulates hippocampal neuronal stem cell fitness." *FENS Abstract,* vol. 5, 091.2, 2010.

Yusuf, S., S. Hawken, S. Ounpuu, T. Dans, A. Avezum, F. Lanas, M. McQueen, A. Budaj, P. Pais, J. Varigos, and L. Lisheng; INTERHEART Study Investigators. "Effect of potentially modifiable risk factors associated with myocardial infarction in 52 countries (the INTERHEART study): case-control study." *Lancet.* September 11–17, 2004, vol. 364, no. 9438: 937–52.

Chapter 2: The New Science of Stress

Ahmed, S., J. F. Passos, M. J. Birket, T. Beckmann, S. Brings, H. Peters, M. A. Birch-Machin, T. von Zglinicki, and G. Saretzki. "Telomerase does not counteract telomere shortening but protects mitochondrial function under oxidative stress." *Journal of Cell Science.* April 1, 2008, vol. 121, pt. 7: 1046–53.

Alder, J. K., J. J. Chen, L. Lancaster, S. Danoff, S. C. Su, J. D. Cogan, I. Vulto, M. Xie, X. Qi, R. M. Tuder, J. A. Phillips 3rd, P. M. Lansdorp, J. E. Loyd, and M. Y. Armanios. "Short telomeres are a risk factor for idiopathic pulmonary fibrosis." *Proceedings of the National Academy of Sciences.* September 2, 2008, vol. 105, no. 35: 13051–6.

Armanios, M. Y., J. J. Chen, J. D. Cogan, J. K. Alder, R. G. Ingersoll, C. Markin, W. E. Lawson, M. Xie, I. Vulto, J. A. Phillips 3rd, P. M. Lansdorp, C. W. Greider, and J. E. Loyd. "Telomerase mutations in families with idiopathic pulmonary fibrosis." *The New England Journal of Medicine.* March 29, 2007, vol. 356, no. 13: 1317–26.

Artandi, S. E. "Telomeres, telomerase, and human disease." *The New England Journal of Medicine.* September 21, 2006, vol. 355, no. 12: 1195–7.

Atzmon, G., M. Cho, R. M. Cawthon, T. Budagov, et al. "Genetic variation in human telomerase is associated with telomere length in Ashkenazi centenarians." *Proceedings of the National Academy of Sciences.* January 2010, vol. 107 (suppl. 1): 1710–1717.

Aubert, G., and P. M. Lansdorp. "Telomeres and aging." *Physiological Reviews.* April 2008, vol. 88, no.2: 557–79.

Aviv, A., A. M. Valdes, and T. D. Spector. "Human telomere biology: pitfalls of moving from the laboratory to epidemiology." *International Journal of Epidemiology.* December 2006, vol. 35, no. 6: 1424–9.

Aviv, A. "Leukocyte telomere length, hypertension, and atherosclerosis: are there potential mechanistic explanations?" *Hypertension.* April 2009, vol. 53, no. 4: 590–1.

Aviv, A. "The epidemiology of human telomeres: faults and promises." *Journals of Gerontology: Biological and Medical Sciences.* September 2008, vol. 63, no. 9: 979–83.

Aviv, A. "Telomeres and human somatic fitness." *Journals of Gerontology: Biological and Medical Sciences.* August 2006, vol. 61, no. 8: 871–3.

Bagheri, S., M. Nosrati, S. Li, S. Fong, et al. "Genes and pathways downstream of telomerase in melanoma metastasis." *Proceedings of the National Academy of Sciences.* July 2006, vol. 103, no. 30:11306–11.

Balaban, R. S., S. Nemoto, and T. Finkel. "Mitochondria, oxidants, and aging." *Cell.* February 2005, vol. 120, no. 4: 483–95.

Beckman, K. B. and B. N. Ames. "The free radical theory of aging matures." *Physiological Reviews.* April 1998, vol. 78, no. 2: 547–81.

Blackburn, E. H., C. W. Greider, and J.W. Szostak. "Telomeres and telomerase: the path from maize, Tetrahymena and yeast to human cancer and aging." *Nature Medicine.* October 2006, vol. 12, no. 10: 1133–8.

Bodnar, A. G., M. Ouellette, M. Frolkis, S. E. Holt, C. P. Chiu, et al. "Extension of lifespan by introduction of telomerase into normal human cells." *Science.* January 1998, vol. 279, no. 5349: 349–52.

Bokov, A., A. Chaudhuri, and A. Richardson. "The role of oxidative damage and stress in aging." *Mechanisms of Ageing and Development.* October–November 2004, vol. 125, nos. 10–11: 811–26.

Campisi, J. "Cancer and ageing: rival demons?" *Nature Reviews Cancer.* May 2003, vol. 3, no. 5: 339–49.

Campisi, J. "Senescent cells, tumor suppression, and organismal aging: good citizens, bad neighbors." *Cell.* February 2005, vol. 120, no. 4: 513–22.

Cawthon, R. M., K. R. Smith, E. O'Brien, A. Sivatchenko, and R. A. Kerber. "Association between telomere length in blood and mortality in people aged 60 years or older." *Lancet.* February 2003, vol. 361, no. 9355: 393-5.

Chang, E. and C. B. Harley. "Telomere length and replicative aging in human vascular tissues." *Proceedings of the National Academy of Sciences.* November 1995, vol. 92, no. 24: 11190-4.

Chang, S. and R. A. DePinho. "Telomerase extracurricular activities." *Proceedings of the National Academy of Sciences.* October 2002, vol. 99, no. 20: 12520-2.

Check, E. "Bush sacks outspoken biologist from ethics council." *Nature.* March 2004, vol. 428. no. 6978: 4.

Chen, W., J. P. Gardner, M. Kimura, M. Brimacombe, et al. "Leukocyte telomere length is associated with HDL cholesterol levels: The Bogalusa heart study." *Atherosclerosis.* August 2009, vol. 205, no. 2: 620–5.

Cherkas, L. F., A. Aviv, A. M. Valdes, J. L. Hunkin, et al. "The effects of social status on biological aging as measured by white-blood-cell telomere length." *Aging Cell.* October 2006, vol. 5, no. 5: 361–5.

Choi, J., S. R. Fauce, and R. B. Effros. "Reduced telomerase activity in human T lymphocytes exposed to cortisol." *Brain, Behavior, and Immunity.* May 2008, vol. 22, no. 4: 600–5.

Davis, T., F. S. Wyllie, M. J. Rokicki, M. C. Bagley, et al. "The role of cellular senescence in Werner syndrome: toward therapeutic intervention in human premature aging." *Annals of the New York Academy of Sciences.* April 2007, vol. 1100: 455–69.

Davis, T. and D. Kipling. "Werner Syndrome as an example of inflammaging: possible therapeutic opportunities for a progeroid syndrome?" *Rejuvenation Research.* Fall 2006, vol. 9, no. 3: 402–7.

Collado, M., M. A. Blasco, and M. Serrano. "Cellular senescence in cancer and aging." *Cell.* July 27 2007, vol. 130, no. 2: 223–33.

"Council member dismissed by White House." *The Journal of the American Medical Association.* May 19 2004, vol. 222, no. 1: 2307.

Damjanovic, A. K., Y. Yang, R. Glaser, J. K. Kiecolt-Glaser, et al. "Accelerated telomere erosion is associated with a declining immune function of caregivers of Alzheimer's disease patients." *Journal of Immunology.* September 15 2007, vol. 179, no. 6: 4249–54.

Dillin, A. and J. Karlseder. "Cellular versus Organismal Aging," in *Telomeres and Telomerase in Ageing, Disease, and Cancer,* by Rudolph, K. L., ed. 2008. Berlin: Springer-Verlag. pp. 3–22.

Dugan, L. L., and K. L. Quick. "Reactive oxygen species and aging: evolving questions." *Science of Aging Knowledge Environment.* June 29 2005, vol. 2005, no. 26: 20.

Effros, R. B. "From Hayflick to Walford: the role of T cell replicative senescence in human aging." *Experimental Gerontology.* June 2004, vol. 39, no. 6: 885–90.

Effros, R. B. "The canary in the coal mine: telomeres and human healthspan." *Journals of Gerontology: Biological and Medical Sciences.* May 2009, vol. 64, no. 5: 511–5.

Effros, R. B. "Replicative senescence of CD8 T cells: potential effects on cancer immune surveillance and immunotherapy." *Canter Immunology, Immunotherapy.* October 2004, vol. 53, no. 10: 925–33.

Effros, R. B. "Role of T lymphocyte replicative senescence in vaccine efficacy." *Vaccine.* January 8 2007, vol. 25, no. 4: 599–604.

Effros, R. B. "Telomerase induction in T cells: a cure for aging and disease?" *Experimental Gerontology.* May 2007, vol. 42, no. 5: 416–20.

Effros, R. B., M. Dagarag, C. Spaulding, and J. Man. "The role of CD8+ T-cell replicative senescence in human aging." *Immunological Reviews.* June 2005, vol. 205: 147–57.

Epel, E. S., E. H. Blackburn, J. Lin, F. S. Dhabhar, et al. "Accelerated telomere shortening in response to life stress." *Proceedings of the National Academy of Sciences.* December 7 2004, vol. 101, no. 49: 17312-5.

Epel, E. S., J. Lin, F. S. Dhabhar, O. M. Wolkowitz, et al. "Dynamics of telomerase activity in response to acute psychological stress." *Brain, Behavior, and Immunity.* May 2010, vol. 24, no. 4: 531–9.

Epel, E. S. "Psychological and metabolic stress: a recipe for accelerated cellular aging?" *Hormones.* January–March 2009, vol. 8, no. 1: 7–22.

Epel, E. S., S. S. Merkin, R. Cawthon, E. H. Blackburn, et al. "The rate of leukocyte telomere shortening predicts mortality from cardiovascular disease in elderly men." *Aging.* December 4 2008, vol. 1, no. 1: 81–8.

Epel, E. S., J. Lin, F. H. Wilhelm, O. M. Wolkowitz, et al. "Cell aging in relation to stress arousal and cardiovascular disease risk factors." *Psychoneuroendocrinology.* April 2006, vol. 31, no. 3: 277–87.

Ershler, W. B., L. Ferrucci, and D. L. Longo. "Hutchinson-Gilford progeria syndrome." *The New England Journal of Medicine.* May 29 2008, vol. 358, no. 22: 2409–10.

Fauce, S. R., B. D. Jamieson, A. C. Chin, R. T. Mitsuyasu, et al. "Telomerase-based pharmacologic enhancement of antiviral function of human CD8+ T lymphocytes." *Journal of Immunology.* November 15 2008, vol. 181, no. 10: 7400-6.

Farzaneh-Far, R., R. M. Cawthon, B. Na, W. S. Browner, et al. "Prognostic value of leukocyte telomere length in patients with stable coronary artery disease: data from the Heart and Soul Study." *Arteriosclerosis, Thrombosis, and Vascular Biology.* July 2008, vol. 28, no. 7: 1379-84.

Farzaneh-Far, R., J. Lin, E. Epel, K. Lapham, et al. "Telomere length trajectory and its determinants in persons with coronary artery disease: longitudinal findings from the heart and soul study." *PLoS One.* January 8 2010, vol. 5, no. 1: 8612.

Feldser, D. M. and C. W. Greider. "Short telomeres limit tumor progression in vivo by inducing senescence." *Cancer Cell.* May 2007, vol. 11, no. 5: 461–9.

Finkel, T., M. Serrano, and M. A. Blasco. "The common biology of cancer and ageing." *Nature.* August 16 2007, vol. 448, no. 7155:767–74.

Fitzpatrick, A. L., R. A. Kronmal, J. P. Gardner, B. M. Psaty, et al. "Leukocyte telomere length and cardiovascular disease in the cardiovascular health study." *American Journal of Epidemiology.* January 1 2007, vol. 165, no. 1: 14–21.

Gilley, D., B. S. Herbert, N. Huda, H. Tanaka, et al. "Factors impacting human telomere homeostasis and age-related disease." *Mechanisms of Ageing and Development.* January-February 2008, vol. 129, nos. 1–2: 27–34.

Giorgio, M., M. Trinei, E. Migliaccio, and P. G. Pelicci. "Hydrogen peroxide: a metabolic by-product or a common mediator of ageing signals?" *Nature Reviews Molecular Cellular Biology.* September 2007, vol. 8, no. 9: 722–8.

Harley, C. B. "Telomerase and cancer therapeutics." *Nature Reviews Cancer.* March 2008, vol. 8, no. 3: 167–79.

Harley, C. B. "Telomerase therapeutics for degenerative diseases." *Current Molecular Medicine.* March 2005, vol. 5, no. 2: 205–11.

Hao, L. Y., M. Armanios, M. A. Strong, B. Karim, D. M. Feldser, et al. "Short telomeres, even in the presence of telomerase, limit tissue renewal capacity." *Cell.* December 2005, vol. 123, no. 6: 1121–31.

Hofer, A. C., R. T. Tran, O. Z. Aziz, W. Wright, et al. "Shared phenotypes among segmental progeroid syndromes suggest underlying pathways of aging." *Journals of Gerontology: Biological and Medical Sciences.* January 2005, vol. 60, no. 1: 10–20.

Huda, N., H. Tanaka, B. S. Herbert, T. Reed, et al. "Shared environmental factors associated with telomere length maintenance in elderly male twins." *Aging Cell.* October 2007, vol. 6, no. 5: 709–13.

Ju, Z., and K. Lenhard Rudolph. "Telomere dysfunction and stem cell ageing." *Biochimie.* January 2008, vol. 90, no. 1: 24–32.

Kawanishi, S. and S. Oikawa. "Mechanism of telomere shortening by oxidative stress." *Annals of the New York Academy of Sciences.* June 2004, vol. 1019: 278–84.

Kiecolt-Glaser, J. K. and R. Glaser. "Psychological stress, telomeres, and telomerase." *Brain, Behavior, and Immunity.* May 2010, vol. 24, no. 4: 529–30.

Kimura, M., L. F. Cherkas, B. S. Kato, S. Demissie, et al. "Offspring's leukocyte telomere length, paternal age, and telomere elongation in sperm." *PLoS Genetics.* February 2008, vol. 4, no. 2: 37.

Kimura, M., J. V. Hjelmborg, J. P. Gardner, L. Bathum, et al. "Telomere length and mortality: a study of leukocytes in elderly Danish twins." *American Journal of Epidemiology.* April 1 2008, vol. 167, no. 7: 799–806.

Kipling, D., D. Wynford-Thomas, C. J. Jones, A. Akbar, et al. "Telomere-dependent senescence." *Nature Biotechnology.* April 1999, vol. 17, no. 4: 313–4.

Korf, B. "Hutchinson-Gilford progeria syndrome, aging, and the nuclear lamina." *The New England Journal of Medicine.* February 7 2008, vol. 358, no. 6: 552–5.

Kotrschal, A., P. Ilmonen, and D. J. Penn. "Stress impacts telomere dynamics." *Biology Letters.* April 22 2007, vol. 3, no. 2: 128–30.

Kurz, D. J., S. Decary, Y. Hong, E. Trivier, et al. "Chronic oxidative stress compromises telomere integrity and accelerates the onset of senescence in human endothelial cells." *Journal of Cell Science.* May 1 2004, vol. 117, no. 11: 2417–26.

Lansdorp, P. M. "Stress, social rank and leukocyte telomere length." *Aging Cell*. December 2006, vol. 5, no. 6: 583–4.

Li, Y., W. Zhi, P. Wareski, and N. P. Weng. "IL-15 activates telomerase and minimizes telomere loss and may preserve the replicative life span of memory CD8+ T cells in vitro." *Journal of Immunology*. April 2005, vol. 174, no. 7: 4019–24.

Liang, Y. and G. Van Zant. "Aging stem cells, latexin, and longevity." *Experimental Cell Research*. June 10 2008, vol. 314, no. 9: 1962–72.

Lin, J., E. Epel, J. Cheon, C. Kroenke, et al. "Analyses and comparisons of telomerase activity and telomere length in human T and B cells: insights for epidemiology of telomere maintenance." *Journal of Immunology* Methods. January 31 2010, vol. 352, nos. 1–2: 71–80.

Martin-Ruiz, C., H. O. Dickinson, B. Keys, E. Rowan, et al. "Telomere length predicts poststroke mortality, dementia, and cognitive decline." *Annals of Neurology*. August 2006, vol. 60, no. 2: 174–80.

Maser, R. S. and R. A. DePinho. "Telomeres and the DNA damage response: why the fox is guarding the henhouse." *DNA Repair*. August-September 2004, vol. 3, nos. 8–9: 979–88.

Merideth, M. A., L. B. Gordon, S. Clauss, V. Sachdev, et al. "Phenotype and course of Hutchinson-Gilford progeria syndrome." *The New England Journal of Medicine*. February 7 2008, vol. 358, no. 6: 592–604.

Miller, R. A. "Extending Life: Scientific prospects and political obstacles." *The Milbank Quarterly*. 2002, vol. 80, no. 1: 155–174.

Muller, F. L., M. S. Lustgarten, Y. Jang, A. Richardson, et al. "Trends in oxidative aging theories." *Free Radical Biology and Medicine*. August 15 2007, vol. 43, no. 4: 477–503.

Nalapareddy, K., H. Jiang, L. M. Guachalla Gutierrez, and K. L. Rudolph. "Determining the influence of telomere dysfunction and DNA damage on stem and progenitor cell aging: what markers can we use?" *Experimental Gerontology*. November 2008, vol. 43, no. 11: 998–1004.

Nishimura, E. K., S. R. Granter, and D. E. Fisher. "Mechanisms of hair graying: incomplete melanocyte stem cell maintenance in the niche." *Science*. February 4, 2005, vol. 307, no. 5710: 720–4.

Njajou, O. T., R. M. Cawthon, C. M. Damcott, S. H. Wu, et al. "Telomere length is paternally inherited and is associated with parental lifespan." *Proceedings of the National Academy of Sciences*. July 17, 2007, vol. 104, no. 29: 12135–9.

Njajou, O. T., W. C. Hsueh, E. H. Blackburn, A. B. Newman, et al. "Association between telomere length, specific causes of death, and years of healthy life in health, aging, and body composition, a population-based cohort study." *Journals of Gerontology: Biological and Medical Sciences*. August 2009, vol. 64, no. 8: 860–4.

Nordfjäll, K., U. Svenson, K. F. Norrback, R. Adolfsson, et al. "The individual blood cell telomere attrition rate is telomere length dependent." *PLoS Genetics*. February 2009, vol. 5, no. 2: 1000375.

Olshansky, S. J., D. Perry, R. A. Miller, and R. N. Butler. "In pursuit of the Longevity Dividend." *The Scientist*. March 2006: 28–36.

Parks, C. G., D. B. Miller, E. C. McCanlies, R. M. Cawthon, et al. "Telomere length, current perceived stress, and urinary stress hormones in women." *Cancer Epidemiology, Biomarkers, and Prevention*. February 2009, vol. 18, no. 2: 551–60.

Passos, J. F., G. Saretzki, and T. von Zglinicki. "DNA damage in telomeres and mitochondria during cellular senescence: is there a connection?" *Nucleic Acids Research*. 2007, vol. 35, no. 22: 7505–13.

Raices, M., H. Maruyama, A. Dillin, and J. Karlseder. "Uncoupling of longevity and telomere length in C. elegans." *PLoS Genetics*. September 2005, vol. 1, no. 3: 30.

Richter, T. and T.von Zglinicki. "A continuous correlation between oxidative stress and telomere shortening in fibroblasts." *Experimental Gerontology*. November 2007, vol. 42, no. 11: 1039–42.

Rudolph, K. L., S. Chang, H. W. Lee, M. Blasco, et al. "Longevity, stress response, and cancer in aging telomerase-deficient mice." *Cell*. March 1999, vol. 96, no. 5: 701–12.

Sapolsky, R. M. "Organismal stress and telomeric aging: an unexpected connection." *Proceedings of the National Academy of Sciences*. December 14, 2004, vol. 101, no. 50: 17323–4.

Sarin, K. Y. and S. E. Artandi. "Aging, graying and loss of melanocyte stem cells." *Stem Cell Reviews*. Fall 2007, vol. 3, no. 3: 212–7.

Sarin, K. Y., P. Cheung, D. Gilison, E. Lee, et al. "Conditional telomerase induction causes proliferation of hair follicle stem cells." *Nature*. August 18, 2005, vol. 436, no. 7053: 1048–52.

Serrano, M. and M. A. Blasco. "Cancer and ageing: convergent and divergent mechanisms." *Nature Reviews Molecular Cellular Biology*. September 2007, vol. 8, no. 9: 715–22.

Sharpless, N. E. and R. A. DePinho. "How stem cells age and why this makes us grow old." *Nature Reviews Molecular Cellular Biology*. September 2007, vol. 8, no. 9: 703–13.

Sherr, C. J. and R. A. DePinho. "Cellular senescence: mitotic clock or culture shock?" *Cell*. August 18 2000, vol. 102, no. 4: 407–10.

Siegl-Cachedenier, I., I. Flores, P. Klatt, and M. A. Blasco. "Telomerase reverses epidermal hair follicle stem cell defects and loss of long-term survival associated with critically short telomeres." *The Journal of Cell Biology*. October 22, 2007, vol. 179, no. 2: 277–90.

Skordalakes, E. "Telomerase and the benefits of healthy living." *Lancet*. November 2008, vol. 9, no. 11: 1023–4.

Song, Z., Z. Ju, and K. L. Rudolph. "Cell intrinsic and extrinsic mechanisms of stem cell aging depend on telomere status." *Experimental Gerontology*. January–February 2009, vol. 44, nos. 1–2: 75–82.

Starr, J. M., P. G. Shiels, S.E. Harris, A. Pattie, et al. "Oxidative stress, telomere length and biomarkers of physical aging in a cohort aged 79 years from the 1932 Scottish Mental Survey." *Mechanisms of Ageing and Development*. December 2008, vol. 129, no. 12: 745–51.

Tomás-Loba, A., I. Flores, P. J. Fernández-Marcos, M. L. Cayuela, et al. "Telomerase reverse transcriptase delays aging in cancer-resistant mice." *Cell*. November 2008, vol. 135, no. 4: 609–22.

Valdes, A. M., T. Andrew, J. P. Gardner, M. Kimura, et al. "Obesity, cigarette smoking, and telomere length in women." *Lancet*. August 20–26, 2005, vol. 366, no. 9486: 662–4.

Van Zant, G. and Y. Liang. "The role of stem cells in aging." *Experimental Hematology*. August 2003, vol. 31, no. 8: 659–72.

Vijg, J., and J. Campisi. "Puzzles, promises and a cure for ageing." *Nature*. August 28 2008, vol. 454, no. 7208: 1065–71.

von Zglinicki, T. and C. M. Martin-Ruiz. "Telomeres as biomarkers for ageing and age-related diseases." *Current Molecular Medicine*. March 2005, vol. 5, no. 2: 197–203.

von Zglinicki, T. "Oxidative stress shortens telomeres." *Trends in Biochemical Sciences*. July 2002, vol. 27, no. 7: 339–44.

Vulliamy, T., R. Beswick, M. Kirwan, A. Marrone, et al. "Mutations in the telomerase component NHP2 cause the premature ageing syndrome dyskeratosis congenita." *Proceedings of the National Academy of Sciences*. June 10 2008, vol. 105, no. 23: 8073–8.

Wallace, D. C. "A mitochondrial paradigm of metabolic and degenerative diseases, aging, and cancer: a dawn for evolutionary medicine." *Annual Review of Genetics*. 2005, vol. 39: 359–407.

Walne, A. J., A. Marrone, and I. Dokal. "Dyskeratosis congenita: a disorder of defective telomere maintenance?" *International Journal of Hematology*. October 2005, vol. 82, no. 3: 184–9.

Warner, H. "Science fact and the SENS agenda: What can we reasonably expect from ageing research." *EMBO Reports*. 2005, vol. 6, no. 11: 1006–1008.

Weng, N. P. "Telomere and adaptive immunity." *Mechanisms of Ageing and Development*. January–February 2008, vol. 129, no. 1–2: 60–6.

Wilmut, I., J. Clark, and C. B. Harley. "Laying hold on eternal life?" *Nature Biotechnology*. June 2000, vol. 18, no. 6: 599–600.

Wolkowitz, O. M., E. S. Epel, V. I. Reus, and S. H. Mellon. "Depression gets old fast: do stress and depression accelerate cell aging?" *Depress Anxiety*. April 2010, vol. 27, no. 4: 327–38.

Wolkowitz, O. M., E. S. Epel, and S. H. Mellon. "When blue turns to grey: do stress and depression accelerate cell aging?" *World Journal of Biological Psychiatry*. 2008, vol. 9, no. 1: 2–5.

Wong, K. K., R. S. Maser, E. Sahin, S. T. Bailey, et al. "Diminished lifespan and acute stress-induced death in DNA-PKcs-deficient mice with limiting telomeres." *Oncogene*. May 3 2007, vol. 26, no. 20: 2815–21.

Xu, L. and E. H. Blackburn. "Human cancer cells harbor T-stumps, a distinct class of extremely short telomeres." *Molecular Cell*. October 26 2007, vol. 28, no. 2: 315–27.

Chapter 3: Your Brain on Stress

Akers, K. G., Z. Yang, D. P. DelVecchio, B. C. Reeb, et al. "Social competitiveness and plasticity of neuroendocrine function in old age: influence of neonatal novelty exposure and maternal care reliability." *PLoS One*. June 30, 2008, vol. 3, no. 7: 2840.

Baran, S. E., A. M. Campbell, J. K. Kleen, C. H. Foltz, et al. "Combination of high fat diet and chronic stress retracts hippocampal dendrites." *NeuroReport*. January 19, 2005, vol. 16, no. 1: 39–43.

Buss, C., C. Lord, M. Wadiwalla, D. H. Hellhammer, et al. "Maternal care modulates the relationship between prenatal risk and hippocampal volume in women but not in men." *The Journal of Neuroscience*. March 7, 2007, vol. 27, no. 10: 2592–5.

Carstensen, L. L. "Growing old or living long: take your pick." *Issues in Science and Technology*. 2007, vol. 23, no. 2: 41–50.

Cavigelli, S. A. and M. K. McClintock. "Fear of novelty in infant rats predicts adult corticosterone dynamics and an early death." *Proceedings of the National Academy of Sciences*. December, 2003, vol. 100, no. 26: 16131–6.

Champagne, F. A. "Epigenetic mechanisms and the transgenerational effects of maternal care." *Frontiers in Neuroendocrinology*. June 2008, vol. 29, no. 3: 386–97.

Champagne, F. A. and M. J. Meaney. "Transgenerational effects of social environment on variations in maternal care and behavioral response to novelty." *Behavioral Neuroscience*. December 2007, vol. 121, no. 6: 1353–63.

Conrad, C. D. "What is the functional significance of chronic stress-induced CA3 dendritic retraction within the hippocampus?" *Behavioral and Cognitive Neuroscience Reviews*. March 2006, vol. 5, no. 1: 41–60.

Conrad, C. D. "Chronic stress-induced hippocampal vulnerability: the glucocorticoid vulnerability hypothesis." *Annual Review of Neuroscience*. 2008, vol. 19, no. 6: 395–411.

Conrad, C. D., K. J. McLaughlin, J. S. Harman, C. Foltz, et al. "Chronic glucocorticoids increase hippocampal vulnerability to neurotoxicity under conditions that produce CA3 dendritic retraction but fail to impair spatial recognition memory." *The Journal of Neuroscience*. August 1, 2007, vol. 27, no. 31: 8278–85.

Conrad, C. D., D. D. MacMillan, S. Tsekhanov, R. L. Wright, et al. "Influence of chronic corticosterone and glucocorticoid receptor antagonism in the amygdala on fear conditioning." *Neurobiology of Learning and Memory*. May 2004, vol. 81, no. 3: 185–99.

Dalla, C., A. S. Whetstone, G. E. Hodes, and T. J. Shors. "Stressful experience has opposite effects on dendritic spines in the hippocampus of cycling versus masculinized females." *Neuroscience Letters*. January 2, 2009, vol. 449, no. 1: 52–6.

Diamond, D. M., C. R. Park, A. M. Campbell, and J. C. Woodson. "Competitive interactions between endogenous LTD and LTP in the hippocampus underlie the storage of emotional memories and stress-induced amnesia." *Hippocampus*. 2005, vol. 15, no. 8: 1006–25.

Diamond, D. M., C. R. Park, and J. C. Woodson. "Stress generates emotional memories and retrograde amnesia by inducing an endogenous form of hippocampal LTP." *Hippocampus*. 2004, vol. 14, no. 3: 281–91.

Diamond, D. M., C. R. Park, A. M. Campbell, J. Halonen, et al. "The temporal dynamics model of emotional memory processing: a synthesis on the neurobiological basis of stress-induced amnesia, flashbulb and traumatic memories, and the Yerkes-Dodson law." *Neural Plasticity*. 2007, vol. 2007: 60803.

Dallman, M. F. "Modulation of stress responses: how we cope with excess glucocorticoids." *Experimental Neurology*. August 2007, vol. 206, no. 2: 179–82.

Draganski, B. and A. May. "Training-induced structural changes in the adult human brain." *Behavioural Brain Research*. September 1 2008, vol. 192, no. 1: 137–42.

Ferguson, D. and R. Sapolsky. "Overexpression of mineralocorticoid and transdominant glucocorticoid receptor blocks the impairing effects of glucocorticoids on memory." *Hippocampus*. 2008, vol. 18, no. 11: 1103–11.

Ferguson, D., S. Lin, and R. Sapolsky. "Viral vector-mediated blockade of the endocrine stress-response modulates non-spatial memory." *Neuroscience Letters*. May 2008, vol. 437, no. 1: 1–4.

Ferrón, S. R., M. A. Marqués-Torrejón, H. Mira, I. Flores, et al. "Telomere shortening in neural stem cells disrupts neuronal differentiation and neuritogenesis." *The Journal of Neuroscience*. November 18, 2009, vol. 29, no. 46: 14394–407.

Fiocco, A. J., R. Joober, and S. J. Lupien. "Education modulates cortisol reactivity to the Trier Social Stress Test in middle-aged adults." *Psychoneuroendocrinology*. September-November 2007, vol. 32, nos. 8–10: 1158–63.

Fiocco, A. J., R. Joober, J. Poirier, and S. Lupien. "Polymorphism of the 5-HT(2A) receptor gene: association with stress-related indices in healthy middle-aged adults." *Behavioral Neuroscience*. 2007, vol. 1: 3.

Finch, C. E. "The neurobiology of middle-age has arrived." *Neurobiology of Aging*. April 2009, vol. 30, no. 4: 515–20.

Fleshner, M., J. Campisi, L. Amiri, and D. M. Diamond. "Cat exposure induces both intra- and extracellular Hsp72: the role of adrenal hormones." *Psychoneuroendocrinology*. October 2004, vol. 29, no. 9: 1142–52.

Gianaros, P. J., S. W. Derbyshire, J. C. May, G. J. Siegle, et al. "Anterior cingulate activity correlates with blood pressure during stress." *Psychophysiology*. November 2005, vol. 42, no. 6: 627–35.

Gianaros, P. J., L. K. Sheu, K. A. Matthews, J. R. Jennings, et al. "Individual differences in stressor-evoked blood pressure reactivity vary with activation, volume, and functional connectivity of the amygdala." *The Journal of Neuroscience*. January 23 2008, vol. 28, no. 4: 990–9.

Gianaros, P. J., J. A. Horenstein, A. R. Hariri, L. K. Sheu, et al. "Potential neural embedding of parental social standing." *Social Cognitive and Affective Neuroscience*. June 2008, vol. 3, no. 2: 91–6.

Gianaros, P. J., J. R. Jennings, L. K. Sheu, P. J. Greer, et al. "Prospective reports of chronic life stress predict decreased grey matter volume in the hippocampus." *Neuroimage*. April 1 2007, vol. 35, no. 2: 795–803.

Gilbertson, M. W., M. E. Shenton, A. Ciszewski, K. Kasai, et al. "Smaller hippocampal volume predicts pathologic vulnerability to psychological trauma." *Nature Neuroscience*. November 2002 , vol. 5. no. 11: 1242–7.

Greenwood, B. N., T. E. Foley, H. E. Day, D. Burhans, et al. "Wheel running alters serotonin (5-HT) transporter, 5-HT1A, 5-HT1B, and alpha 1b-adrenergic receptor mRNA in the rat raphe nuclei." *Biological Psychiatry*. March 1, 2005, vol. 57, no. 5: 559–68.

Herbert, J., I. M. Goodyer, A. B. Grossman, M. H. Hastings, et al. "Do corticosteroids damage the brain?" *Journal of Neuroendocrinology*. June 2006, vol. 18, no. 6: 393–411.

Jessberger, S. and F. H. Gage. "Stem-cell-associated structural and functional plasticity in the aging hippocampus." *Psychology and Aging*. December 2008, vol. 23, no. 4: 684–91.

Kern, S., T. R. Oakes, C.K. Stone, E. M. McAuliff, et al. "Glucose metabolic changes in the prefrontal cortex are associated with HPA axis response to a psychosocial stressor." *Psychoneuroendocrinology*. May 2008, vol. 33, no. 4: 517–29.

Kleen, J. K., M. T. Sitomer, P. R. Killeen, and C. D. Conrad. "Chronic stress impairs spatial memory and motivation for reward without disrupting motor ability and motivation to explore." *Behavioral Neuroscience*. August 2006, vol. 120, no. 4: 842–51.

Koo, J. W. and R. S. Duman. "IL-1beta is an essential mediator of the antineurogenic and anhedonic effects of stress." *Proceedings of the National Academy of Sciences*. January 15, 2008, vol. 105, no. 2: 751–6.

Kozorovitskiy, Y., C. G. Gross, C. Kopil, L. Battaglia, et al. "Experience induces structural and biochemical changes in the adult primate brain." *Proceedings of the National Academy of Sciences*. November 29 2005, vol. 102, no. 48: 17478–82.

Lachman, M. E. "Perceived control over aging-related declines: Adaptive beliefs and behaviors." *Current Directions in Psychological Science*. 2006, vol. 15, no. 6: 282–286.

Lee, J., Y. S. Jo, Y. H. Sung, I. K. Hwang, et al. "Telomerase deficiency affects normal brain functions in mice." *Neurochemical Research*. February 2010, vol. 35, no. 2: 211–8.

Lee, T., T. Jarome, S. J. Li, J. J. Kim, et al. "Chronic stress selectively reduces hippocampal volume in rats: a longitudinal magnetic resonance imaging study." *NeuroReport.* November 25 2009, vol. 20, no. 17: 1554–8.

Leuner, B., E. R. Glasper, and E. Gould. "A rewarding experience enhances structural plasticity in the adult hippocampus and is anxiolytic despite elevated glucocorticoid levels" in *Neuroscience Meeting Planner.* 2008. Chicago, IL: Society for Neuroscience.

Leuner, B., Y. Kozorovitskiy, C. G. Gross, E. Gould. "Diminished adult neurogenesis in the marmoset brain precedes old age." *Proceedings of the National Academy of Sciences.* October 23, 2007, vol. 104, no. 43: 17169–73.

Leuner, B., E. Gould, T. J. Shors. "Is there a link between adult neurogenesis and learning?" *Hippocampus.* 2006, vol. 16, no. 3: 216–24.

Leuner, B., S. Mendolia-Loffredo, Y. Kozorovitskiy, D. Samburg, et al. "Learning enhances the survival of new neurons beyond the time when the hippocampus is required for memory." *The Journal of Neuroscience.* August 25, 2004, vol. 24, no. 34: 7477–81.

Lightman, S. L. "The neuroendocrinology of stress: a never ending story." *Journal of Neuroendocrinology.* June 2008, vol. 20, no. 6: 880–4.

Liston, C., B. S. McEwen, and B. J. Casey. "Psychosocial stress reversibly disrupts prefrontal processing and attentional control." *Proceedings of the National Academy of Sciences.* January 20, 2009, vol. 106, no. 3: 912–7.

Liston, C., M. M. Miller, D. S. Goldwater, J. J. Radley, et al. "Stress-induced alterations in prefrontal cortical dendritic morphology predict selective impairments in perceptual attentional set-shifting." *The Journal of Neuroscience.* July 26 2006, vol. 26, no. 30: 7870–4.

Lupien, S. J. "Brains under stress." *Canadian Journal of Psychiatry.* January 2009, vol. 54, no. 1: 4–5.

Lupien, S. J., B. S. McEwen, M. R. Gunnar, and C. Heim. "Effects of stress throughout the lifespan on the brain, behaviour and cognition." *Nature Reviews Neuroscience.* June 2009, vol. 10, no. 6: 434–45.

Lupien, S. J., A. Evans , C. Lord, J. Miles, et al. "Hippocampal volume is as variable in young as in older adults: implications for the notion of hippocampal atrophy in humans." *Neuroimage.* January 15, 2007, vol. 34, no. 2: 479–85.

Lupien, S. J., A. Fiocco, N. Wan, F. Maheu, et al. "Stress hormones and human memory function across the lifespan." *Psychoneuroendocrinology.* April 2005, vol. 30,no. 3: 225–42.

Lupien, S. J. and N. Wan. "Successful ageing: from cell to self." *Philosophical Transactions of the Royal Society of London B: Biological Sciences.* September 29, 2004, vol. 359, no. 1449: 1413–26.

Lupien, S. J. and T. E. Schramek. "The differential effects of stress on memory consolidation and retrieval: a potential involvement of reconsolidation?" *Behavioral Neuroscience.* June 2006, vol. 120, no. 3: 735–8.

Lupien, S. J., F. Maheu, M. Tu, A. Fiocco, et al. "The effects of stress and stress hormones on human cognition: Implications for the field of brain and cognition." *Brain and Cognition.* December 2007, vol. 65, no. 3: 209–37.

Mahncke, H. W., B. B.Connor, J. Appelman, O. N. Ahsanuddin, et al. "Memory enhancement in healthy older adults using a brain plasticity-based training program: a randomized, controlled study." *Proceedings of the National Academy of Sciences.* August 15, 2006, vol. 103, no. 33: 12523–8.

Marsland, A. L., P. J. Gianaros, S. M. Abramowitch, S. B. Manuck, et al. "Interleukin-6 covaries inversely with hippocampal grey matter volume in middle-aged adults." *Biological Psychiatry*. September 15, 2008, vol. 64, no. 6: 484–90.

Mattson, M. P., S. L. Chan, and W. Duan. "Modification of brain aging and neurodegenerative disorders by genes, diet, and behavior." *Physiological Reviews*. July 2002, vol. 82, no. 3: 637–72.

Maya Vetencourt, J. F., A. Sale, A. Viegi, L. Baroncelli, et al. "The antidepressant fluoxetine restores plasticity in the adult visual cortex." *Science*. April 18, 2008, vol. 320, no. 5874: 385–8.

McCann, J. C. and B. N. Ames. "Is there convincing biological or behavioral evidence linking vitamin D deficiency to brain dysfunction?" *FASEB Journal*. April 2008, vol. 22, no. 4: 982–1001.

McEwen, B. S. "Central effects of stress hormones in health and disease: Understanding the protective and damaging effects of stress and stress mediators." *European Journal of Pharmacology*. April 2008, vol. 583, no. 2-3: 174–85.

McEwen, B. S. "Physiology and neurobiology of stress and adaptation: central role of the brain." *Physiological Reviews*. July 2007, vol. 87, no. 3: 873–904.

McEwen, B. S. "Protective and damaging effects of stress mediators: central role of the brain." *Dialogues in Clinical NeuroSciences*. 2006, vol. 8, no. 4: 367–81.

McEwen, B. S. and P. J. Gianaros. "Central role of the brain in stress and adaptation: links to socioeconomic status, health, and disease." *Annals of the New York Academy of Sciences*. February 2010, vol. 1186: 190–222.

McEwen, B. S. "Protective and damaging effects of stress mediators." *The New England Journal of Medicine*. January 15, 1998, vol. 338, no. 3: 171–9.

McEwen, B. S. "The neurobiology of stress: from serendipity to clinical relevance." *Brain Research*. December 15, 2000, vol. 886, nos. 1–2: 172–189.

McEwen, B. S. "Understanding the potency of stressful early life experiences on brain and body function." *Metabolism*. October 2008, vol. 57, Suppl. 2: S11–5.

McIntosh L. J. and R. M. Sapolsky. "Glucocorticoids increase the accumulation of reactive oxygen species and enhance adriamycin-induced toxicity in neuronal culture." *Experimental Neurology*. October 1996, vol. 141, no. 2: 201–6.

McIntosh, L. J., K. E. Hong, and R. M. Sapolsky. "Glucocorticoids may alter antioxidant enzyme capacity in the brain: baseline studies." *Brain Research*. April 1998, vol. 791, nos. 1–2: 209–14.

McLaughlin, K. J., J. L. Gomez, S. E. Baran, and C. D. Conrad. "The effects of chronic stress on hippocampal morphology and function: an evaluation of chronic restraint paradigms." *Brain Research*. August 3 2007, vol. 1161: 56–64.

Miller, A. H. "Inflammation versus glucocorticoids as purveyors of pathology during stress: have we reached the tipping point?" *Biological Psychiatry*. August 15, 2008, vol. 64, no. 4: 263–5.

Mitra, R., R. M. Sapolsky. "Acute corticosterone treatment is sufficient to induce anxiety and amygdaloid dendritic hypertrophy." *Proceedings of the National Academy of Sciences*. April 8, 2008, vol. 105, no. 14: 5573–8.

Mitra, R. and R. M. Sapolsky. "Expression of chimeric estrogen-glucocorticoid-receptor in the amygdala reduces anxiety." *Brain Research*. April 7, 2010.

Park, C. R., P. R. Zoladz, C. D. Conrad, M. Fleshner, et al. "Acute predator stress impairs the consolidation and retrieval of hippocampus-dependent memory in male and female rats." *Learn & Memory*. April 7, 2008, vol. 15, no. 4: 271–80.

Park, C. R., A. M. Campbell, J. C. Woodson, T. P. Smith, et al. "Permissive influence of stress in the expression of a u-shaped relationship between serum corticosterone levels and spatial memory errors in rats." *Dose Response.* June 20, 2006, vol. 4, no. 1: 55–74.

Payne, J. D., E. D. Jackson, L. Ryan, S. Hoscheidt, et al. "The impact of stress on neutral and emotional aspects of episodic memory." *Memory.* January 2006, vol. 14, no. 1: 1–16.

Pittenger, C. and R. S. Duman. "Stress, depression, and neuroplasticity: a convergence of mechanisms." *Neuropsychopharmacology.* January 2008, vol. 33, no. 1: 88–109.

Price, J. L. "What does it take to stay healthy past 100?: Commentary on 'No disease in the brain of a 115-year-old woman'." *Neurobiology of Aging.* August 2008, vol. 29, no. 8: 1140–2.

Pruessner, J. C., K. Dedovic, N. Khalili-Mahani, V. Engert, et al. "Deactivation of the limbic system during acute psychosocial stress: evidence from positron emission tomography and functional magnetic resonance imaging studies." *Biological Psychiatry.* January 15, 2008, vol. 63, no. 2: 234–40.

Pruessner, J. C., K. Dedovic, M. Pruessner, C. Lord, et al. "Stress regulation in the central nervous system: evidence from structural and functional neuroimaging studies in human populations." *Psychoneuroendocrinology.* January 2010, vol. 35, no. 1: 179–91.

Radley, J. J., A. B. Rocher, A. Rodriguez, D. B. Ehlenberger, et al. "Repeated stress alters dendritic spine morphology in the rat medial prefrontal cortex." *The Journal of Comparative Neurology.* March 1, 2008, vol. 507, no. 1: 1141–50.

Romeo, R. D., F. S. Ali, I. N. Karatsoreos, R. Bellani, et al. "Glucocorticoid receptor mRNA expression in the hippocampal formation of male rats before and after pubertal development in response to acute or repeated stress." *Neuroendocrinology.* 2008, vol. 87, no. 3: 160–7.

Ryff, C. D. and H. Burton. "Know thyself and become what you are: A eudaimonic approach to psychological well-being." *Journal of Happiness Studies.* 2008, vol. 9, no. 1: 13–39.

Sapolsky, R. M., L. M. Romero, and A. U. Munck. "How do glucocorticoids influence stress responses? Integrating permissive, suppressive, stimulatory, and preparative actions." *Endocrine Reviews.* February 2000, vol. 21, no. 1: 55–89.

Sapolsky, R. M. "Why stress is bad for your brain." *Science.* August 1996 , vol. 273, no. 5276: 749-50.

Shors, T. J. "From stem cells to grandmother cells: how neurogenesis relates to learning and memory." *Cell Stem Cell.* September 11, 2008, vol. 3, no. 3: 253–8.

Shors, T. J., G. Miesegaes, A. Beylin, M. Zhao, et al. "Neurogenesis in the adult is involved in the formation of trace memories." *Nature.* March 15 2001, vol. 410, no. 6826: 372–6.

Simon, N. M., J. . Smoller, K. L. McNamara, R. S. Maser, et al. "Telomere shortening and mood disorders: preliminary support for a chronic stress model of accelerated aging." *Biological Psychiatry.* September 2006, vol. 60, no. 5: 432–5.

Sorrells, S. F. and R. M. Sapolsky. "An inflammatory review of glucocorticoid actions in the CNS." *Brain, Behavior, and Immunity.* March 2007, vol. 21, no. 3: 259–72.

Spinelli, S., S. Chefer, S. J. Suomi, J. D. Higley, et al. "Early-life stress induces long-term morphologic changes in primate brain." *Archives of General Psychiatry.* June 2009, vol. 66, no. 6: 658–65.

Steptoe, A., C. H. van Jaarsveld, C. Semmler, R. Plomin, et al. "Heritability of daytime cortisol levels and cortisol reactivity in children." *Psychoneuroendocrinology.* February 2009, vol. 34, no. 2: 273–80.

Szyf, M., P. McGowan, and M. J. Meaney. "The social environment and the epigenome." *Environmental and Molecular Mutagenesis*. January 2008, vol. 49, no. 1: 46–60.

Terry, D. F., V. G. Nolan, S. L. Andersen, T. T. Perls, et al. "Association of longer telomeres with better health in centenarians." *Journals of Gerontology: Biological and Medical Sciences*. August 2008, vol. 63, no. 8: 809–12.

Teter, B. and C. E. Finch. "Caliban's heritance and the genetics of neuronal aging." *Trends in Neurosciences*. October 2004, vol. 27, no. 10: 627–32.

Thomas, R. M., G. Hotsenpiller, and D. A. Peterson. "Acute psychosocial stress reduces cell survival in adult hippocampal neurogenesis without altering proliferation." *The Journal of Neuroscience*. March 2007, vol. 27, no. 11: 2734–43.

Thuret, S., N. Toni, S. Aigner, G. W. Yeo, et al. "Hippocampus-dependent learning is associated with adult neurogenesis in MRL/MpJ mice." *Hippocampus*. July 2009, vol. 19, no. 7: 658–69.

Tyrka, A. R., L. H. Price, H. T. Kao, B. Porton, et al. "Childhood maltreatment and telomere shortening: preliminary support for an effect of early stress on cellular aging." *Biological Psychiatry*. March 15, 2010, vol. 67, no. 6: 531–4.

Uchida, S., A. Nishida, K. Hara, T. Kamemoto, et al. "Characterization of the vulnerability to repeated stress in Fischer 344 rats: possible involvement of microRNA-mediated down-regulation of the glucocorticoid receptor. " *The Journal of Neuroscience*. May 2008, vol. 27, no. 9: 2250–61.

Valdes, A. M., I.J. Deary, J. Gardner, M. Kimura, et al. "Leukocyte telomere length is associated with cognitive performance in healthy women." *Neurobiology of Aging*. June 2010, vol. 31, no. 6: 986–92.

Walker, T. "Renewable source of stem cells identified in the hippocampus" in *Neuroscience Meeting Planner*. 2008. Chicago, IL: Society for Neuroscience.

Weekes, N.Y., R.S. Lewis, S.G. Goto, J. Garrison-Jakel, et al. "The effect of an environmental stressor on gender differences on the awakening cortisol response." *Psychoneuroendocrinology*. July 2008, vol. 33, no. 6: 766–72.

Wood, G. E., E. H. Norris, E. Waters, J. T. Stoldt, et al. "Chronic immobilization stress alters aspects of emotionality and associative learning in the rat." *Behavioral Neuroscience*. April 2008, vol. 122, no. 2: 282–92.

Wright R. L., and C. D. Conrad. "Enriched environment prevents chronic stress-induced spatial learning and memory deficits." *Behavioural Brain Research*. February 2008, vol. 187, no. 1:41–7.

Yehuda, R., S. Brand, and R. K. Yang. "Plasma neuropeptide Y concentrations in combat exposed veterans: relationship to trauma exposure, recovery from PTSD, and coping." *Biological Psychiatry*. April 2006, vol. 59, no. 7: 660–3.

Zhao, C., W. Deng, and F. H. Gage. "Mechanisms and functional implications of adult neurogenesis." *Cell*. February 22, 2008, vol. 132, no. 4: 645–60.

Zoladz, P. R., C. D. Conrad, M. Fleshner, and D.M. Diamond. "Acute episodes of predator exposure in conjunction with chronic social instability as an animal model of post-traumatic stress disorder." *Stress*. 2008, vol. 11, no. 4: 259–81.

Chapter 4: Stress and Diet

Adam, T. C., and E. S. Epel. "Stress, eating and the reward system." *Physiology and Behavior*. July 24 2007, vol. 91, no. 4: 449–58.

Ali, R. E., and S. I. Rattan. "Curcumin's biphasic hormetic response on proteasome activity and heat-shock protein synthesis in human keratinocytes." *Annals of the New York Academy of Sciences.* May 2006, vol. 1067: 394–9.

Ames, B. N. "Low micronutrient intake may accelerate the degenerative diseases of aging through allocation of scarce micronutrients by triage." *Proceedings of the National Academy of Sciences.* November 21, 2006, vol. 103, no. 47: 17589–94.

Andreoli, A., S. Lauro, N. Di Daniele, R. Sorge, et al. "Effect of a moderately hypoenergetic Mediterranean diet and exercise program on body cell mass and cardiovascular risk factors in obese women." *European Journal of Clinical Nutrition.* July 2008, vol. 62, no. 7: 892–7.

Baur, J. A., K. J. Pearson, N. L. Price, H. A. Jamieson, et al. "Resveratrol improves health and survival of mice on a high-calorie diet." *Nature.* November 16, 2006, vol. 444, no. 7117: 337–42.

Benetou, V., A. Trichopoulou, P. Orfanos, A. Naska, et al. "Conformity to traditional Mediterranean diet and cancer incidence: the Greek EPIC cohort." *British Journal of Cancer.* July 2008, vol. 99, no. 1: 191–5.

Berge, U., P. Kristensen, and S. I. Rattan. "Hormetic modulation of differentiation of normal human epidermal keratinocytes undergoing replicative senescence in vitro." *Experimental Gerontology.* July 2008, vol. 43, no. 7: 658–62.

Bickford, P. C., J. Tan, R. D. Shytle, C. D. Sanberg, et al. "Nutraceuticals synergistically promote proliferation of human stem cells." *Stem Cells and Development.* February 2006, vol. 15, no. 1: 118–23.

Bravata, D. M., L. Sanders, J. Huang, H. M. Krumholz, et al. "Efficacy and safety of low-carbohydrate diets: a systematic review." *The Journal of the American Medical Association.* April 2003, vol. 289, no. 14: 1837–50.

Brehm B. J., and D. A. D'Alessio. "Weight loss and metabolic benefits with diets of varying fat and carbohydrate content: separating the wheat from the chaff." *Nature Clinical Practice Endocrinology & Metabolism.* March 2008, vol. 4, no. 3: 140–6.

Brydon, L., C. E. Wright, K. O'Donnell, I. Zachary, et al. "Stress-induced cytokine responses and central adiposity in young women." *International Journal of Obesity.* March 2008, vol. 32, no. 3: 443–50.

Cangemi, R., A. J. Friedmann, J. O. Holloszy, and L. Fontana. "Long-term effects of calorie restriction on serum sex-hormone concentrations in men." *Aging Cell.* April 2010, vol. 9, no. 2: 236–42.

Chronwall, B. M., and Z. Zukowska. "Neuropeptide Y, ubiquitous and elusive." *Peptides.* March 2004 , vol. 25, no. 3: 359–63.

Cook, R., and E. J. Calabrese. "The importance of hormesis to public health." *Environmental Health Perspectives.* November 2006, vol. 114, no. 11: 1631–5.

Conklin, S. M., J. I. Harris, S. B. Manuck, J. K. Yao, et al. "Serum omega-3 fatty acids are associated with variation in mood, personality and behavior in hypercholesterolemic community volunteers." *Psychiatry Research.* July 2007, vol. 152, no. 1: 1–10.

Dallman, M. F., N. C. Pecoraro, and S. E. la Fleur. "Chronic stress and comfort foods: self-medication and abdominal obesity." *Brain, Behavior, and Immunity.* July 2005, vol. 19, no. 4: 275–80.

Dallman, M. F., N. C. Pecoraro, S. F. Akana, S. E. la Fleur, et al. "Chronic stress and obesity: a new view of 'comfort food'." *Proceedings of the National Academy of Sciences.* September 2003, vol. 100, no. 20: 11696–701.

Dallman, M. F., J. P. Warne, M. T. Foster, and N. C. Pecoraro. "Glucocorticoids and insulin both modulate caloric intake through actions on the brain." *The Journal of Physiology.* September 2007, vol. 583, no. 2: 431–6.

Dallman, M. F., N. C. Pecoraro, S. E. La Fleur, J. P. Warne, et al. "Glucocorticoids, chronic stress, and obesity." *Progress in Brain Research.* 2006, vol. 153: 75–105.

Dallman, M. F., S. F. Akana, N. C. Pecoraro, J. P. Warne, et al. "Glucocorticoids, the etiology of obesity and the metabolic syndrome." *Current Alzheimer Research.* April 2007, vol. 4. no. 2: 199–204.

D'Anci, K. E., K. L. Watts, R. B. Kanarek, and H. A. Taylor. "Low-carbohydrate weight-loss diets: Effects on cognition and mood." *Appetite.* February 2009, vol. 52, no. 1: 96–103.

Daubenmier, J., L. Yglecias, M. Kuwata, N. Maninger, et al. "Effects of mindfulness meditation training on eating behavior, cortisol and body fat distribution."Abstract presented at *American Psychosomatic Society,* Baltimore, MD, March 12–15, 2008.

Dewell, A., G. Weidner, M. D. Sumner, C. S. Chi, et al. "A very-low-fat vegan diet increases intake of protective dietary factors and decreases intake of pathogenic dietary factors." *Journal of the American Dietetic Association.* February 2008, vol. 108, no. 2: 347–56.

Dewell, A., G. Weidner, M. D. Sumner, R. J. Barnard, et al. "Relationship of dietary protein and soy isoflavones to serum IGF-1 and IGF binding proteins in the Prostate Cancer Lifestyle Trial." *Nutrition and Cancer.* 2007, vol. 58, no. 1: 35–42.

Duffy, K. B., E. L. Spangler, B. D. Devan, Z. Guo, et al. "A blueberry-enriched diet provides cellular protection against oxidative stress and reduces a kainate-induced learning impairment in rats." *Neurobiology of Aging.* November 2008, vol. 29. no. 11: 1680–9.

Epel, E., S. Jimenez, K. Brownell, L. Stroud, et al. "Are stress eaters at risk for the metabolic syndrome?" *Annals of the New York Academy of Sciences.* December 2004, vol. 1032: 208–10.

Epel, E., N. Adler, J. Ickovics, and B. McEwen. "Social status, anabolic activity, and fat distribution." *Annals of the New York Academy of Sciences.* 1999, vol. 896: 424–6.

Epel, E., R. Lapidus, B. McEwen, and K. Brownell. "Stress may add bite to appetite in women: a laboratory study of stress-induced cortisol and eating behavior." *Psychoneuroendocrinology.* January 2001, vol. 26, no. 1: 37–49.

Epel, E. S., B. McEwen, T. Seeman, K. Matthews, et al. "Stress and body shape: stress-induced cortisol secretion is consistently greater among women with central fat. *Psychosomatic Medicine.* September-October 2000, vol. 62, no. 5: 623–32.

Farzaneh-Far, R., J. Lin, E. S. Epel, W. S. Harris, et al. "Association of marine omega-3 fatty acid levels with telomeric aging in patients with coronary heart disease." *The Journal of the American Medical Association.* January 2010, vol. 303, no. 3: 250–7.

Fontana, L. "The scientific basis of caloric restriction leading to longer life." *Current Opinion in Gastroenterology.* March 2009, vol. 25, no. 2: 144–50.

Foster, M. T., J. P. Warne, A. B. Ginsberg, H. F. Horneman et al. "Palatable foods, stress, and energy stores sculpt corticotropin-releasing factor, adrenocorticotropin, and corticosterone concentrations after restraint." *Endocrinology.* May 2009, vol. 150, no. 5: 2325–33.

Freeman, M. P., J. R. Hibbeln, K. L. Wisner, J. M. Davis, et al. "Omega-3 fatty acids: evidence basis for treatment and future research in psychiatry." *Journal of Clinical Psychiatry.* December 2006 , vol. 67, no. 12: 1954–67.

Gebauer, S. K., S. G. West, C. D. Kay, P. Alaupovic, et al. "Effects of pistachios on cardiovascular disease risk factors and potential mechanisms of action: a dose-response study." *American Journal of Clinical Nutrition*. September 2008, vol. 88, no. 3: 651–9.

Gebauer, S. K., T. L. Psota, W. S. Harris, and P. M. Kris-Etherton. "n-3 fatty acid dietary recommendations and food sources to achieve essentiality and cardiovascular benefits." *American Journal of Clinical Nutrition*. June 2006, vol. 83, no. 6, Suppl.: 1526S–1535S.

Gems, D., and L. Partridge. "Stress-response hormesis and aging: 'that which does not kill us makes us stronger'." *Cell Metabolism*. March 2008, vol. 7, no. 3: 200–3.

Gesta, S., Y. H. Tseng, and C. R. Kahn. "Developmental origin of fat: tracking obesity to its source." *Cell*. October 19, 2007, vol. 131, no. 2: 242–56.

Gibson, E. L. "Emotional influences on food choice: sensory, physiological and psychological pathways." *Physiology and Behavior*. August 30, 2006, vol. 89, no. 1: 53–61.

Gómez-Pinilla, F. "Brain foods: the effects of nutrients on brain function." *Nature Reviews Neuroscience*. July 2008, vol. 9, no. 7: 568–78.

Grigson, P. S. "Like drugs for chocolate: separate rewards modulated by common mechanisms?" *Physiology and Behavior*. July 2002, vol. 76, no. 3: 389–95.

Harrison, D. E., R. Strong, Z. D. Sharp, J. F. Nelson, et al. "Rapamycin fed late in life extends lifespan in genetically heterogeneous mice." *Nature*. July 2009, vol. 460. no. 7253: 392–5.

Hayes, D. P. "Nutritional hormesis." *European Journal of Clinical Nutrition*. February 2007, vol. 61, no. 2: 147–59.

Heilig, M. "The NPY system in stress, anxiety and depression." *Neuropeptides*. August 2004, vol. 38, no. 4: 213–24.

Hibbeln, J. R. "Depression, suicide and deficiencies of omega-3 essential fatty acids in modern diets." *World Review of Nutrition and Dietetics*. 2009, vol. 99: 17–30.

Hibbeln, J. R. "From homicide to happiness--a commentary on omega-3 fatty acids in human society." *Nutrition and Health*. 2007, vol. 19, nos. 1–2: 9–19.

Hilpert, K. F., P. M. Kris-Etherton, and S. G. West. "Lipid response to a low-fat diet with or without soy is modified by C-reactive protein status in moderately hypercholesterolemic adults." *Journal of Nutrition*. May 2005, vol. 135, no. 5: 1075–9.

Holloszy, J. O., and L. Fontana. "Caloric restriction in humans." *Experimental Gerontology*. August 2007, vol. 42, no. 8: 709–12.

Jakulj, F., K. Zernicke, S. L. Bacon, L. E. van Wielingen, et al. "A high-fat meal increases cardiovascular reactivity to psychological stress in healthy young adults." *Journal of Nutrition*. April 2007, vol. 137, no. 4: 935–9.

Jefremov, V., M. Zilmer, K. Zilmer, N. Bogdanovic, et al. "Antioxidative effects of plant polyphenols: from protection of G protein signaling to prevention of age-related pathologies." *Annals of the New York Academy of Sciences*. January 2007, vol. 1095: 449–57.

Joseph, J. A., B. Shukitt-Hale, and F. C. Lau. "Fruit polyphenols and their effects on neuronal signaling and behavior in senescence." *Annals of the New York Academy of Sciences*. April 2007, vol. 1100: 470–85.

Joseph, J. A., B. Shukitt-Hale, and L. M. Willis. "Grape juice, berries, and walnuts affect brain aging and behavior." *Journal of Nutrition*. September 2009, vol. 139, no. 9: 1813S–7S.

Joseph, J. A., B. Shukitt-Hale, and G. Casadesus. "Reversing the deleterious effects of aging on neuronal communication and behavior: beneficial properties of fruit poly-phenolic compounds." *American Journal of Clinical Nutrition*. January 2005, vol. 81, no. 1, Suppl.: 313S–316S.

Kaeberlein, M., and B. K. Kennedy. "Ageing: A midlife longevity drug?" *Nature*. July 2009, vol. 460. no. 7253: 331–2.

Kaeberlein, M. "Resveratrol and rapamycin: are they anti-aging drugs?" *Bioessays*. February 2010, vol. 32, no. 2: 96–9.

Katan, M. B. "Weight-loss diets for the prevention and treatment of obesity." *The New England Journal of Medicine*. February 26, 2009, vol. 360, no. 9: 923–5.

Katic, M., and C. R. Kahn. "The role of insulin and IGF-1 signaling in longevity." *Cellular and Molecular Life Sciences*. February 2005, vol. 62, no. 3: 320–43.

Kay, C. D., P. M. Kris-Etherton, and S. G. West. "Effects of antioxidant-rich foods on vascular reactivity: review of the clinical evidence." *Current Atherosclerosis Reports*. November 2006, vol. 8, no. 6: 510–22.

Kelley, A. E., V. P. Bakshi, S. N. Haber, T. L. Steininger, et al. "Opioid modulation of taste hedonics within the ventral striatum." *Physiology and Behavior*. July 2002, vol. 76, no. 3: 365–77.

Kiefer, A., J. Lin, E. Blackburn, and E. Epel. "Dietary restraint and telomere length in pre- and postmenopausal women." *Psychosomatic Medicine*. October 2008, vol. 70, no. 8: 845–9.

Kim, S., C. G. Parks, L. A. DeRoo, H. Chen, et al. "Obesity and weight gain in adulthood and telomere length." *Cancer Epidemiology, Biomarkers, and Prevention*. March 2009, vol. 18, no. 3: 816–20.

Knasmuller, S., D. M. DeMarini, I. Johnson, J. Gerhauser, eds. *Chemoprevention of Cancer and DNA Damage by Dietary Factors*. Foreword: "Prevention of cancer and the other degenerative disease of aging, through nutrition," by B. N. Ames and J. C. McCann. 2009. Germany: Wiley-Blackwell/Verlag GmbH. 2009: xxxi–xxxviii.

Kos, K., A. L. Harte, S. James, and D. R. Snead. "Secretion of neuropeptide Y in human adipose tissue and its role in maintenance of adipose tissue mass." *American Journal of Physiology: Endocrinology and Metabolism*. November 2007, vol. 293, no. 5: E1335–40.

Krikorian, R., M. D. Shidler, T. A. Nash, W. Kalt, et al. "Blueberry supplementation im-proves memory in older adults." *Journal of Agricultural and Food Chemistry*. April 2010, vol. 58, no. 7: 3996–4000.

Krikorian, R., M. D. Shidler, T. A. Nash, B. Shukitt-Hale, et al. "Concord grape juice supplementation improves memory function in older adults with mild cognitive im-pairment." *British Journal of Nutrition*. March 2010, vol. 103. no. 5: 730–4.

Kris-Etherton, P. M., A. E. Griel, T. L. Psota, S. K. Gebauer, et al. "Dietary stearic acid and risk of cardiovascular disease: intake, sources, digestion, and absorption." *Lipids*. December 2005 , vol. 40, no. 12: 1193–200.

Kos, K., A. L. Harte, S. James, D. R. Snead, et al. "Secretion of neuropeptide Y in human adipose tissue and its role in maintenance of adipose tissue mass." *American Journal of Physiology: Endocrinology and Metabolism*. November 2007, vol. 293, no. 5: E1335–40.

Kuo, L. E., M. Czarnecka, J. B. Kitlinska, J. U. Tilan, et al. "Chronic stress, combined with a high-fat/high-sugar diet, shifts sympathetic signaling toward neuropeptide Y and leads to obesity and the metabolic syndrome." *Annals of the New York Academy of Sciences*. December 2008, vol. 1148: 232–7.

Kuo, L. E., J. B. Kitlinska, J. U. Tilan, L. Li, et al. "Neuropeptide Y acts directly in the periphery on fat tissue and mediates stress-induced obesity and metabolic syndrome." *Nature Medicine.* July 2007, vol. 13, no. 7: 803–11.

Lau, F. C., B. Shukitt-Hale, and J. A. Joseph. "The beneficial effects of fruit polyphenols on brain aging." *Neurobiology of Aging.* December 2005, vol. 26, suppl. 1: 128–32.

Ludwig, D. S., J. A. Majzoub, A. Al-Zahrani, G. E. Dallal, et al. "High glycemic index foods, overeating, and obesity." *Pediatrics.* March 1999, vol. 103, no. 3: E26.

Lutter, M., I. Sakata, S. Osborne-Lawrence, S. A. Rovinsky, et al. "The orexigenic hormone ghrelin defends against depressive symptoms of chronic stress." *Nature Neuroscience.* July 2008, vol. 11 no. 7: 752–3.

May, Y., J. R. Hébert, W. Li, E. R. Bertone-Johnson, et al. "Association between dietary fiber and markers of systemic inflammation in the Women's Health Initiative Observational Study." *Nutrition.* October 2008, vol. 24, no. 10: 941–9.

Markus, C. R. "Dietary amino acids and brain serotonin function; implications for stress-related affective changes." *NeuroMolecular Medicine.* 2008, vol. 10, no. 4: 247–58.

Mather, M. and L. L. Carstensen. "Aging and motivated cognition: the positivity effect in attention and memory.: *Trends in Cognitive Sciences.* October 2005, vol. 9, no. 10: 496–502.

Mather, M., T. Canli, T. English, S. Whitfield, et al. "Amygdala responses to emotionally valenced stimuli in older and younger adults." *Psychological Science.* April 2004, vol. 15, no. 4: 259–63.

Mattson, M. P. "Hormesis defined." *Ageing Research Reviews.* January 2008, vol. 7, no. 1: 1–7.

McCann, J. C., and B. N. Ames. "Vitamin K, an example of triage theory: is micronutrient inadequacy linked to diseases of aging?" *American Journal of Clinical Nutrition.* October 2009, vol. 90, no. 4: 889–907.

Mikels, J. A., C. E. Löckenhoff, S. J. Maglio, L. L. Carstensen, et al. "Following your heart or your head: focusing on emotions versus information differentially influences the decisions of younger and older adults." *Journal of Experimental Psychology: Applied.* March 2010, vol. 16, no. 1: 87–95.

Muzumdar, R., D. B. Allison, D. M. Huffman, X. Ma, et al. "Visceral adipose tissue modulates mammalian longevity." *Aging Cell.* June 2008, vol. 7, no. 3: 438–40.

Naleid, A. M., J. W. Grimm, D. A. Kessler, A. J. Sipols, et al. "Deconstructing the vanilla milkshake: the dominant effect of sucrose on self-administration of nutrient-flavor mixtures." *Appetite.* January 2008 , vol. 50, no. 1: 128–38.

O'Hare, E., D. L. Shaw, K. J. Tierney, A. S. Levine, et al. "Behavioral and neurochemical mechanisms of the action of mild stress in the enhancement of feeding." *Behavioral Neuroscience.* February 2004, vol. 118, no. 1: 173–7.

Ornish, D. "Mostly plants." *American Journal of Cardiology.* October 1 2009, vol. 104, no. 7: 957–8.

Ornish, D. "Was Dr. Atkins right?" *Journal of the American Dietetic Association.* April 2004, vol. 104 no. 4: 537–42.

Pani, L., A. Porcella, and G. L. Gessa. "The role of stress in the pathophysiology of the dopaminergic system." *Molecular Psychiatry.* January 2000, vol. 5, no. 1: 14–21.

Pecoraro, N., F. Reyes, F. Gomez, A. Bhargava, et al. "Chronic stress promotes palatable feeding, which reduces signs of stress: feedforward and feedback effects of chronic stress." *Endocrinology.* August 2004, vol. 145, no. 8: 3754–62.

Piché, M. E., A. Lapointe, S. J. Weisnagel, L. Corneau, et al. "Regional body fat distribution and metabolic profile in postmenopausal women." *Metabolism.* August 2008, vol. 57, no. 8: 1101–7.

Pischon, T., H. Boeing, K. Hoffmann, M. Bergmann, et al. "General and abdominal adiposity and risk of death in Europe." *The New England Journal of Medicine.* November 2008, vol. 359, no. 20: 2105–20.

Psota, T. L., B. Lohse, and S. G. West. "Associations between eating competence and cardiovascular disease biomarkers." *Journal of Nutrition Education and Behavior.* September-October 2007, vol. 39, no. 5 Suppl.: S171–8.

Psota, T. L., S. K. Gebauer, and P. Kris-Etherton. "Dietary omega-3 fatty acid intake and cardiovascular risk." *American Journal of Cardiology.* August 21, 2006, vol. 98, no. 4A: 3i–18i.

Raffaghello, L., C. Lee, F. M. Safdie, M. Wei, et al. "Starvation-dependent differential stress resistance protects normal but not cancer cells against high-dose chemotherapy." *Proceedings of the National Academy of Sciences.* June 17, 2008, vol. 105, no. 24: 8215–20.

Rattan, S. I., R. A. Fernandes, D. Demirovic, B. Dymek, et al. "Heat stress and hormetin-induced hormesis in human cells: effects on aging, wound healing, angiogenesis, and differentiation." *Dose Response.* 2009, vol. 7, no. 1: 90–103.

Rattan, S. I., and D. Demirovic. "Hormesis can and does work in humans." *Dose Response.* December 10 2009, vol. 8, no. 1: 58–63.

Rattan, S. I. "Hormesis in aging." *Ageing Research Reviews.* January 2008, vol. 7, no. 1: 63–78.

Rattan, S.I. and R. E. Ali. "Hormetic prevention of molecular damage during cellular aging of human skin fibroblasts and keratinocytes." *Annals of the New York Academy of Sciences.* April 2007, vol. 1100: 424–30.

Rattan, S. I. "Increased molecular damage and heterogeneity as the basis of aging." *The Journal of Biological Chemistry.* March 2008, vol. 389, no. 3: 267–72.

Rattan, S. I., H. Sejersen, R. A. Fernandes, and W. Luo. "Stress-mediated hormetic modulation of aging, wound healing, and angiogenesis in human cells." *Annals of the New York Academy of Sciences.* November 2007, vol. 1119: 112–21.

Rattan, S. I. "Theories of biological aging: genes, proteins, and free radicals." *Free Radical Research.* December 2006, vol. 40, no. 12: 1230–8.

Reis, L. C., and J. R. Hibbeln. "Cultural symbolism of fish and the psychotropic properties of omega-3 fatty acids." *Prostaglandins, Leukotrienes, and Essential Fatty Acids.* October-November 2006, vol. 75, nos. 4–5: 227–36.

Robson, L. G., S. Dyall, D. Sidloff, and A. T. Michael-Titus. "Omega-3 polyunsaturated fatty acids increase the neurite outgrowth of rat sensory neurons throughout development and in aged animals." *Neurobiology of Aging.* April 2010, vol. 31, no. 4: 678–87.

Rosmond, R. "Role of stress in the pathogenesis of the metabolic syndrome." *Psychoneuroendocrinology.* January 2005, vol. 30. no. 1: 1–10.

Roth, G. S., D. K. Ingram, and J. A. Joseph. "Nutritional interventions in aging and age-associated diseases." *Annals of the New York Academy of Sciences.* October 2007, vol. 1114: 369–71.

Russell, S. J., and C. R. Kahn. "Endocrine regulation of ageing." *Nature Reviews Molecular Cellular Biology.* September 2007, vol. 8, no. 9: 681–91.

Russo, S., I. P. Kema, M. R. Fokkema, J. C. Boon, et al. "Tryptophan as a link between psychopathology and somatic states." *Psychosomatic Medicine.* July-August 2003, vol. 65, no. 4: 665–71.

Sacks, F. M., G.A. Bray, V. J. Carey, S. R. Smith, et al. "Comparison of weight-loss diets with different compositions of fat, protein, and carbohydrates." *The New England Journal of Medicine.* February 26, 2009, vol. 360, no. 9: 859–73.

Safdie, F. M., T. Dorff, D. Quinn, L. Fontana, et al. "Fasting and cancer treatment in humans: A case series report." *Aging.* December 31 2009, vol. 1, no. 12: 988–1007.

Shai, I., D. Schwarzfuchs, Y. Henkin, D. R. Shahar, et al. "Weight loss with a low-carbohydrate, Mediterranean, or low-fat diet." *The New England Journal of Medicine.* July 17, 2008, vol. 359, no. 3: 229–41.

Shively, C. A., T. C. Register, and T. B. Clarkson. "Social stress, visceral obesity, and coronary artery atherosclerosis: product of a primate adaptation." *American Journal of Primatology.* September 2009, vol. 71, no. 9: 742–51.

Shukitt-Hale, B., F. C. Lau, and J. A. Joseph. "Berry fruit supplementation and the aging brain." *Journal of Agricultural and Food Chemistry.* February 2008, vol. 56, no. 3: 636–41.

Shytle, R. D., J. Ehrhart, J. Tan, J. Vila, et al. "Oxidative stress of neural, hematopoietic, and stem cells: protection by natural compounds." *Rejuvenation Research.* June 2007, vol. 10, no. 2: 173–8.

Sinha, R. "Chronic stress, drug use, and vulnerability to addiction." *Annals of the New York Academy of Sciences.* October 2008, vol. 1141: 105–30.

Son, T. G., S. Camandola, and M. P. Mattson. "Hormetic dietary phytochemicals." *NeuroMolecular Medicine.* 2008, vol. 10, no. 4: 236–46.

Stephenson, J. "Low-carb, low-fat diet gurus face off - Interview: Atkins RC, Ornish D, Wadden T." *The Journal of the American Medical Association.* April 9, 2003, vol. 289, no. 14: 1767–8, 1773.

Spiegel, K., R. Leproult, M. L'hermite-Balériaux, G. Copinschi, et al. "Leptin levels are dependent on sleep duration: relationships with sympathovagal balance, carbohydrate regulation, cortisol, and thyrotropin." *Journal of Clinical Endocrinology and Metabolism.* November 2004, vol. 89, no. 11: 5762–71.

Sucajtys-Szulc, E., E. Goyke, J. Korczynska, E. Stelmanska, et al. "Chronic food restriction differentially affects NPY mRNA level in neurons of the hypothalamus and in neurons that innervate liver." *Neuroscience Letters.* March 15, 2008, vol. 433, no. 3: 174–7.

Teegarden, S. L., and T. L. Bale. "Decreases in dietary preference produce increased emotionality and risk for dietary relapse." *Biological Psychiatry.* May 1 2007, vol. 61, no. 9: 1021–9.

Teegarden, S. L., A. N. Scott, and T. L. Bale. "Early life exposure to a high fat diet promotes long-term changes in dietary preferences and central reward signaling." *Neuroscience.* September 2009, vol. 162, no. 4: 924–32.

Teegarden, S. L., and T. L. Bale. "Effects of stress on dietary preference and intake are dependent on access and stress sensitivity." *Physiology and Behavior.* March 18, 2008, vol. 93, nos. 4–5: 713–23.

Tomiyama, A. J., T. Mann, D. Vinas, J. M. Hunger, et al. "Low-calorie dieting increases cortisol." *Psychosomatic Medicine.* April 5, 2010 [in pre-publication].

Traustadóttir, T., S. S. Davies, A. A. Stock, Y. Su et al. "Tart cherry juice decreases oxidative stress in healthy older men and women." *Journal of Nutrition.* October 2009, vol. 139, no. 10: 1896–900.

Valdes, A. M., T. Andrew, J. P. Gardner, M. Kimura, et al. "Obesity, cigarette smoking, and telomere length in women." *Lancet.* August 20–26, 2005, vol. 366, no. 9486: 662–4.

Wand, G. S., L. M. Oswald, M. E. McCaul, D. F. Wong, et al. "Association of amphetamine-induced striatal dopamine release and cortisol responses to psychological stress." *Neuropsychopharmacology*. November 2007, vol. 32, no. 11: 2310–20.

Warne, J. P., and M. F. Dallman. "Stress, diet and abdominal obesity: Y?" *Nature Medicine*. July 2007, vol. 13, no. 7: 781–3.

West, S. G., K. F. Hilpert, V. Juturu, P. L. Bordi, et al. "Effects of including soy protein in a blood cholesterol-lowering diet on markers of cardiac risk in men and in postmenopausal women with and without hormone replacement therapy." *Journal of Women's Health*. April 2005, vol. 14, no. 3: 253–62.

West, S. G., A. Likos-Krick, P. Brown, and F. Mariotti. "Oral L-arginine improves hemodynamic responses to stress and reduces plasma homocysteine in hypercholesterolemic men." *Journal of Nutrition*. February 2005, vol. 135, no. 2: 212–7.

Whitmer, R. A., D. R. Gustafson, E. Barrett-Connor, M.N. Haan, et al. "Central obesity and increased risk of dementia more than three decades later." *Neurology*. September 2008, vol. 71, no. 14: 1057–64.

Willis, L. M., B. Shukitt-Hale, V. Cheng, and J. A. Joseph. "Dose-dependent effects of walnuts on motor and cognitive function in aged rats." *British Journal of Nutrition*. April 2009, vol. 101, no. 8: 1140–4.

Willis, L. M., B. Shukitt-Hale, and J. A. Joseph. "Recent advances in berry supplementation and age-related cognitive decline." *Current Opinion in Clinical Nutrition and Metabolic Care*. January 2009, vol. 12, no. 1: 91–4.

Xu, Q., C. G. Parks, L. A. DeRoo, R. M. Cawthon, D. P. Sandler, et al. "Multivitamin use and telomere length in women." *American Journal of Clinical Nutrition*. June 2009, vol. 89, no. 6: 1857–63.

Xu, Y., D. Lin, S. Li, G. Li et al. "Curcumin reverses impaired cognition and neuronal plasticity induced by chronic stress." *Neuropharmacology*. September 2009, vol. 57, no. 4: 463–71.

Yang, K., H. Guan, E. Arany, D. J. Hill, et al. "Neuropeptide Y is produced in visceral adipose tissue and promotes proliferation of adipocyte precursor cells via the Y1 receptor." *FASEB Journal*. July 2008, vol. 22, no. 7: 2452–64.

Zellner, D. A., S. Loaiza, Z. Gonzalez, J. Pita, et al. "Food selection changes under stress." *Physiology and Behavior*. April 15, 2006, vol. 87, no. 4: 789–93.

Chapter 5: Stress and Exercise

Brown, D. A., M.S. Johnson, C. J. Armstrong, L. M. Lynch, et al. "Short-term treadmill running in the rat: what kind of stressor is it?" *Journal of Applied Physiology*. December 2007, vol. 103, no. 6: 1979–85.

Brownley, K. A., A. L. Hinderliter, S. G. West, S. S. Girdler, et al. "Sympathoadrenergic mechanisms in reduced hemodynamic stress responses after exercise." *Medicine and Science in Sports and Exercise*. June 2003, vol. 35, no. 6: 978–86.

Campeau, S., T. J. Nyhuis, S. K. Sasse, E. M. Kryskow, et al. "Hypothalamic pituitary adrenal axis responses to low intensity stressors are reduced following voluntary wheel running in rats." *Journal of Neuroendocrinology*. April 16, 2010. [Epub ahead of print]

Cherkas, L. F., J. L. Hunkin, B. S. Kato, J. B. Richards, et al. "The association between physical activity in leisure time and leukocyte telomere length." *Archives of Internal Medicine*. January 28, 2008, vol. 168, no. 2: 154–8.

Colcombe, S. J., K. I. Erickson, P. E. Scalf, J. S. Kim et al. "Aerobic exercise training increases brain volume in aging humans." *Journals of Gerontology: Biological and Medical Sciences.* November 2006, vol. 61, no. 11: 1166–70.

Cotman, C. W., N. C. Berchtold, and L. A. Christie. "Exercise builds brain health: key roles of growth factor cascades and inflammation." *Trends in Neurosciences.* September 2007, vol. 30, no. 9: 464–72.

Devries, M. C., M. J. Hamadeh, A. W. Glover, S. Raha, et al. "Endurance training without weight loss lowers systemic, but not muscle, oxidative stress with no effect on inflammation in lean and obese women." *Free Radical Biology and Medicine.* August 15, 2008, vol. 45, no. 4: 503–11.

Dishman, R. K., H. R. Berthoud, F. W. Booth, C. W. Cotman, et al. "Neurobiology of exercise." *Obesity.* March 2006, vol. 14, no. 3: 345–56.

Duman, C. H., L. Schlesinger, D. S. Russell, and R. S. Duman. "Voluntary exercise produces antidepressant and anxiolytic behavioral effects in mice." *Brain Research.* March 14, 2008, vol. 1199: 148–58.

Emery, C. F., J. K. Kiecolt-Glaser, R. Glaser, W. B. Malarkey, et al. "Exercise accelerates wound healing among healthy older adults: a preliminary investigation." *Journals of Gerontology: Biological and Medical Sciences.* November 2005, vol. 60, no. 11: 1432–6.

Erickson, K. I., R. S. Prakash, M. W. Voss, L. Chaddock, et al. "Aerobic fitness is associated with hippocampal volume in elderly humans." *Hippocampus.* October 2009, vol. 19, no. 10: 1030–9.

Fleshner, M., J. Campisi, T. Deak, B. N. Greenwood, et al. "Acute stressor exposure facilitates innate immunity more in physically active than in sedentary rats." *American Journal of Physiology: Regulatory, Integrative, and Comparative Physiology.* June 2002, vol. 282, no. 6: 1680–6.

Fleshner, M., J. Campisi, and J. D. Johnson. "Can exercise stress facilitate innate immunity? A functional role for stress-induced extracellular Hsp72." *Exercise Immunology Reviews.* 2003, vol. 9: 6–24.

Fleshner, M. "Physical activity and stress resistance: sympathetic nervous system adaptations prevent stress-induced immunosuppression." *Exercise Sport Science Review.* July 2005, vol. 33, no. 3: 120–6.

Fleshner, M., C. M. Charkey, M. Nickerson, and J. D. Johnson. "Endogenous extracellular Hsp72 release is an adaptive feature of the acute stress response" in *Psychoneuroimmunology*, Vol. 2, 4th Ed. by R. Ader (ed.) 2006. Oxford, UK: Academic Press/Elsevier: 1–23.

Foley, T. E., and M. Fleshner. "Neuroplasticity of dopamine circuits after exercise: implications for central fatigue." *NeuroMolecular Medicine.* 2008, vol. 10, no. 2: 67–80.

Gibala, M. J., J. P. Little, M. van Essen, G. P. Wilkin, et al. "Short-term sprint interval versus traditional endurance training: similar initial adaptations in human skeletal muscle and exercise performance." *The Journal of Physiology.* September 2006, vol. 575, pt. 3: 901–11.

Grant, R. W., R. A. Mariani, V. J. Vieira, M. Fleshner, et al. "Cardiovascular exercise intervention improves the primary antibody response to keyhole limpet hemocyanin (KLH) in previously sedentary older adults." *Brain, Behavior, and Immunity.* August 2008, vol. 22, no. 6: 923–32.

Greenwood, B. N., P. V. Strong, T. E. Foley, and M. Fleshner. "A behavioral analysis of the impact of voluntary physical activity on hippocampus-dependent contextual conditioning." *Hippocampus*. October 2009, vol. 19, no. 10: 988–1001.

Greenwood, B. N., and M. Fleshner. "Exercise, learned helplessness, and the stress-resistant brain." *NeuroMolecular Medicine*. 2008, vol. 10, no. 2: 81–98.

Greenwood, B. N., P. V. Strong, A. A. Dorey, and M. Fleshner. "Therapeutic effects of exercise: wheel running reverses stress-induced interference with shuttle box escape." *Behavioral Neuroscience*. October 2007, vol. 121. no. 5: 992–1000.

Greenwood, B. N., T. E. Foley, D. Burhans, S. F. Maier, et al. "The consequences of uncontrollable stress are sensitive to duration of prior wheel running." *Brain Research*. February 8 2005, vol. 1033, no. 2: 164–78.

Gazda, L. S., T. Smith, L. R. Watkins, S. F. Maier, et al. "Stressor exposure produces long-term reductions in antigen-specific T and B cell responses." *Stress*. December 2003, vol. 6, no. 4: 259–67.

Hillman, C.H., K. I. Erickson, and A. F. Kramer. "Be smart, exercise your heart: exercise effects on brain and cognition." *Nature Reviews Neuroscience*. January 2008, vol. 9, no. 1: 58–65.

Hu, S., Z. Ying, F. Gomez-Pinilla, and S. A. Frautschy. "Exercise can increase small heat shock proteins (sHSP) and pre- and post-synaptic proteins in the hippocampus." *Brain Research*. January 16 2009, vol. 1249: 191–201.

Ji, L. L., M. C. Gomez-Cabrera, and J. Vina. "Exercise and hormesis: activation of cellular antioxidant signaling pathway." *Annals of the New York Academy of Sciences*. May 2006, vol. 1067: 425–35.

Kadi, F., and E. Ponsot. "The biology of satellite cells and telomeres in human skeletal muscle: effects of aging and physical activity." *Scandinavian Journal of Medicine and Science in Sports*. September 17, 2009.

Kadi, F., E. Ponsot, K. Piehl-Aulin, A. Mackey, et al. "The effects of regular strength training on telomere length in human skeletal muscle." *Medicine and Science in Sports and Exercise*. January 2008, vol. 40, no. 1: 82–7.

Kennedy, S. L., T. P. Smith, and M. Fleshner. "Resting cellular and physiological effects of freewheel running." *Medicine and Science in Sports and Exercise*. January 2005, vol. 37, no. 1: 79–83.

Khaw, K. T., R. Jakes, S. Bingham, A. Welch, et al. "Work and leisure time physical activity assessed using a simple, pragmatic, validated questionnaire and incident cardiovascular disease and all-cause mortality in men and women: The European Prospective Investigation into Cancer in Norfolk prospective population study." *International Journal of Epidemiology*. August 2006, vol. 35, no. 4: 1034–43.

Kramer, A. F. and K. I. Erickson. "Capitalizing on cortical plasticity: influence of physical activity on cognition and brain function." *Trends in Cognitive Sciences*. August 2007, vol. 11, no. 8: 342–8.

Kramer, A. F., K. I., Erickson, and S. J. Colcombe. "Exercise, cognition, and the aging brain." *Journal of Applied Physiology*. October 2006, vol. 101, no. 4: 1237–42.

Kramer, A. F., S. J. Colcombe, E. McAuley, P. E. Scalf, et al. "Fitness, aging and neurocognitive function." *Neurobiology of Aging*. December 2005, vol. 26, suppl. 1: 124–7.

Lautenschlager, N. T., F. L. Cox, L. Flicker, J. K. Foster, et al. "Effect of physical activity on cognitive function in older adults at risk for Alzheimer disease: a randomized trial." *The Journal of the American Medical Association*. September 3, 2008, vol. 300, no. 9: 1027–37.

Little, J. P., A. Safdar, G. P. Wilkin, M. A. Tarnopolsky, et al. "A practical model of low-volume high-intensity interval training induces mitochondrial biogenesis in human skeletal muscle: potential mechanisms." *The Journal of Physiology*. March 15, 2010, vol. 588, pt. 6: 1011–22.

Ludlow, A. T., J. B. Zimmerman, S. Witkowski, J. W. Hearn, et al. "Relationship between physical activity level, telomere length, and telomerase activity." *Medicine and Science in Sports and Exercise*. October 2008, vol. 40, no. 10: 1764–71.

Marcell, T. J., K. A. McAuley, and T. Traustadóttir. "Exercise training is not associated with improved levels of C-reactive protein or adiponectin." *Metabolism*. April 2005, vol. 54, no. 4: 533–41.

McArdle, A., and M. J. Jackson. "Exercise, oxidative stress and ageing." *Journal of Anatomy*. November 2000, vol. 197, pt. 4: 539–41.

Melov, S., M. A. Tarnopolsky, K. Beckman, K. Felkey, et al. "Resistance exercise reverses aging in human skeletal muscle." *PLoS One*. May 23, 2007, vol. 2, no. 5: e465.

Mirabello, L., W. Y. Huang, J. Y. Wong, N. Chatterjee, et al. "The association between leukocyte telomere length and cigarette smoking, dietary and physical variables, and risk of prostate cancer." *Aging Cell*. August 2009, vol. 8, no. 4: 405–13.

Moraska, A., T. Deak, R. L. Spencer, D. Roth, et al. "Treadmill running produces both positive and negative physiological adaptations in Sprague-Dawley rats." *American Journal of Physiology: Regulatory, Integrative, and Comparative Physiology*. October 2000, vol. 279, no. 4: R1321–9.

Oguma ,Y., H. D. Sesso, R. S. Paffenbarger Jr., and I. M. Lee. "Physical activity and all cause mortality in women: a review of the evidence." *British Journal of Sports Medicine*. June 2002, vol. 36, no. 3: 162–72.

Parise, G., A. N. Brose, and M. A. Tarnopolsky. "Resistance exercise training decreases oxidative damage to DNA and increases cytochrome oxidase activity in older adults." *Experimental Gerontology*. March 2005, vol. 40, no. 3: 173–80.

Ponsot, E., J. Lexell, and F. Kadi. "Skeletal muscle telomere length is not impaired in healthy physically active old women and men." *Muscle Nerve*. April 2008, vol. 37, no. 4: 467–72.

Puterman, E., J. Lin, E. Blackburn, A. O'Donovan, et al. *The Power of Exercise: Buffering the Effect of Chronic Stress on Telomere Length*. In press.

Rimmele, U., R. Seiler, B. Marti, P. H. Wirtz, et al. "The level of physical activity affects adrenal and cardiovascular reactivity to psychosocial stress." *Psychoneuroendocrinology*. February 2009, vol. 34, no. 2: 190–8.

Rovio, S., G. Spulber, L. J. Nieminen, E. Niskanen, et al. "The effect of midlife physical activity on structural brain changes in the elderly." *Neurobiology of Aging*. December 3, 2008.

Sasse, S. K., B. N. Greenwood, C. V. Masini, T. J. Nyhuis, et al. "Chronic voluntary wheel running facilitates corticosterone response habituation to repeated audiogenic stress exposure in male rats." *Stress*. 2008, vol. 11, no. 6: 425–37.

Smith, T. P., S. L. Kennedy, and M. Fleshner. "Influence of age and physical activity on the primary in vivo antibody and T cell-mediated responses in men." *Journal of Applied Physiology*. August 2004, vol. 97, no. 2: 491–8.

Stranahan, A. M., D. Khalil, and E. Gould. "Running induces widespread structural alterations in the hippocampus and entorhinal cortex." *Hippocampus*. 2007, vol. 17, no. 11: 1017–22.

Tarnopolsky, M., A. Zimmer, J. Paikin, A. Safdar, et al. "Creatine monohydrate and conjugated linoleic acid improve strength and body composition following resistance exercise in older adults. *PLoS One.* October 3, 2007: vol. 2, no. 10: e991.

Tarnopolsky, M. A., C. D. Rennie, H. A. Robertshaw, S. N. Fedak-Tarnopolsky, et al. "Influence of endurance exercise training and sex on intramyocellular lipid and mitochondrial ultrastructure, substrate use, and mitochondrial enzyme activity." *American Journal of Physiology: Regulatory, Integrative, and Comparative Physiology.* March 2007, vol. 292, no. 3: R1271–8.

Tarnopolsky, M. A. "Mitochondrial DNA shifting in older adults following resistance exercise training." *Applied Physiology, Nutrition, and Metabolism.* June 2009, vol. 34, no. 3: 348–54.

Tarnopolsky, M. A., and A. Safdar. "The potential benefits of creatine and conjugated linoleic acid as adjuncts to resistance training in older adults." *Applied Physiology, Nutrition, and Metabolism.* February 2008, vol. 33, no. 1: 213–27.

Traustadóttir, T., P. R. Bosch, T. Cantu, and K. S. Matt. "Hypothalamic-pituitary-adrenal axis response and recovery from high-intensity exercise in women: effects of aging and fitness." *Journal of Clinical Endocrinology and Metabolism.* July 2004, vol. 89, no. 7: 3248–54.

Traustadóttir, T., P. R. Bosch, and K. S. Matt. "The HPA axis response to stress in women: effects of aging and fitness." *Psychoneuroendocrinology.* May 2005, vol. 30, no. 4: 392–402.

van Praag, H., T. Shubert, C. Zhao, and F. H. Gage. "Exercise enhances learning and hippocampal neurogenesis in aged mice." *The Journal of Neuroscience.* September 2005, vol. 25, no. 38: 8680–5.

Werner, C., M. Hanhoun, T. Widmann, A. Kazakov, et al. "Effects of physical exercise on myocardial telomere-regulating proteins, survival pathways, and apoptosis." *Journal of the American College of Cardiology.* August 5, 2008, vol. 52, no. 6: 470–82.

Wilkinson, S. B., S. M. Phillips, P. J. Atherton, R. Patel, et al. "Differential effects of resistance and endurance exercise in the fed state on signalling molecule phosphorylation and protein synthesis in human muscle." *The Journal of Physiology.* August 1, 2008, vol. 586, pt. 15: 3701–17.

Chapter 6: *Stress and the Mind*

Atkinson, N. L., and R. Permuth-Levine. "Benefits, barriers, and cues to action of yoga practice: a focus group approach." *American Journal of Health Behavior.* January–February 2009, vol. 33, no. 1: 3–14.

Brefczynski-Lewis, J. A., A. Lutz, H. S. Schaefer, D. B. Levinson, et al. "Neural correlates of attentional expertise in long-term meditation practitioners." *Proceedings of the National Academy of Sciences.* July 3, 2007, vol. 104, no. 27: 11483–8.

Carmody ,J., S. Crawford, and L. Churchill. A pilot study of mindfulness-based stress reduction for hot flashes. *Menopause.* September–October 2006, vol. 13, no. 5: 760–9.

Carmody, J., R. A. Baer, L. B. Lykins, and N. Olendzki. "An empirical study of the mechanisms of mindfulness in a mindfulness-based stress reduction program." *Journal of Clinical Psychology.* June 2009, vol. 65, no. 6: 613–26.

Carmody, J., G. Reed, J. Kristeller, and P. Merriam. "Mindfulness, spirituality, and health-related symptoms." *Journal of Psychosomatic Research.* April 2008, vol. 64, no. 4: 393–403.

Carmody, J., and R. A. Baer. "Relationships between mindfulness practice and levels of mindfulness, medical and psychological symptoms and well-being in a mindfulness-based stress reduction program." *Journal of Behavioral Medicine.* February 2008, vol. 31, no. 1: 23–33.

Carmody, J. "Evolving conceptions of mindfulness in clinical settings." *Journal of Cognitive Psychotherapy. An International Quarterly.* 2009, vol. 23, no 3: 270–280.

Carver, C. S., M. F. Scheier, and S. C. Segerstrom. "Optimism." *Clinical Psychology Review.* February 1, 2010.

Chida, Y., A. Steptoe, and L. H. Powell. "Religiosity/spirituality and mortality. A systematic quantitative review." *Psychotherapy and Psychosomatics.* 2009, vol. 78. no. 2: 81–90.

Chida, Y., and A. Steptoe. "Positive psychological well-being and mortality: a quantitative review of prospective observational studies." *Psychosomatic Medicine.* September 2008, vol. 70, no. 7: 741–56.

Creswell, J. D., H. F. Myers, S. W. Cole, and M. R. Irwin. "Mindfulness meditation training effects on CD4+ T lymphocytes in HIV-1 infected adults: a small randomized controlled trial." *Brain, Behavior, and Immunity.* February 2009, vol. 23, no. 2: 184–8.

Creswell, J. D., B. M. Way, N. I. Eisenberger, and M. D. Lieberman. "Neural correlates of dispositional mindfulness during affect labeling." *Psychosomatic Medicine.* July–August 2007, vol. 69, no. 6: 560–5.

Daubenmier, J. J., G. Weidner, M. D. Sumner, N. Mendell, et al. "The contribution of changes in diet, exercise, and stress management to changes in coronary risk in women and men in the multisite cardiac lifestyle intervention program." *Annals of Behavioral Medicine.* February 2007, vol. 33, no. 1: 57–68.

Davidson, R. J., J. Kabat-Zinn, J. Schumacher, M. Rosenkranz, et al. "Alterations in brain and immune function produced by mindfulness meditation." *Psychosomatic Medicine.* July–August 2003, vol. 65, no. 4: 564–70.

Davidson, R. J., and A. Lutz. "Buddha's brain: Neuroplasticity and meitation." *IEEE Signal Processing Magazine.* September 2007: 172–176.

Dunn, E. W., L. B. Aknin, and M. I. Norton. "Spending money on others promotes happiness." *Science.* March 21, 2008, vol. 319, no. 5870: 1687–8.

Dusek, J. A., H. H. Otu, A. L.Wohlhueter, M. Bhasin, et al. "Genomic counter-stress changes induced by the relaxation response." *PLoS One.* July 2008, vol. 3, no. 7: e2576.

Dusek, J. A., and H. Benson. "Mind-body medicine: a model of the comparative clinical impact of the acute stress and relaxation responses." *Minnesota Medicine.* May 2009, vol. 92, no. 5: 47–50.

Epel, E., J. Daubenmier, J. T. Moskowitz, S. Folkman, et al. "Can meditation slow rate of cellular aging? Cognitive stress, mindfulness, and telomeres." *Annals of the New York Academy of Sciences.* August 2009, vol. 1172: 34–53.

Feldman, G., A. Hayes, S. Kumar, J. Greeson, et al. "Mindfulness and emotion regulation: The development and initial validation of the cognitive and affective mindfulness scale—revised (CAMS-R)." *Journal of Psychopathology and Behavioral Assessment.* 2007, vol. 29: 177–190.

Galvin, J.A., H. Benson, G. R. Deckro, G. L. Fricchione, et al. "The relaxation response:

reducing stress and improving cognition in healthy aging adults." *Complementary Therapies in Clinical Practice*. August 2006, vol. 12, no. 3: 186–91.

Giltay, E. J., M. H. Kamphuis, S. Kalmijn, F. G. Zitman, et al. "Dispositional optimism and the risk of cardiovascular death: the Zutphen Elderly Study." *Archives of Internal Medicine*. February 27, 2006, vol. 166, no. 4: 431–6.

Giltay, E. J., J. M. Geleijnse, F. G. Zitman, B. Buijsse et al. "Lifestyle and dietary correlates of dispositional optimism in men: The Zutphen Elderly Study." *Journal of Psychosomatic Research*. November 2007, vol. 63, no. 5: 483–90.

Hartfield N., J. Havenhand, S. B. Khalsa, G. Clarke, et al. "The effectiveness of yoga for the improvement of well-being and resilience to stress in the workplace." *Scandinavian Journal of Work, Environment, and Health*. April 6, 2010. [Epub ahead of print]

Harvard Mental Health Letter. "Yoga for anxiety and depression: Studies suggest that this practice modulates the stress response." April 2009.

Hölzel, B. K., J. Carmody, K. C. Evans, E. A. Hoge, et al. "Stress reduction correlates with structural changes in the amygdala." *Social Cognitive and Affective Neuroscience*. March 2010, vol. 5, no. 1: 11–7.

Kabat-Zinn, J. "Bringing mindfulness to medicine: an interview with Jon Kabat-Zinn, PhD. Interview by Karolyn Gazella." *Advances in Mind-Body Medicine*. Summer 2005, vol. 21, no. 2: 22–7.

Kabat-Zinn, J., E. Wheeler, T. Light, A. Skillings, et al. "Influence of a mindfulness meditation-based stress reduction intervention on rates of skin clearing in patients with moderate to severe psoriasis undergoing phototherapy (UVB) and photochemotherapy (PUVA)." *Psychosomatic Medicine*. September–October 1998, 60, no. 5: 625–32.

Kabat-Zinn, J. "Mindfulness-based interventions in context: Past, present, and future. Commentaries on Baer." *Clinical Psychology: Science and Practice*. Summer 2003, vol. 10, no. 2: 144–156.

Kalin, N. H., S. E. Shelton, and R. J. Davidson. "Role of the primate orbitofrontal cortex in mediating anxious temperament." *Biological Psychiatry*. November 2007, vol. 62, no. 10: 1134–9.

Khalsa, S. B. "Treatment of chronic insomnia with yoga: a preliminary study with sleep-wake diaries." *Applied Psychophysiology and Biofeedback*. December 2004, vol. 29, no. 4: 269–78.

Khalsa, S. B. "Yoga as a therapeutic intervention: a bibliometric analysis of published research studies." *The Journal of Physiology*. July 2004, vol. 48, no. 3: 269–85.

Kiecolt-Glaser, J. K., L. Christian, H. Preston, C. R. Houts, et al. "Stress, inflammation, and yoga practice." *Psychosomatic Medicine*. February 2010, vol. 72, no. 2: 113–21.

Kubzansky, L. D., R. J. Wright, S. Cohen, S. Weiss, et al. "Breathing easy: a prospective study of optimism and pulmonary function in the normative aging study." *Annals of Behavioral Medicine*. Fall 2002 , vol. 24, no. 4: 345–53.

Kubzansky, L. D., and R. C. Thurston. "Emotional vitality and incident coronary heart disease: benefits of healthy psychological functioning." *Archives of General Psychiatry*. December 2007, vol. 64, no. 12: 1393–401.

Kubzansky, L. D., D. Sparrow, P. Vokonas, and I. Kawachi. "Is the glass half empty or half full? A prospective study of optimism and coronary heart disease in the normative aging study." *Psychosomatic Medicine*. November–December 2001, vol. 63, no. 6: 910–6.

Kubzansky, L. D., P. E. Kubzansky, and J. Maselko. "Optimism and pessimism in the context of health: bipolar opposites or separate constructs?" *Psychology Bulletin*. August 2004, vol. 30, no. 8: 943-56.

Kubzansky, L. D.. "Sick at heart: the pathophysiology of negative emotions." *Cleveland Clinic Journal of Medicine*. February 2007, vol. 74, suppl. 1: S67-72.

Lambert, C. "The science of happiness." *Harvard Magazine*. January-February 2007.

Lazar, S. W., G. Bush, R. L. Gollub, G. L. Fricchione, et al. "Functional brain mapping of the relaxation response and meditation." *NeuroReport*. May 15, 2000, vol. 11, 7: 1581–5.

Lazar, S. W., C. E. Kerr, R. H. Wasserman, J. R. Gray, et al. "Meditation experience is associated with increased cortical thickness." *NeuroReport*. November 28 2005, vol. 16, no. 17: 1893–7.

Luders, E., A. W. Toga, N. Lepore, and C. Gaser. "The underlying anatomical correlates of long-term meditation: larger hippocampal and frontal volumes of gray matter." *Neuroimage*. April 15, 2009, vol. 45, no. 3: 672–8.

Ludwig, D. S., and J. Kabat-Zinn. "Mindfulness in medicine." *The Journal of the American Medical Association*. September 17, 2008, vol. 300, no. 11: 1350–2.

Lutz, A., H. A. Slagter, J. D. Dunne, and R. J. Davidson. "Attention regulation and monitoring in meditation." *Trends in Cognitive Sciences*. April 2008, vol. 12, no. 4: 163-9.

Lutz, A., L. L. Greischar, D. M. Perlman, and R. J. Davidson. "BOLD signal in insula is differentially related to cardiac function during compassion meditation in experts vs. novices." *Neuroimage*. September 2009, vol. 47, no. 3: 1038–46.

Lutz, A., H. A. Slagter, N. B. Rawlings, A. D. Francis, et al. "Mental training enhances attentional stability: neural and behavioral evidence." *The Journal of Neuroscience*. October 21 2009, vol. 29, no. 42: 13418–27.

Lutz, A., J. Brefczynski-Lewis, T. Johnstone, and R. J. Davidson. "Regulation of the neural circuitry of emotion by compassion meditation: effects of meditative expertise." *PLoS One*. March 26, 2008, vol. 3, no. 3: e1897.

Maninger, N., O. M. Wolkowitz, V. I. Reus, E. S. Epel, et al. "Neurobiological and neuropsychiatric effects of dehydroepiandrosterone (DHEA) and DHEA sulfate (DHEAS)." *Frontiers in Neuroendocrinology*. January 2009, vol. 30, no. 1: 65–91.

Moskowitz, J. T., E. S. Epel, and M. Acree. "Positive affect uniquely predicts lower risk of mortality in people with diabetes." *Health Psychology*. January 2008, vol. 27, no. 1: S73–82.

O'Donnell, K., L. Brydon, C. E. Wright, A. Steptoe. "Self-esteem levels and cardiovascular and inflammatory responses to acute stress." *Brain, Behavior, and Immunity*. November 2008, vol. 22, no. 8: 1241–7.

O'Donovan, A., J. Lin, F. S. Dhabhar, O. Wolkowitz, et al. "Pessimism correlates with leukocyte telomere shortness and elevated interleukin-6 in post-menopausal women." *Brain, Behavior, and Immunity*. May 2009, vol. 23, no. 4: 446–9.

Ospina, M. B., K. Bond, M. Karkhaneh, L. Tjosvold, et al. "Meditation practices for health: state of the research." *Evidence Report – Technology Assessment*. June 2007, no. 155: 1–263.

Ostir, G. V., I. M. Berges, K. S. Markides, and K. J. Ottenbacher. "Hypertension in older adults and the role of positive emotions." *Psychosomatic Medicine*. September-October 2006, vol. 68, no. 5: 727–33.

Ostir, G. V., K. J. Ottenbacher, and K. S. Markides. Onset of frailty in older adults and the protective role of positive affect. *Psychology and Aging*. September 2004, vol. 19, no. 3: 402–8.

Ostir, G. V., K. S. Markides, M. K. Peek, and J. S. Goodwin. "The association between emotional well-being and the incidence of stroke in older adults." *Psychosomatic Medicine.* March-April 2001, vol. 63, no. 2: 210–5.

Pace, T. W., L. T. Negi, D. D. Adam, S. P. Cole, et al. "Effect of compassion meditation on neuroendocrine, innate immune and behavioral responses to psychosocial stress." *Psychoneuroendocrinology.* January 2009, vol. 34, no. 1: 87–98.

Pagnoni, G., M. Cekic, and Y. Guo. "'Thinking about not-thinking': neural correlates of conceptual processing during Zen meditation." *PLoS One.* September 2008, vol. 3, no. 9: e3083.

Rasmussen, H. N., M. F. Scheier, and J. B. Greenhouse. "Optimism and physical health: a meta-analytic review." *Annals of Behavioral Medicine.* June 2009, vol. 37, no. 3: 239–56.

Scheier, M. F., C. S. Carver, and M. W. Bridges. "Distinguishing optimism from neuroticism (and trait anxiety, self-mastery, and self-esteem): a reevaluation of the Life Orientation Test." *Journal of Personality and Social Psychology.* December 1994, vol. 67, no. 6: 1063–78.

Segerstrom, S. C. "Optimism and immunity: do positive thoughts always lead to positive effects?" *Brain, Behavior, and Immunity.* May 2005, vol. 19, no. 3: 195–200.

Segerstrom, S. C. "Optimism and resources: Effects on each other and on health over 10 years." *Journal of Research in Personality.* August 2007, vol. 41, no. 4: 772–786.

Shapiro, S. L., D. Oman, C. E. Thoresen, T. G. Plante, et al. "Cultivating mindfulness: effects on well-being." *Journal of Clinical Psychology.* July 2008, vol. 64, no. 7: 840–62.

Sherman, D. K., D. P. Bunyan, J. D. Creswell, and L. M. Jaremka. "Psychological vulnerability and stress: the effects of self-affirmation on sympathetic nervous system responses to naturalistic stressors." *Health Psychology.* September 2009, vol. 28, no. 5: 554–62.

Slagter, H. A., A. Lutz, L. L. Greischar, A. D. Francis, et al. "Mental training affects distribution of limited brain resources." *PLoS Biology.* June 2007, vol. 5, no. 6: e138.

Steptoe, A., C. Wright, S.R. Kunz-Ebrecht, and S. Iliffe. "Dispositional optimism and health behaviour in community-dwelling older people: associations with healthy ageing." *British Journal of Health Psychology.* February 2006, vol. 11, pt. 1: 71–84.

Steptoe, A., K. O'Donnell, E. Badrick, M. Kumari, et al. "Neuroendocrine and inflammatory factors associated with positive affect in healthy men and women: the Whitehall II study." *American Journal of Epidemiology.* January 2008, vol. 167, no. 1: 96–102.

Steptoe, A., J. Wardle, and M. Marmot. "Positive affect and health-related neuroendocrine, cardiovascular, and inflammatory processes." *Proceedings of the National Academy of Sciences.* May 2005, vol. 102, no. 18: 6508–12.

Tang, Y. Y., Y. Ma, Y. Fan, H. Feng, et al. "Central and autonomic nervous system interaction is altered by short-term meditation." *Proceedings of the National Academy of Sciences.* June 2 2009, vol. 106, no. 22: 8865–70.

Tang, Y. Y., Y. Ma, Y. Fan, H. Feng, et al. "Short-term meditation training improves attention and self-regulation." *Proceedings of the National Academy of Sciences.* October 23, 2007, vol. 104, no. 43: 17152–6.

Tindle, H. A., Y. F. Chang, L. H. Kuller, J. E. Manson, et al. "Optimism, cynical hostility, and incident coronary heart disease and mortality in the Women's Health Initiative." *Circulation.* August 2009, vol. 120, no. 8: 656–62.

Walton, K. G., R. H. Schneider, S. I. Nidich, J. W. Salerno, et al. "Psychosocial stress and cardiovascular disease Part 2: effectiveness of the Transcendental Meditation program in treatment and prevention." *Behavioral Medicine.* Fall 2002, vol. 28, no. 3: 106–23.

Walton, K. G., R. H. Schneider, S. I. Nidich, and J. W. Salerno. "Psychosocial stress and cardiovascular disease. Part 3: Clinical and policy implications of research on the transcendental meditation program." *Behavioral Medicine.* Winter 2005, vol. 30, no. 4: 173–83.

Chapter 7: Stress and Social Support

Allen, K., J. Blascovich, and W. B. Mendes. "Cardiovascular reactivity and the presence of pets, friends, and spouses: the truth about cats and dogs." *Psychosomatic Medicine.* September-October 2002, vol. 64, no. 5: 727–39.

Baumgartner, T., M. Heinrichs, A. Vonlanthen, U. Fischbacher, et al. "Oxytocin shapes the neural circuitry of trust and trust adaptation in humans." *Neuron.* May 22, 2008, vol. 58, no. 4: 639–50.

Berkman, L. F. "Assessing the physical health effects of social networks and social support." *Annual Review of Public Health.* 1984, vol. 5: 413–32.

Berkman, L. F. "Looking beyond age and race: the structure of networks, functions of support, and chronic stress." *Epidemiology.* September 1997, vol. 8, no. 5: 469–70.

Berkman, L. F. "Which influences cognitive function: living alone or being alone?" *Lancet.* April 2000, vol. 355, no. 9212: 1291–2.

Carlson, M. C., K. I. Erickson, A. F. Kramer, M. W. Voss, et al. "Evidence for neurocognitive plasticity in at-risk older adults: the experience corps program." *Journals of Gerontology: Biological and Medical Sciences.* December 2009, vol. 64, no. 12: 1275–82.

Carter, C. S., H. Pournajafi-Nazarloo, K. M. Kramer, T. E. Ziegler, et al. "Oxytocin: behavioral associations and potential as a salivary biomarker." *Annals of the New York Academy of Sciences.* March 2007, vol. 1098: 312–22.

Carter, C. S., A. J. Grippo, H. Pournajafi-Nazarloo, M. G. Ruscio, et al. "Oxytocin, vasopressin and sociality." *Progress in Brain Research.* 2008, vol. 170: 331–6.

Costa, D. L., and M. E. Kahn. "Health, wartime stress, and unit cohesion: evidence from Union Army veterans." *Demography.* February 2010, vol. 47, no. 1: 45–66.

Crocker, J., and A. Canevello. "Creating and undermining social support in communal relationships: the role of compassionate and self-image goals." *Journal of Personality and Social Psychology.* September 2008, vol. 95, no. 3: 555–75.

Ditzen, B., I. D. Neumann, G. Bodenmann, B. von Dawans, et al. "Effects of different kinds of couple interaction on cortisol and heart rate responses to stress in women." *Psychoneuroendocrinology.* June 2007, vol. 32, no. 5: 565–74.

Ditzen, B., M. Schaer, B. Gabriel, G. Bodenmann, et al. "Intranasal oxytocin increases positive communication and reduces cortisol levels during couple conflict." *Biological Psychiatry.* May 2009, vol. 65, no. 9: 728–31.

Donaldson, Z. R., and L. J. Young. "Oxytocin, vasopressin, and the neurogenetics of sociality." *Science.* November 7, 2008, vol. 322, no. 5903: 900–4.

Dykema, R. "'Don't talk to me now, I'm scanning for danger.' How your nervous system sabotages your ability to relate. An interview with Stephen Porges about his polyvagal theory." *NEXUS.* March/April 2006: 30–35.

Eisenberger, N. I., M. D. Lieberman, and K. D. Williams. "Does rejection hurt? An FMRI study of social exclusion." *Science.* October 10, 2003, vol. 302, no. 5643: 290–2.

Eisenberger, N. I., and M. D. Lieberman. "Why rejection hurts: a common neural alarm system for physical and social pain." *Trends in Cognitive Sciences*. July 2004, vol. 8, no. 7: 294–300.

Eisenberger, N. I., S. E. Taylor, S. L. Gable, C. J. Hilmert, et al. "Neural pathways link social support to attenuated neuroendocrine stress responses." *Neuroimage*. May 1, 2007, vol. 35, no. 4: 1601–12.

Eisenberger, N. I., B. M. Way, S. E. Taylor, W. T. Welch, et al. "Understanding genetic risk for aggression: clues from the brain's response to social exclusion." *Biological Psychiatry*. May 1 2007, vol. 61, no. 9: 1100–8.

Ertel, K. A., M. M. Glymour, and L. F. Berkman. "Effects of social integration on preserving memory function in a nationally representative US elderly population." *American Journal of Public Health*. July 2008, vol. 98, no. 7: 1215–20.

Fried, L. P., M. C. Carlson, M. Freedman, K. D. Frick, et al. "A social model for health promotion for an aging population: initial evidence on the Experience Corps model." *Journal of Urban Health*. March 2004, vol. 81, no. 1: 64-78.

Glass, T. A., M. Freedman, M. C. Carlson, J. Hill, et al. "Experience Corps: design of an intergenerational program to boost social capital and promote the health of an aging society." *Journal of Urban Health*. March 2004, vol. 81, no. 1: 94–105.

Heinrichs, M., B. von Dawans, and G. Domes. "Oxytocin, vasopressin, and human social behavior." *Frontiers in Neuroendocrinology*. October 2009, vol. 30, no. 4: 548–57.

Kiecolt-Glaser, J. K., J. P. Gouin, and L. Hantsoo. "Close relationships, inflammation, and health." *Neuroscience and Biobehavioral Reviews*. September 12 2009. [Epub ahead of print]

Kim, H.S., D. K. Sherman, and S. E. Taylor. "Culture and social support." *American Psychologist*. September 2008, vol. 63, no. 6: 518–26.

Kubzansky, L.D., W. B. Mendes, A. Appleton, J. Block, et al. "Protocol for an experimental investigation of the roles of oxytocin and social support in neuroendocrine, cardiovascular, and subjective responses to stress across age and gender." *BMC Public Health*. December 21, 2009, vol. 9: 481.

Kumari, M., E. Badrick, T. Chandola, N. E. Adler, et al. "Measures of social position and cortisol secretion in an aging population: findings from the Whitehall II study." *Psychosomatic Medicine*. January 2010, vol. 72, no. 1: 27–34.

Lemay, E. P., Jr., and M. S. Clark. "How the head liberates the heart: projection of communal responsiveness guides relationship promotion." *Journal of Personality and Social Psychology*. April 2008, vol. 94, no. 4: 647–71.

Lieberman, M. D. and N. I. Eisenberger. "Neuroscience: Pains and pleasures of social life." *Science*. February 13, 2009, vol. 323, no. 5916: 890–1.

Lount, R. B., Jr. "The impact of positive mood on trust in interpersonal and intergroup interactions." *Journal of Personality and Social Psychology*. March 2010, vol. 98, no. 3: 420–33.

Master, S. L., N. I. Eisenberger, S. E. Taylor, B. D. Naliboff, et al. "A picture's worth: partner photographs reduce experimentally induced pain." *Psychological Science*. November 2009, vol. 20, 11: 1316–8.

Master, S. L., D. M. Amodio, A. L. Stanton, C. M. Yee, et al. "Neurobiological correlates of coping through emotional approach." *Brain, Behavior, and Immunity*. January 2009, vol. 23, no. 1: 27–35.

Mickelson, K. D., and L. D. Kubzansky. "Social distribution of social support: the mediating role of life events." *American Journal of Community Psychology.* December 2003, vol. 32, nos. 3–4: 265–81.

Moll, J., F. Krueger, R. Zahn, M. Pardini, et al. "Human fronto-mesolimbic networks guide decisions about charitable donation." *Proceedings of the National Academy of Sciences.* October 17, 2006, vol. 103, no. 42: 15623–8.

O'Donnell, K., E. Badrick, M. Kumari, and A. Steptoe. "Psychological coping styles and cortisol over the day in healthy older adults." *Psychoneuroendocrinology.* June 2008, vol. 33, no. 5: 601–11.

Petrovic, P., R. Kalisch, T. Singer, and R. J. Dolan. "Oxytocin attenuates affective evaluations of conditioned faces and amygdala activity." *The Journal of Neuroscience.* June 25, 2008, vol. 28, no. 26: 6607–15.

Porges, S. W. "The polyvagal perspective." *Biological Psychology.* February 2007, vol. 74, no. 2: 116–43.

Porges, S. W. "The polyvagal theory: new insights into adaptive reactions of the autonomic nervous system." *Cleveland Clinic Journal of Medicine.* April 2009, vol. 76, suppl. 2: S86–90.

Rimmele, U., K. Hediger, M. Heinrichs, and P. Klaver. "Oxytocin makes a face in memory familiar." *The Journal of Neuroscience.* January 7, 2009, vol. 29, no. 1: 38–42.

Schulz, U., C. R. Pischke, G. Weidner, J. Daubenmier, et al. "*Psychology, Health, and Medicine.* August 2008, vol. 13, no. 4: 423–37.

Seeman, T. E., L. F. Berkman, P. A. Charpentier, D. G. Blazer, et al. "Behavioral and psychosocial predictors of physical performance: MacArthur studies of successful aging." *Journals of Gerontology: Biological and Medical Sciences.* July 1995, vol. 50, no. 4: M177–83.

Seeman, T. E., and E. Crimmins. "Social environment effects on health and aging: integrating epidemiologic and demographic approaches and perspectives." *Annals of the New York Academy of Sciences.* December 2001, vol. 954: 88–117.

Seeman, T. E., B. H. Singer, C. D. Ryff, G. Dienberg Love, et al. "Social relationships, gender, and allostatic load across two age cohorts." *Psychosomatic Medicine.* May-June 2002, vol. 64, no. 3: 395–406.

Seeman, T. E., T. M. Lusignolo, M. Albert, and L. Berkman. "Social relationships, social support, and patterns of cognitive aging in healthy, high-functioning older adults: MacArthur studies of successful aging." *Health Psychology.* July 2001, vol. 20, no. 4: 243–55.

Taylor S. E., L. C. Klein, B. P. Lewis, T. L. Gruenewald, et al. "Biobehavioral responses to stress in females: tend-and-befriend, not fight-or-flight." *Psychological Review.* July 2000, vol. 107, no. 3: 411–29.

Taylor S. E., W. T. Welch, H. S. Kim, and D. K. Sherman. "Cultural differences in the impact of social support on psychological and biological stress responses." *Psychological Science.* September 2007, vol. 18, no. 9: 831–7.

Taylor S. E., B. M. Way, W. T. Welch, C. J. Hilmert, et al. "Early family environment, current adversity, the serotonin transporter promoter polymorphism, and depressive symptomatology." *Biological Psychiatry.* October 1, 2006, vol. 60, no. 7: 671–6.

Taylor S. E., T. E. Seeman, N. I. Eisenberger, T. A. Kozanian, et al. "Effects of a supportive or an unsupportive audience on biological and psychological responses to stress." *Journal of Personality and Social Psychology.* January 2010, vol. 98, no. 1: 47–56.

Taylor S. E., L. J. Burklund, N. I. Eisenberger, B. J. Lehman, et al. "Neural bases of moderation of cortisol stress responses by psychosocial resources." *Journal of Personality and Social Psychology*. July 2008, vol. 95, no. 1: 197–211.

Taylor S. E., N. I. Eisenberger, D. Saxbe, B. J. Lehman, et al. "Neural responses to emotional stimuli are associated with childhood family stress." *Biological Psychiatry*. August 1, 2006, vol. 60, no. 3: 296–301.

Taylor S. E., B. J. Lehman, C. I. Kiefe, and T. E. Seeman. "Relationship of early life stress and psychological functioning to adult C-reactive protein in the coronary artery risk development in young adults study." *Biological Psychiatry*. October 15, 2006, vol. 60, no. 8: 819–24.

Taylor S. E., G. C. Gonzaga, L. C. Klein, P. Hu, et al. "Relation of oxytocin to psychological stress responses and hypothalamic-pituitary-adrenocortical axis activity in older women." *Psychosomatic Medicine*. March-April 2006, vol. 68, no. 2: 238–45.

Taylor S. E. "Tend and befriend: Biobehavioral bases of affiliation under stress." *Current Directions in Psychological Science*. 2006, vol. 15, no. 6: 273–277.

Thurston, R. C. and L. D. Kubzansky. "Women, loneliness, and incident coronary heart disease." *Psychosomatic Medicine*. October 2009, vol. 71, no. 8: 836–42.

Chapter 8: Stress and Sleep

Banks, S., and D. F. Dinges. "Behavioral and physiological consequences of sleep restriction." *Journal of Clinical Sleep Medicine*. August 15, 2007, vol. 3, no. 5: 519–28.

Basner, M., and D. F. Dinges. "Dubious bargain: trading sleep for Leno and Letterman." *Sleep*. June 2009, vol. 32, no. 6: 747–52.

Bixler, E. O., M. N. Papaliaga, A. N. Vgontzas, H. M. Lin, et al. "Women sleep objectively better than men and the sleep of young women is more resilient to external stressors: effects of age and menopause." *Journal of Sleep Research*. June 2009, vol. 18, no. 2: 221–8.

CBSNews. *60 Minutes*. Transcript. "The Science of Sleep." March 16, 2008.

Centers for Disease Control and Prevention (CDC), et al. "Perceived insufficient rest or sleep among adults—United States, 2008. MMWR Morbidity Mortality Weekly Report, *The Journal of the American Medical Association*. 2009, vol. 302, no. 23: 2532–2539.

Cho, K., A. Ennaceur, J. C. Cole, C. K. Suh. "Chronic jet lag produces cognitive deficits." *The Journal of Neuroscience*. March 15, 2000, vol. 20, no. 6: RC66.

Cho, K. "Chronic 'jet lag' produces temporal lobe atrophy and spatial cognitive deficits." *Nature Neuroscience*. June 2001, 4, no. 6: 567–8.

Cohen, D. A., W. Wang, J. K. Wyatt, R. E. Kronauer, et al. "Uncovering residual effects of chronic sleep loss on human performance." *Science Translational Medicine*. January 2010, vol. 2, no. 4: 14ra3.

Ellenbogen, J. M., P. T. Hu, J.D. Payne, D. Titone, et al. "Human relational memory requires time and sleep." *Proceedings of the National Academy of Sciences*. May 1, 2007, vol. 104, no. 18: 7723–8.

Ellenbogen, J. M., J. D. Payne, and R. Stickgold. "The role of sleep in declarative memory consolidation: passive, permissive, active or none?" *Current Opinion in Neurobiology*. December 2006, vol. 16, no. 6: 716–22.

Frey, D. J., M. Fleshner, and K. P. Wright, Jr. "The effects of 40 hours of total sleep deprivation on inflammatory markers in healthy young adults." *Brain, Behavior, and Immunity*. November 2007, vol. 21, no. 8: 1050–7.

Friedman, E. M., M. S. Hayney, G. D. Love, H. L. Urry, et al. "Social relationships, sleep quality, and interleukin-6 in aging women." *Proceedings of the National Academy of Sciences*. December 2005, vol. 102, no. 51: 18757–62.

Friedman, E. M., G. D. Love, M. A. Rosenkranz, H. L. Urry, et al. "Socioeconomic status predicts objective and subjective sleep quality in aging women." *Psychosomatic Medicine*. September–October 2007, vol. 69, no. 7: 682–91.

Gilpin, H., D. Whitcomb, and K. Cho. "Atypical evening cortisol profile induces visual recognition memory deficit in healthy human subjects." *Molecular Brain*. August 2008, vol. 1, no. 1: 4.

Goel, N., H. Rao, J. S. Durmer, and D. F. Dinges. "Neurocognitive consequences of sleep deprivation." *Seminars in Neurology*. September 2009, vol. 29, no. 4: 320–39.

Gujar, No. , S. S. Yoo, P. Hu, and M. P. Walker. "The unrested resting brain: sleep deprivation alters activity within the default-mode network." *Journal of Cognitive Neuroscience*. August 24, 2009.

Hairston, I. S., M. T. Little, M. D. Scanlon, M. T. Barakat, et al. "Sleep restriction suppresses neurogenesis induced by hippocampus-dependent learning. *Journal of Neurophysiology*. December 2005, vol. 94, no. 6: 4224–33.

Irwin, M. R., R. Olmstead, and S. J. Motivala. "Improving sleep quality in older adults with moderate sleep complaints: A randomized controlled trial of Tai Chi Chih." *Sleep*. July 1 2008, vol. 31, no. 7: 1001–8.

Knutson, K. L., and E. Van Cauter. "Associations between sleep loss and increased risk of obesity and diabetes." *Annals of the New York Academy of Sciences*. 2008, vol. 1129: 287–304.

Knutson, K. L., A. M. Ryden, B. A. Mander, and E. Van Cauter. "Role of sleep duration and quality in the risk and severity of type 2 diabetes mellitus." *Archives of Internal Medicine*. September 2006, vol. 166, no. 16: 1768–74.

Knutson, K. L., K. Spiegel, P. Penev, and E. Van Cauter. "The metabolic consequences of sleep deprivation." *Sleep Medicine Reviews*. June 2007, vol. 11, no. 3:163–78.

Mander, B. A., S. Santhanam, and M. P. Walker. "Sleep restores the human brain capacity to learn." *Abstract presentation at 2010 AAAS Annual Meeting*. February 2010.

McEwen, B. S. "Sleep deprivation as a neurobiologic and physiologic stressor: Allostasis and allostatic load." *Metabolism*. October 2006, vol. 55, no. 10, suppl. 2: S20–3.

Meerlo. P., R. E. Mistlberger, B. L. Jacobs, H. C. Heller, et al. "New neurons in the adult brain: the role of sleep and consequences of sleep loss." *Sleep Medicine Reviews*. June 2009, vol. 13, no. 3: 187–94.

Mirescu, C., J. D. Peters, L. Noiman, and E. Gould. "Sleep deprivation inhibits adult neurogenesis in the hippocampus by elevating glucocorticoids." *Proceedings of the National Academy of Sciences*. December 12, 2006, vol. 103, no. 50: 19170–5.

Morin, C. M., R. R. Bootzin, D. J. Buysse, J. D. Edinger, et al. "Psychological and behavioral treatment of insomnia: update of the recent evidence (1998–2004)." *Sleep*. November 1, 2006, vol. 29, no. 11: 1398–414.

NOVA *ScienceNow*, July 10, 2007. Transcript.

Payne, J. D., and L. Nadel. "Sleep, dreams, and memory consolidation: the role of the stress hormone cortisol." *Learn & Memory*. November–December 2004, vol. 11, no. 6: 671–8.

Payne, J. D., R. Stickgold, K. Swanberg, and E. A. Kensinger. "Sleep preferentially enhances memory for emotional components of scenes." *Psychological Science*. August 2008, vol. 19, no. 8: 781–8.

Payne, J. D., E. D. Jackson, S. Hoscheidt, L. Ryan, et al. "Stress administered prior to encoding impairs neutral but enhances emotional long-term episodic memories." *Learn & Memory*. December 17, 2007, vol. 14, no. 12: 861–8.

Rajaratnam, S. M., M. H. Polymeropoulos, D. M. Fisher, T. Roth, et al. "Melatonin agonist tasimelteon (VEC-162) for transient insomnia after sleep-time shift: two randomised controlled multicentre trials." *Lancet*. February 7, 2009, vol. 373, no. 9662: 482–91.

Ritterband, L. M., F. P. Thorndike, L. A. Gonder-Frederick, J. C. Magee, et al. "Efficacy of an Internet-based behavioral intervention for adults with insomnia." *Archives of General Psychiatry*. July 2009, vol. 66, no. 7: 692–8.

Schutte-Rodin, S., L. Broch, D. Buysse, C. Dorsey, et al. "Clinical guideline for the evaluation and management of chronic insomnia in adults." *Journal of Clinical Sleep Medicine*. October 15, 2008, vol. 4, no. 5: 487–504.

Simpson, N. and D. F. Dinges. "Sleep and inflammation." *Nutrition Reviews*. December 2007, vol. 65, no. 12, pt. 2: S244–52.

Sivertsen, B., S. Omvik, S. Pallesen, B. Bjorvatn, et al. "Cognitive behavioral therapy vs zopiclone for treatment of chronic primary insomnia in older adults: a randomized controlled trial." *The Journal of the American Medical Association*. June 28, 2006, vol. 295, no. 24: 2851–8.

Spiegel, K., R. Leproult, M. L'hermite-Balériaux, G. Copinschi, et al. "Leptin levels are dependent on sleep duration: relationships with sympathovagal balance, carbohydrate regulation, cortisol, and thyrotropin." *Journal of Clinical Endocrinology and Metabolism*. November 2004, vol. 89, no. 11: 5762–71.

Spiegel, K., K. Knutson, R. Leproult, E. Tasali, et al. "Sleep loss: a novel risk factor for insulin resistance and Type 2 diabetes." *Journal of Applied Physiology*. November 2005, vol. 99, no. 5: 2008–19.

Steptoe, A., K. O'Donnell, M. Marmot, and J. Wardle. "Positive affect, psychological well-being, and good sleep." *Journal of Psychosomatic Research*. April 2008, vol. 64, no. 4: 409–15.

Stickgold, R. and M. P. Walker. "Memory consolidation and reconsolidation: what is the role of sleep?" *Trends in Neurosciences*. August 2005, vol. 28, no. 8: 408–15.

Thorndike, F. P., D. K. Saylor, E. T. Bailey, L. Gonder-Frederick et al. "Development and perceived utility and impact of an internet intervention for insomnia." *E-Journal of Applied Psychology*. 2008, vol. 4, no. 2: 32-42.

Van Cauter, E., U. Holmback, K. Knutson, R. Leproult, et al. "Impact of sleep and sleep loss on neuroendocrine and metabolic function." *Hormonal Research*. 2007, vol. 67, suppl. 1: 2–9.

Van Cauter, E., K. Spiegel, E. Tasali, and R. Leproult. "Metabolic consequences of sleep and sleep loss." *Sleep Medicine*. September 2008, vol. 9, suppl. 1: S23–8.

Van Cauter E. and K. L. Knutson. "Sleep and the epidemic of obesity in children and adults." *European Journal of Endocrinology*. December 2008, vol. 159, suppl. 1: S59–66.

Vgontzas A. N., C. Tsigos, E. O. Bixler, C. A. Stratakis, et al. "Chronic insomnia and activity of the stress system: a preliminary study." *Journal of Psychosomatic Research*. July 1998, vol. 45, spec no. 1: 21–31.

Vgontzas A. N., S. Pejovic, E. Zoumakis, H. M. Lin, et al. "Daytime napping after a night of sleep loss decreases sleepiness, improves performance, and causes beneficial changes in cortisol and interleukin-6 secretion." *American Journal of Physiology: Endocrinology and Metabolism*. January 2007, vol. 292, no.1: E253–61.

Vgontzas A. N., D. Liao, E. O. Bixler, G. P. Chrousos, et al. "Insomnia with objective short sleep duration is associated with a high risk for hypertension." *Sleep*. April 1, 2009, vol. 32, no. 4: 491–7.

Vgontzas A. N., D. Liao, S. Pejovic, S. Calhoun, et al. "Insomnia with objective short sleep duration is associated with type 2 diabetes: A population-based study." *Diabetes Care*. November 2009, vol, 32, no. 11: 1980–5.

Vgontzas A. N., E. O. Bixler, G. P. Chrousos, and S. Pejovic. "Obesity and sleep disturbances: meaningful sub-typing of obesity." *Archives of Physiology and Biochemistry*. October 2008, vol. 114, no. 4: 224–36.

Vgontzas A. N., H. M. Lin, M. Papaliaga, S. Calhoun, et al. "Short sleep duration and obesity: the role of emotional stress and sleep disturbances." *International Journal of Obesity*. May 2008, vol. 32, no. 5: 801–9.

Vgontzas A. N., G. Mastorakos, E. O. Bixler , A. Kales, et al. "Sleep deprivation effects on the activity of the hypothalamic-pituitary-adrenal and growth axes: potential clinical implications." *Clinical Endocrinology*. August 1999, vol. 51, no.2: 205–15.

Walker M. P., and R. Stickgold. "Sleep, memory, and plasticity." *Annual Review of Psychology*. 2006, vol. 57: 139–66.

Walker M. P. "The role of sleep in cognition and emotion." *Annals of the New York Academy of Sciences*. March 2009, vol.1156: 168–97.

Walker M. P., and E. van der Helm. "Overnight therapy? The role of sleep in emotional brain processing." *Psychology Bulletin*. September 2009, vol. 135, no.5: 731–48.

Walker M. P. "The role of slow wave sleep in memory processing." *Journal of Clinical Sleep Medicine*. April 15, 2009, vol. 5, suppl. 2: S20–6.

Yoo S. S., P. T. Hu, N. Gujar, F. A. Jolesz, et al. "A deficit in the ability to form new human memories without sleep." *Nature Neuroscience*. March 2007, vol. 10, no. 3: 385–92.

Yoo S. S., N. Gujar, P. Hu, F. A. Jolesz, et al. "The human emotional brain without sleep—a prefrontal amygdala disconnect." *Current Biology*. October 23, 2007, vol. 17, no. 20: R877–8.

Conclusion: I Should Have Danced All Night

Asbury, C., and R. Barbara, eds. *Learning, Arts, and the Brain. The Dana Consortium Report on Arts and Cognition*. New York: Dana Press, 2008.

Berens, M. S., I. Kovelman, K.S. White, M. H. Shalinsky, et al. "Cognitive benefits and neural processing following early and continued arts education in Dance." *Abstracts for the Cognitive Neuroscience Society*, May 5–8, 2007.

Berens, M. S., J. K. Nelson, L. Petitto, and N. Dunbar. "Identification of potentially influential genes in pursuing expertise in the performing arts." *Neuroscience Meeting Planner*. Chicago, IL: Society for Neuroscience, 2008.

Conrad C., H. Niess, K. W. Jauch, C. J. Bruns, et al. "Overture for growth hormone: Requiem for interleukin-6?" *Critical Care Medicine*. October 23, 2007.

Blasing, B. "The cognitive structure of movements in classical dance." *Psychology of Sport and Exercise*. 2009, vol. 10, no. 3: 350–360.

Brown, S., and L. M. Parsons. "The neuroscience of dance." *Scientific American*. July 2008, vol. 299, no. 1: 78–83.

Brown S., M. J. Martinez, and L. M. Parsons. "The neural basis of human dance." *Cerebral Cortex*. August 2006, vol. 16, no. 8: 1157–67.

Calvo-Merino B., D. E. Glaser, J. Grèzes, R. E. Passingham, et al. "Action observation and acquired motor skills: an FMRI study with expert dancers." *Cerebral Cortex*. August 2005, vol. 15, no. 8: 1243–9.

Calvo-Merino B., S. Ehrenberg, D. Leung, and P. Haggard. "Experts see it all: configural effects in action observation." *Psychological Research*. October 25, 2009.

Calvo-Merino B., J. Grèzes, D. E. Glaser, R. E. Passingham, et al. "Seeing or doing? Influence of visual and motor familiarity in action observation." *Current Biology*. October 10, 2006, vol. 16, no. 19: 1905–10.

Cross E. S., A. F. Hamilton, and S. T. Grafton. "Building a motor simulation de novo: observation of dance by dancers." *Neuroimage*. July 1, 2006, vol. 31, no. 3: 1257–67.

Cross E. S., A. F. Hamilton, D. J. Kraemer, W. M. Kelley, et al. "Dissociable substrates for body motion and physical experience in the human action observation network." *The Journal of Neuroscience*. October 2009, vol. 30, no. 7: 1383–92.

Feder A., E. J. Nestler, and D. S. Charney. "Psychobiology and molecular genetics of resilience." *Nature Reviews Neuroscience*. June 2009, vol. 10, no. 6: 446–57.

Hui E., B. T. Chui, and J. Woo. "Effects of dance on physical and psychological well-being in older persons." *Archives of Gerontological Geriatrics*. July–August 2009 , vol. 49, no. 1: e45–50.

Marder E., and P. L. Strick. "Motor systems. Editorial Overview." *Current Opinion in Neurobiology*. December 2006, vol. 16, no. 6: 601–3.

Nelson A., W. Hartl, K. W. Jauch, G. L. Fricchione, et al. "The impact of music on hypermetabolism in critical illness." *Current Opinion in Clinical Nutrition and Metabolic Care*. November 2008, vol. 11, no. 6: 790–4.

Ornish D., J. Lin, J. Daubenmier, G. Weidner, et al. "Increased telomerase activity and comprehensive lifestyle changes: a pilot study." *Lancet Oncology*. November 2008, vol. 9, no. 11: 1048–57.

Rizzolatti G., and L. Craighero. "The mirror-neuron system." *Annual Review of Neuroscience*. 2004, vol. 27: 169–92.

Singer, T. "The quality of Merce: Fifty years in the company of a modern dance great." *Boston Magazine*, August 2003: 301.

Singer, T. "A window into a world of movement." *The Boston Globe*. July 29, 2008: E2.

Smith B. W., J. Dalen, K. Wiggins, E, Tooley, et al. "The brief resilience scale: assessing the ability to bounce back." *International Journal of Behavioral Medicine*. 2008, vol. 15, no. 3: 194–200.

Smith B. W., B.M. Shelley, J. Dalen, K. Wiggins, et al. "A pilot study comparing the effects of mindfulness-based and cognitive-behavioral stress reduction." *Journal of Alternative Complementary Medicine*. April 2008, vol. 14, no. 3: 251–8.

Stranahan A. M., D. Khalil, and E. Gould. "Social isolation delays the positive effects of running on adult neurogenesis." *Nature Neuroscience*. April 2006, vol. 9, no. 4: 526–33.

Urgesi C., B. Calvo-Merino, P. Haggard, and S. M. Aglioti. "Transcranial magnetic stimulation reveals two cortical pathways for visual body processing." *The Journal of Neuroscience*. July 25, 2007, vol. 27, no. 30: 8023–30.

SOURCES

TEST SOURCES

pp. 3–4: Drentea and Lavrakas. 2000. "Over the Limit: The Association Among Health, Race, and Debt." *Social Science and Medicine.* 50: 517–529.

pp. 31–33: Cohen, S., T. Kamarck., and R. Mermelstein. "A global measure of perceived stress." *Journal of Health and Social Behavior*, vol. 24, 1983: 385–396.

pp. 66–67: Crook, Feher, and Larrabee. "Assessment of Memory Complaint in Age-Associated Memory Impairment: The MAC-Q." *International Psychogeriatrics*, 1992, vol. 4, no. 2: 165–176.

pp. 93–94: Power of Food scale © 2006 Drexel University. All Rights Reserved. No part of this work may be reproduced or used in any form without the prior written permission of the copyright holder or the author, Michael R. Lowe, Ph.D.

pp. 135–136: Sallis, J. F., R. B. Pinski, R. M. Grossman, T. L. Patterson, and P. R. Nader. "The development of self-efficacy scales for health-related diet and exercise behaviors." *Health Education Research*, 1998, vol. 3: 283–292.

pp. 168–169: Feldman, G. C., A. M. Hayes, S. M. Kumar, J. M. Greeson, and J. P. Laurenceau. "Mindfulness and Emotion Regulation: The Development and Initial Validation of the Cognitive and Affective Mindfulness Scale—Revised (CAMS-R)." *Journal of Psychopathology and Behavioral Assessment*, 2007, vol. 29: 177–190.

pp. 179–180: Scheier, M. F., C. S. Carver, and M. W. Bridges. "Distinguishing optimism from neuroticism (and trait anxiety, self-mastery, and self-esteem): A re-evaluation of the Life Orientation Test." *Journal of Personality and Social Psychology*, 1994, vol. 67: 1063–1078.

pp. 197–200: Seeman, T. E., B. S. McEwen, J. W. Rowe, and B. H. Singer. "Allostatic load as a marker of cumulative biological risk: MacArthur studies of successful aging." *Proceedings of the National Academy of Sciences*, 2001, vol. 98: 4770–4775.

pp. 223–224: Buysse, D. J., C. F. Reynolds, T. H. Monk, S. R. Berman, and D. J. Kupfer. "The Pittsburgh Sleep Quality Index (PQSI): A new instrument for psychiatric research and practice." *Psychiatry Research*, 1998, vol. 28, no. 2: 193–213.

pp. 253–254: Smith, Bruce W., Jeanne Dalen, Kathryn Wiggins, Erin Tooley, Paulette Christopher, and Jennifer Bernard. "The Brief Resilience Scale: Assessing the Ability to Bounce Back." *International Journal of Behavioral Medicine*, 2008, vol. 15, no. 3: 194–200.

INDEX

Note: Page numbers in *italics* refer to illustrations. Page numbers followed by an *n* refer to notes at the bottom of the page.